Handbook of Hernia

Handbook of Hernia

Editor: Hugh Bryant

MURPHY & MOORE
www.murphy-moorepublishing.com

www.murphy-moorepublishing.com

MURPHY & MOORE

Cataloging-in-Publication Data

Handbook of hernia / edited by Hugh Bryant.
p. cm.
Includes bibliographical references and index.
ISBN 978-1-63987-282-4
1. Hernia. 2. Abdomen--Diseases. 3. Pathology. I. Bryant, Hugh.
RD621 .H36 2022
617.559 059--dc23

Murphy & Moore Publishing,
1 Rockefeller Plaza,
New York City, NY 10020, USA

ISBN 978-1-63987-282-4 (Hardback)

Contents

Preface

I am honored to present to you this unique book which encompasses the most up-to-date data in the field. I was extremely pleased to get this opportunity of editing the work of experts from across the globe. I have also written papers in this field and researched the various aspects revolving around the progress of the discipline. I have tried to unify my knowledge along with that of stalwarts from every corner of the world, to produce a text which not only benefits the readers but also facilitates the growth of the field.

The medical condition in which a fatty tissue or organ squeezes through a weak spot in a muscle or connective tissue is known as a hernia. There are various types of hernia, such as inguinal, femoral, umbilical, incisional and hiatal. Hernias occur when pressure is applied through a weakened fascia or muscle. This abnormal pressure could be applied by diarrhea, coughing, constipation, sneezing or lifting heavy objects without supporting the muscles in the abdomen. The diagnosis of a hernia involves a physical examination as well as imaging techniques such as X-rays and ultrasound. The most common treatment for hernias is through a hernia-repair surgery. If left untreated, the hernia might become strangulated and cause serious complications. Different approaches, evaluations, methodologies and management strategies of hernia have been included in this book. Its aim is to present researches that have transformed the research on this medical condition and aided its advancement. The book is appropriate for students seeking detailed information in this area as well as for experts.

Finally, I would like to thank all the contributing authors for their valuable time and contributions. This book would not have been possible without their efforts. I would also like to thank my friends and family for their constant support.

Editor

1

Congenital Diaphragmatic Hernia: Part 1

Adrian Claudiu Ratiu

Abstract

Over the past 20 years, prenatal detection of congenital diaphragmatic hernia (CDH) has improved worldwide, reaching up to 60% in Europe. Pulmonary hypoplasia and persistent pulmonary hypertension are the two main determinants of neonatal mortality and morbidity, so new tools have been focused on their evaluation. Fetal surgery for severe cases requires proper evaluation of the prognosis of fetuses with CDH. It is very important to identify reliable prenatal prognostic factors that can be used worldwide for several reasons: patient counseling is more accurate; the results of pre- and postnatal treatments will be comparable across different institutions; fetuses eligible for fetal surgery will be selected correctly; and a woman expecting a child with a very poor prognosis can prepare herself for the postnatal demise of her baby or, in some countries, opt for termination of pregnancy.

Keywords: congenital diaphragmatic hernia, thoracic anomalies, diaphragm anomalies

1. Introduction

Congenital diaphragmatic hernia (CDH) consists of a defect in variable size in the fetal diaphragm. It occurs more often on the left side and abdominal organs herniate into the thoracic cavity. Most if the time the diagnosis is made during the second trimester fetal morfology ultrasound examination. Diagnosis is based mainly on finding abdominal organs such as stomach, bowel, and liver in the chest cavity or in the presence of a chest mass which pushes the heart toward the lateral thoracic wall.

Although the surgical repair offers excellent results from the technical point of view, the problem with these patients are related to the impaired development of the lungs and their vasculature, therefore, the mortality and morbidity of these babies remain high even after surgery.

2. Spectrum of disease

2.1. Definition

Congenital diaphragmatic hernia (CDH) is defined by the presence of an orifice in the diaphragm that permits the herniation of abdominal contents into the thorax.

2.2. Epidemiology

CDH is a rare condition that occurs in <1–5:10,000 births [1]. The most common anatomic type encountered is the left-sided posterolateral hernia (Bochdalek hernia), including the vast majority of cases 85–90%, while the anterior hernia of Morgagni is rare. A bilateral defect accounts for 15–20% of cases; tissue defect involving most of the hemidiaphragm is called agenesis [2].

2.3. Causes

2.3.1. Environmental causes

No cases of CDH in humans have been unequivocally attributed to teratogenic or environmental exposures. Recently, a potential association with the immunosuppressive drug mycophenylate mofetil has been made, but the mechanism by which this drug could cause diaphragmatic defect is unknown [3].

2.3.2. Heritable causes

About 10% of all individuals with CDH have a chromosome abnormality. The most common abnormalities are trisomy 18 and isochromosome 12p (Pallister-Killian syndrome or PKS), although many additional abnormalities have been reported (**Table 1**). Some of the more common monogenic syndromes in which CDH occurs are listed in (**Tables 2** and **3**) [4].

2.4. Classification

There are six types of CHD (**Figure 1**):

1. Posterolateral defect (Bochdalek hernia) occurs most often on the left side and contains stomach, bowel, and spleen, and if right-sided, contains liver.

2. Parasternal defect (Morgagni hernia), located on anterior retrosternal or parasternal portion of the diaphragm, is rare and more often right-sided or bilateral and usually contains liver or bowel.

3. Other anterior hernias associated with Pentalogy of Cantrell are rare findings but are usually severe, probably derived from septum transversum. These cases are usually associated with Pentalogy of Cantrell (including defects in the midline abdominal wall supraumbilical, lower sternum, diaphragmatic pericardium, and heart).

Chromosome abnormality/locus	Frequency of congenital diaphragmatic hernia	
	Found in this disorder	Attributed to this disorder
Pallister-Killian syndrome/ (isochromosome or tetrasomy 12p)	~30%	? < 5%
Trisomy 13	Rare	Very rare
Trisomy 18	?1–2%	Rare among all CDH; most common chromosome abnormality in prenatally diagnosed CDH
Trisomy 21	Rare (Morgagni hernias > Bochdalek hernias)	Very rare
Del(4)(p16) (Wolf-Hirschhorn syndrome)	Rare	Very rare
+der (22) t(11;22)(q23;q11)	5–10%	Very rare
Del(15)(q26.2)	Unknown (?but possibly majority)	Unknown
Del(1)(q41-q42)	Unknown	Unknown
Del(8)(p23.1)	?30%	Unknown

Table 1. Common chromosome anomalies associated with CDH.

4. Central hernia is rare; the diaphragm defect involves the central tendinous (amuscular) part of the diaphragm. In these cases, the entire rim of diaphragmatic musculature is found to be present.
5. Hiatal hernia, extremely rare, occurs through a congenitally large esophageal orifice.
6. Diaphragmatic eventration is defined as an elevation or abnormal upward displacement of a part or entire normal diaphragm into the chest cavity. This rare type of CDH is caused by the existence of a thinner part of diaphragm which allows the upward displacement of abdominal organs.

For practical reasons regarding the imaging approach and counseling, it was proposed to classify CDH as intrapleural and mediastinal.

Intrapleural hernias occur through defects in the muscular diaphragm, which may result from deficient fusion of the pleuroperitoneal membranes and abdominal wall musculature or absence of the pleuroperitoneal membranes. Intrapleural hernia contents cause compressions on intrathoracic visceras, causing pulmonary hypoplasia and contralateral mediastinal shift. This category includes the traditionally classified Bochdalek hernias.

Mediastinal hernias can be classified into two types: retrosternal and central. Retrosternal hernias are categorized as Morgagni hernias, although a true Morgagni hernia is only a small anatomic located in the space between the sternal and costal heads of the diaphragm. True Morgagni hernia is considered to be a subtype of retrosternal mediastinal hernias, with larger

Syndrome	Frequency of CDH in this disorder	Mode of inheritance	Gene
Cornelia de Lange syndrome	?up to 5%	AD	*NIPBL*
			SMC3
	Unknown	XL	*SMC1A*
Craniofrontonasal syndrome	Rare	XL (but males less severely affected than females)	*EFNB1*
Denys-Drash syndrome	Rare	AD	*WT1*
Donnai-Barrow syndrome	~70%	AR	*LRP2*
Fryns syndrome	>80% (but ascertainment may be biased)	AR	Unknown (possible etiologic heterogeneity)
Matthew-Wood syndrome	~50%	AR	*STRA6*
Spondylocostal dysostosis (SCDO)	Rare	AR	*DLL3*
	Rare		*MESP2*
	Rare		*LFNG*
	Rare		*HES7*
Simpson-Golabi-Behmel syndrome	Rare	XL	*GPC3*

Table 2. Selected syndromes in which CDH is a feature.

ventral hernias which are defects in the central tendon stemming from septum transversum impaired development. Hiatal hernias, as their name shows, develop more through the esophageal hiatus and do not involve the central tendon. Differentiating ventral mediastinal hernias from intrapleural hernias is important because the intrapleural hernias, usually, do not lead to pulmonary hypoplasia, which is the major complication of CHD [5] (**Table 4**).

2.5. Embriology

The diaphragm starts to develop at approximately 4 weeks of gestation. It develops from several structures. The anterior central tendon develops from an infolding of the ventral body wall: the septum transversum. Another infolding on the posterolateral sides establishes the pleuroperitoneal membranes. Closure of the pleuroperitoneal canals occurs when the septum transversum fuses to the structures surrounding the esophagus, the esophageal mesentery, and connects to the pleuroperitoneal membranes. Closure of the pleuroperitoneal canals normally occurs around the eighth week of gestation in humans. The right side of the diaphragm closes before the left side [6].

The central portion and possibly anterior regions are thought to develop from the septum transversum, which is initially fused to the liver during development and becomes the unmuscularized central tendon of the diaphragm [7].

The posterolateral section, the place where Bochdalek hernia occurs, develops from the pleuroperitoneal folds (PPFs), which are triangular structures derived from mesoderm that form in

Syndrome	Gene (locus)
Apert syndrome	*FGFR2*
Beckwith-Wiedemann syndrome	Dysregulation of imprinted genes on 11p15.5
CHARGE syndrome	*CHD7*
C (trigonocephaly) syndrome	*CD96*
Coffin-Siris syndrome	Unknown
Czeizel-Losonci syndrome	Unknown
Gershoni-Baruch syndrome	Unknown
Goltz syndrome (focal dermal hypoplasia)	*PORCN*
Kabuki syndrome	Unknown
Marfan syndrome	*FBN1*
Mathieu syndrome	Unknown
Meacham syndrome	*WT1*
Microphthalmia with linear skin lesions syndrome	*HCCS*
PAGOD syndrome	Unknown
Pentalogy of Cantrell	Unknown
Poland anomaly	Unknown
Swyer syndrome	Unknown
Thoraco-abdominal schisis	Unknown

Table 3. Syndromes in which CDH is less frequently a feature.

the thorax in the early development of the diaphragm. These PPFs are part of the diaphragmatic connective tissue. The membranous diaphragm is later muscularized by migrating muscle precursor cells to the PPF from the cervical somites. This phenomenon happens before these cells proliferate, differentiate, and migrate onto the membranous diaphragm [8, 9]. The hypothesis is that a Bochdalek hernia occurs if the PPFs do not fuse with the septum transversum and the dorsal mesentery of the esophagus by the 10th week of gestation [4].

The lung originates as an outpouch of the ventral wall of the posterior end of the laryngotracheal tube and divides into two bronchial buds at 3–4 weeks of gestation [10]. As the two buds elongate, the primitive tubular foregut tube begins to pinch into two tubes, namely, the dorsal esophagus and the ventral trachea [11]. Further outgrowth of the lung-buds produces the secondary bronchi. In humans, the right lung has three lobes, whereas, the left lung is composed of two lobes. The branching of the primary bronchial buds are monopodial. Every secondary bronchus then undergoes progressive dichotomous branching as each branch bifurcates repeatedly. Reproducible branching in humans is completed at 16 generations in 16 weeks of gestation [12]. The last seven generations of airway are completed during the last part of gestation. Alveolization starts after 28–30 weeks in humans and is completed in postnatal period [13]. Reid [14] presented this process in her laws of development of the human lung:

1. The bronchial tree is completed by the 16th gestational weeks.
2. Alveoli, developed after birth, increase in number until 8 years of age and in size until the chest wall finishes growing.
3. Blood vessels are remodeled and increase, as new alveoli form, probably until the chest growth is complete.

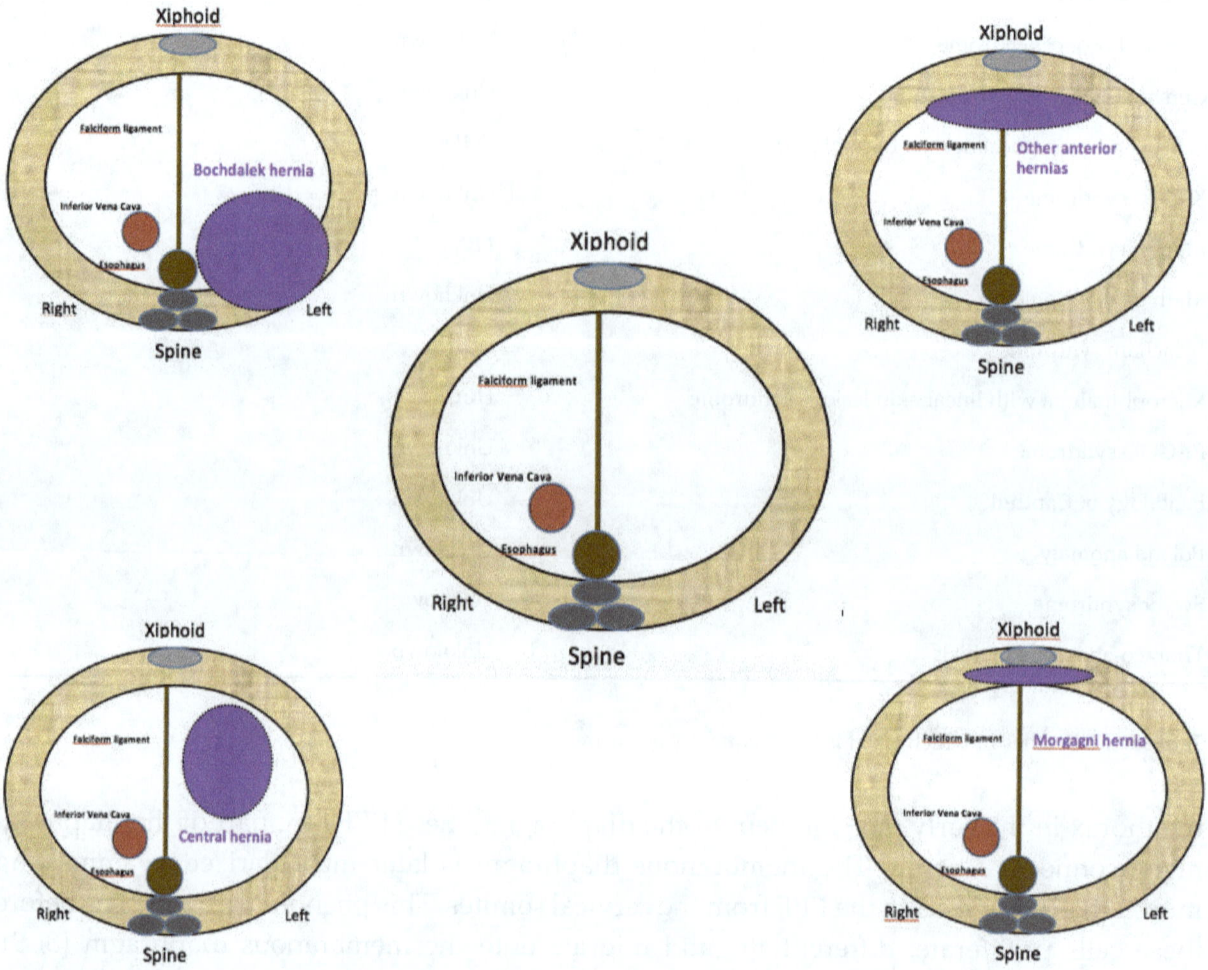

Figure 1. Types of congenital diaphragmatic hernia.

Hernia type	Location	Contents	Associated findings
Intrapleural	Lateral, usually left-sided	Stomach, bowel, spleen, variable-sized portions of the liver	Pulmonary hypoplasia
Mediastinal			
Ventral	Anterior and central	Liver, bowel	Pericardial effusion, pentalogy of Cantrell
Morgagni	Anteromedial, small, typically isolated	Liver, bowel	No pericardial communication
Hiatal	Posterior and central	Stomach, sometimes other organs	Congenital short esophagus

Table 4. Texas Children's Fetal Center classification of CDH.

2.6. Pathogenesis

The pathogenesis of CDH is poorly understood. The diaphragmatic defect is caused by delayed or impaired separation of the two compartments: thoracic and abdominal. This is due to closure of embryonic pleuroperitoneal canals influenced by the growth of the post-hepatic mesenchymal plate and of the pleuroperitoneal folds [15, 16]. In CDH, respiratory failure at birth is the result of pulmonary hypoplasia (PH), reduced airway branching, and surfactant deficiency. Extensive muscularization of the pulmonary vessels may result in persistent pulmonary hypertension (PPH) of the newborn. Historically, PH was believed to be the result of compression of the lungs by the herniating intrathoracic abdominal organs. However, our understanding of abnormal pulmonary development in relation to CDH has significantly improved and we know that pulmonary development is already affected prior to development of the diaphragmatic hernia, implicating that the lungs are primarily disturbed in their development before mechanical compression can happen [17, 18].

2.7. Associated anomalies

The most common associated anomalies are cardiovascular in 40–60% of live-born infants and in 95% of fetal demise; therefore, a detailed ultrasound examination must be performed in every case diagnosed with CDH [19] (**Table 5**).

2.8. Ultrasound diagnosis

Ultrasound evaluation of the thorax can be carried out easily until 25–26 weeks of gestation; after this period, the increased mineralization of the ribs limits the display of intrathoracic organs, especially for coronal or sagittal views. A number of thoracic anomalies evolve; they can appear only in the third trimester or they can regress before birth. Therefore, if an initial assessment of the thorax can be performed as early as at the 12th week of gestation, in order to follow up abnormal cases, late third-trimester scans may be needed.

Scanning planes: the most important view for the assessment of intrathoracic anatomy is the classic *four chamber view* of the fetal heart. In this plane, most thoracic viscera can be visualized, including the ribs, the sternum, and the cutaneous outline. The *midsagittal* and *parasagittal views* allow display of the diaphragm as a hypoechoic line below the lungs and the heart and above the liver and the stomach. The diaphragm shows a curved outline, convex toward the thorax.

Cardiovascular	VSD, ASD, tetralogy of fallot, hypoplastic left heart syndrome
Gastrointestinal abnormalities	Meckel diverticulum, anal atresia
Central nervous system	Neural tube defects, hydrocephalus, agenesis of corpus callosum
Limb abnormalities	Absence defects, polydactyly, syndactyly
Genitourinary abnormalities	Cryptorhydia, absent testes, ectopic kidney, horseshoe kidney
Eye abnormalities	Microphtalmia and anophtalmia

Table 5. Asociated anomalies.

Axial four-chamber view: the following structures should be checked: the two lungs appear as solid, homogeneous; weakly hyperechogenic that almost completely surrounds the heart, right larger than left lung; thoracic aorta behind the left atrium; the heart oriented toward the left; the ribs and overlaying cutaneous tissue; and posterior, the spine (**Figure 2**).

Three-vessel view: allows visualization of the thymus and its relationship with the great vessels and appears as a well-defined roundish solid structure interposed between the great vessels and the sternum. It is weakly hypoechogenic in comparison with the surrounding lungs. In front of the spine and behind the three vessels, the trachea, and, with some difficulty, the esophagus can be seen (**Figure 3**).

Midsagittal view: does not give significant information regarding the lungs because it is occupied mainly by the heart.

Right parasagittal view: the diaphragmatic hypoechogenic layer can be seen below the right lung.

Left parasagittal view: the diaphragmatic hypoechogenic layer can be seen below the left lung and the heart and allows to demonstrate that the stomach is located below the diaphragm.

The ultrasound diagnosis of CDH is, in general, indirect: the abnormal intrathoracic position of the stomach and/or the other migrated viscera and the displacement of the heart and the mediastinum is detected (**Figure 4**).

Left posterolateral CDH: in the *four-chamber view*, the stomach is in the left hemithorax or in the mediastinum (**Figure 5**).

Frequently, a few small bowel loops can be visualized near the stomach, while the heart and the mediastinum are pushed contralaterally. Much more rarely, the spleen and/or the left liver lobe may migrate as well. In few cases, only some ileal loops and/or the left hepatic

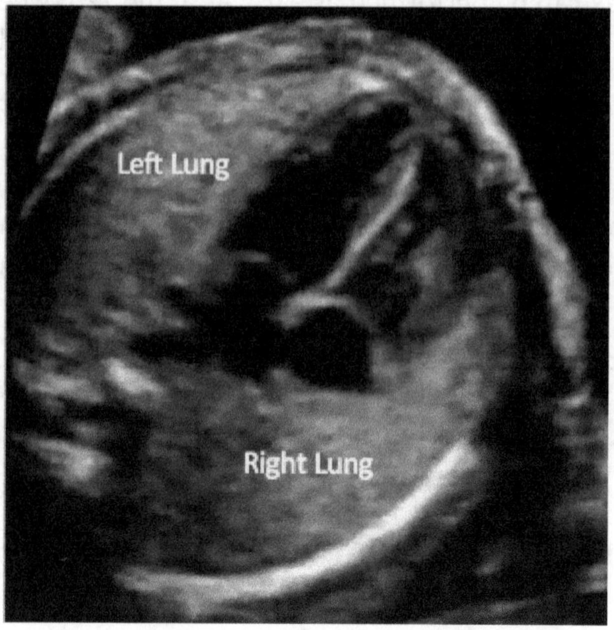

Figure 2. Four chamber view.

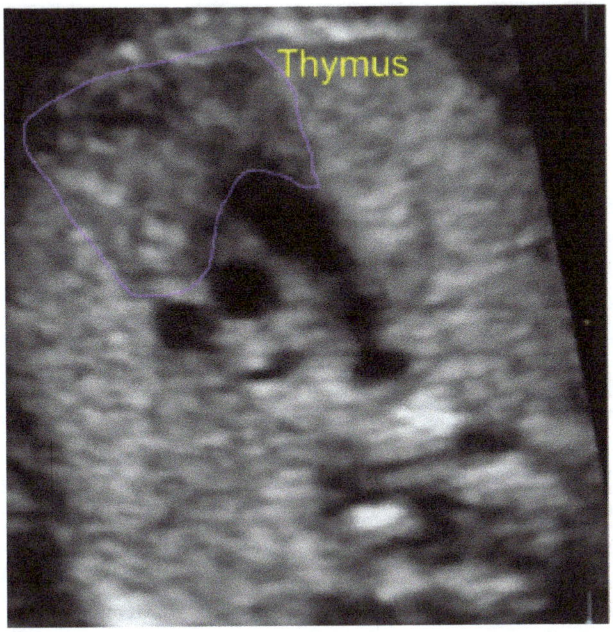

Figure 3. Three-vessel view. Note the thymus slightly hypoechogenic than lungs.

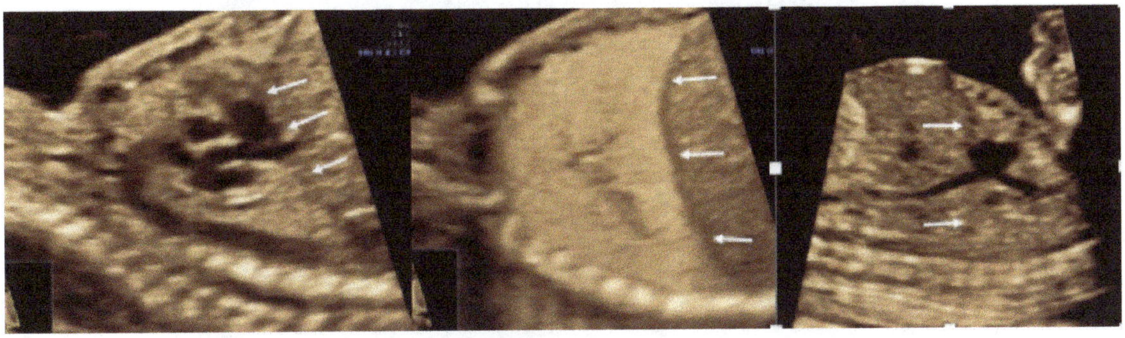

Figure 4. Sagittal view. Note the different echogenicity between lungs and abdominal viscera. Diaphragm appears as a hypoechogenic thin line.

lobe migrate into the thorax; therefore, the diagnosis is based only on dextrocardia and the unusual inhomogeneous appearance of the left hemithorax (**Figure 6**).

Kinking of the sinus venosus is a reliable sign in case of herniated left liver lobe; the bowing of the umbilical segment of the portal vein (portal sinuses) to the left of the midline and coursing of portal vessels to the lateral segment of the left hepatic lobe toward or above the diaphragm is considered the best predictor for liver herniation [20] (**Figure 7**).

It must be kept in mind that even though the diaphragmatic defect occurs in the first trimester, the visceral herniation is variable in time, from early second trimester to the first hour of life.

The sagittal views allow to detect some additional features that help confirm the diagnosis; the evidence of intrathoracic viscera on the four-chamber view is the basic requirement for a correct diagnosis of CDH.

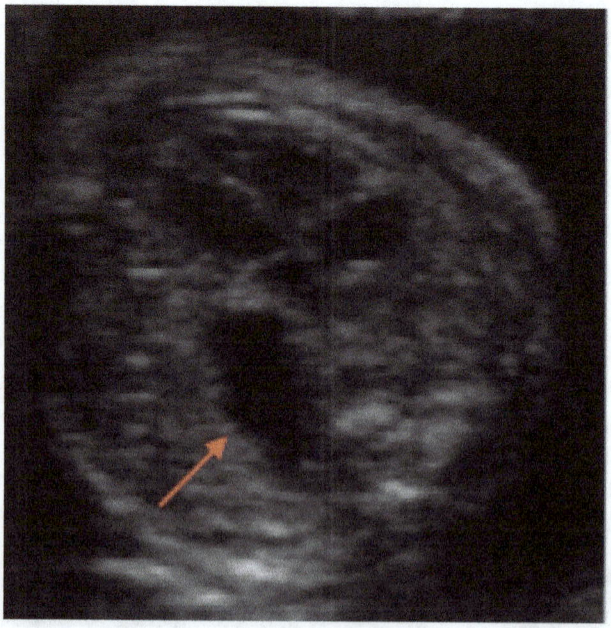

Figure 5. Left congenital diaphragmatic hernia. The stomach is in the left hemithorax and the heart is displaced to the right.

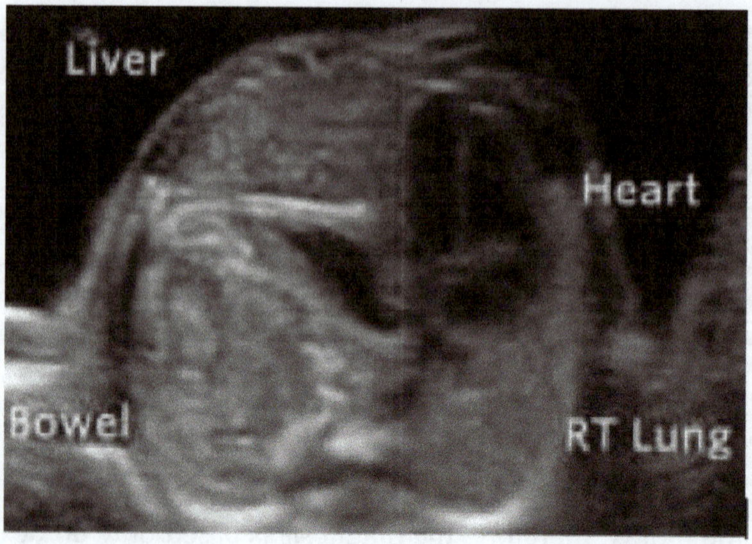

Figure 6. Left CDH. Herniation of left liver lobe and bowel loops. The heart is displaced to the right hemithorax.

Right-sided CDH: the diagnosis is difficult because the main feature, the intrathoracic displacement of the stomach, is absent because the defect is on the other side of the diaphragm. There are several indirect signs that lead to diagnosis. One is the leftward rotation of the heart with increase of the cardiac axis (**Figure** 8) and the upward displacement of the right hepatic lobe into the right hemithorax. This sign is best observed using color Doppler to identify the suprahepatic veins in the thorax because of the similar echogenicity of the lung and liver. Right-sided intrapleural hernias are less common, always contain liver, and may contain variable amounts of bowel and stomach. Rarely, intrapleural hernias may be bilateral; these tend to be associated with severe pulmonary hypoplasia. The midline position of the heart, the lack of

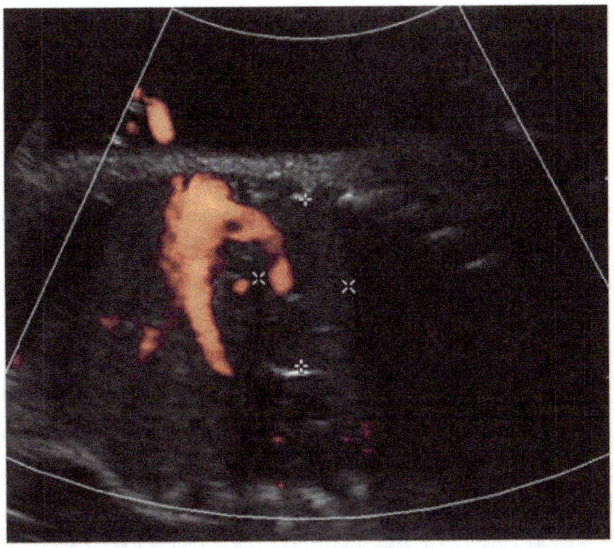

Figure 7. Portal vessels extending into the thorax. Left liver lobe (markers).

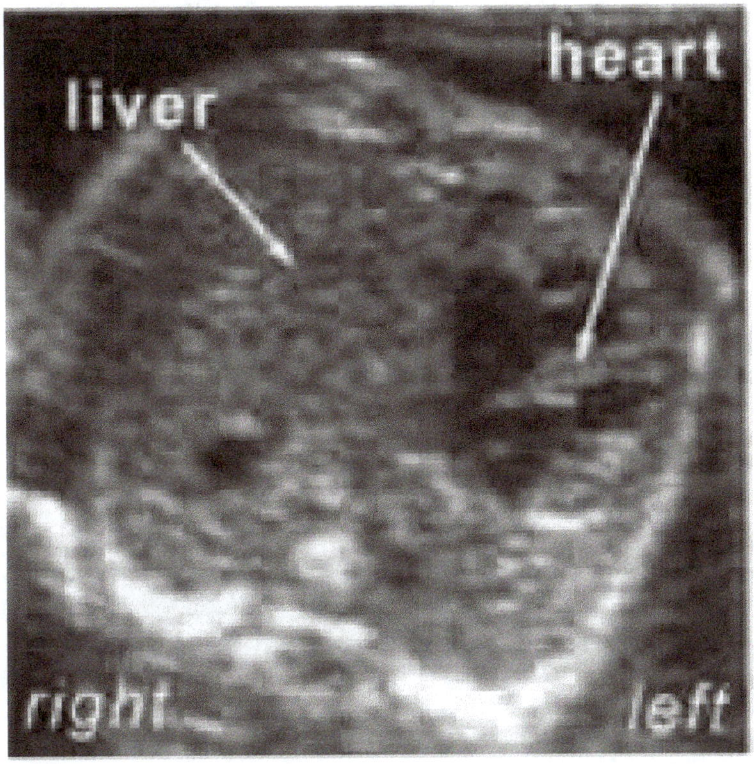

Figure 8. Leftward rotation of the heart with increase of the cardiac axis and upward displacement of the right hepatic lobe into the right hemithorax.

cardiomediastinal shift in cases of suspected intrapleural hernia should raise suspicion for the presence of bilateral intrapleural hernias.

Anterior and central CDH: the ventral type appears anteriorly because of the central tendons' defect. The central tendon of the diaphragm on his upper surface and the pericardium are communicating, if there is a defect at this site a pericardial effusion may develop. Ventral hernias may push the heart posteriorly but do not tend to cause pulmonary hypoplasia (**Figure 9**).

The smaller Morgagni hernia, usually is an isolated anterior defect and given its small size and location does not cause compression of thoracic organs. Morgagni hernias do not communicate with the pericardial space; therefore, this feature is a key element in differentiation from mediastinal hernias (**Table 6**).

Hiatal CDH: on ultrasound examination, it may appear as a hypoechogenic image behind the fetal heart in the posterior mediastinum, anterior to the vertebral body in continuity with a small fetal stomach located in the abdominal cavity just below the diaphragm in a median position. Parasagittal sonographic sections of the fetal thorax show an intact diaphragm on both sides. During the examination, stomach peristalsis may be visualized or the up and down movements of the stomach into the fetal thorax [21, 22]. The absence of liver in a hiatal hernia should help distinguish it from a right-sided intrapleural hernia.

The diagnosis of diaphragmatic hernia is rare during the first trimester. Early diagnosis has been associated with poor prognosis and the presence of additional defects [23, 24]. A diagnosis of CDH is suggestive if a displacement of the fetal heart in association with an intrathoracic mass having the appearance of the liver or stomach is detected.

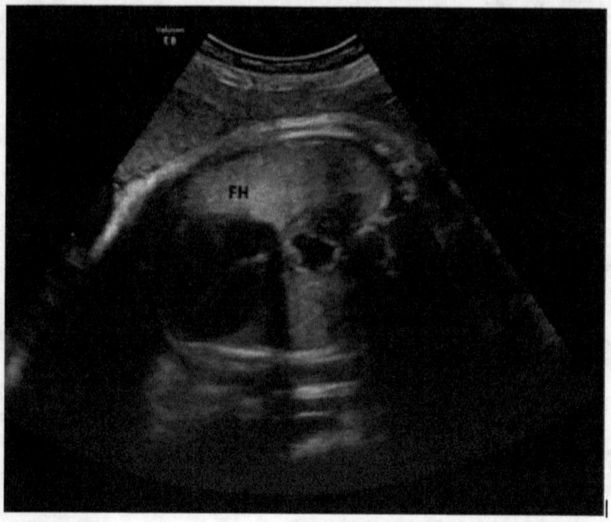

Figure 9. Transverse view of the fetal thorax with an anechogenic mass behind the heart; FH—fetal heart; Ao—aorta; S—stomach.

- Thoracic mass with mediastinal shift.
- Left-sided CHD: stomach is in thorax seen in *four-chamber view*, almost half of the cases have liver herniation.
- Right-sided CHD: almost always have liver herniation which is difficult to see; diagnosis is suspected in case of left mediastinal shift and Doppler reveals abnormal course of hepatic vessels.
- Polyhydramnios secondary to esophageal compression.

Table 6. Key sonographic features.

It was reported in a prospective study on 78,000 pregnancies at first trimester screening for chromosomal abnormalities by nuchal translucency thickness, 19 chromosomally normal fetuses with diagnosis of congenital diaphragmatic hernia. Only one of them was diagnosed in the first trimester; diagnosis was based on the visualization of the stomach in the thorax. In about one-third of the cases of diaphragmatic hernia, they found increased nuchal translucency. In the majority of the infants (83%) who died in the neonatal period due to pulmonary hypoplasia, nuchal translucency was increased, while the respective percentage for the survivors was 22%. The authors hypothesized that the accumulated nuchal fluid may be caused by venous congestion determined by intrathoracic compression due to early herniation of the abdominal organs [25].

The compression of herniated organs on esophagus or gastic outlet obstruction causes polyhydramnios which may became visible later in pregnancy. Another cause of polyhydramnios in cases with CDH is esophageal atresia with tracheoesophageal fistula, which may be very difficult to diagnose because the visualization of the proximal esophageal pouch is dependent on its being distended by swallowed amniotic fluid.

2.9. Differential diagnosis

Bronchogenic cysts (*foregut duplication*) contain several components of the bronchi, including respiratory epithelia, mucous glands, and cartilage and may occur anywhere along the length of the trachea or esophagus [26]. Most are diagnosed incidentally or if large enough, can compress the esophagus and/or trachea.

Congenital cystic adenomatoid malformation (CCAM): a developmental abnormality of the lung resulting from abnormal cell proliferation and decreased programmed cell death of lung tissue. Type I CCAM is most common and is distinguished by relatively large cysts and mucin production.

Cystic teratomas are benign tumors most often found in the anterior mediastinum. They consist of several differentiated cell types derived from endoderm, ectoderm, and/or mesoderm [27, 28].

Neurogenic tumors are the most common lesion found in the posterior mediastinum. They are likely to be of neural crest origin; the majority is benign: neurilemoma, neurofibroma, ganglioneuroma, pheochromocytoma, and neuroblastoma.

Pulmonary agenesis refers to partial or complete absence of lung tissue that is caused by failure of lung bud development.

Pulmonary sequestration results from primitive lung tissue that is not connected to the tracheobronchial tree. Sequestration may be intrapulmonary, occurring within the pleura of the normal lung or extrapulmonary, occurring outside the normal lung within its own pleural sac.

2.10. Prognostic indicators

The best validated measurement is contralateral lung area assessed by 2D ultrasound through the so-called lung area/head circumference ratio (LHR) [29]. Different methods for measuring were described but the most reproducible and accurate method involves tracing the lung contours.

Normal lung area develops four times more than the head circumference between week 12 and 32; therefore, the LHR needs to be adjusted according to gestational age. The effect of gestational age on LHR can be minimized by expressing the observed LHR as a ratio to the expected mean LHR for that gestational age.

2.10.1. *The lung area to head circumference ratio*

The lung-to-head circumference ratio (LHR) is a sonographic measure proposed to identify fetuses with congenital diaphragmatic hernia (CDH) that have a poor prognosis. The lung area contralateral to the CDH is measured at the level of *four-chamber view* by manual tracing of the lung which appears to be the most reproducible way of measuring the lung area [30]. The product is divided by the head circumference (HC) to obtain the LHR.

The lung area to head circumference ratio (LHR) = lung area/head circumference.

2.10.2. *Observed/expected lung-to-head ratio*

The observed LHR may be expressed as a percentage of the expected mean for gestational age as the observed/expected lung-to-head ratio O/E LHR [31, 32].

O/E LHR = (observed LHR/expected LHR) × 100

There has been proposed a four-step stratification of fetuses based on their observed/expected (O/E) LHR wherein it was also taken into account their liver position.

- Fetuses with an O/E LHR <15% have extreme pulmonary hypoplasia and there are no survivors reported.
- Fetuses with an O/E LHR between 15 and 25% have severe pulmonary hypoplasia and survival prediction is about 20%, those with the liver down having better prognosis than those with liver up in the thorax.
- Fetuses with an O/E LHR between 26 and 35% and those with an O/E LHR between 36 and 45% but with the liver up have moderate hypoplasia. They have an expected survival rate between 30 and 60%, which depends on the lung size.
- Fetuses with an O/E LHR between 36 and 45% with the liver down and those with an O/E LHR >45% have mild hypoplasia and have better prognosis, >75% survival rate [33, 34] (**Table 7**).

• Prenatal prediction of postnatal outcome in CDH patients is based on ultrasound measurement of contralateral lung size and magnetic resonance total lung volumetry.
• The ratio of observed to predicted lung/head ratio is the most validated predictor for postnatal outcome; the liver position is also predictive.
• Fetal tracheal occlusion has been shown safe and feasible by minimally invasive means.

Table 7. Key points.

2.10.3. Fetal lung volumes

On fetal MR imaging there are several methods described for estimation of fetal pulmonary hypoplasia. All of these methods include the measuring of total fetal lung volume (TFLV). MR volumetry is considered the most accurate method for measuring ipsilateral lung and, therefore, for best estimation of fetal lung volumes, compared to three-dimensional ultrasound [35].

2.10.4. Fetal intervention

Because CDH is an anomaly with poor prognosis that can be identified in the prenatal period, it is justified to perform an intervention which improves lung function. Di Fiore and Wilson studied the concept of triggering lung growth by tracheal occlusion [36]. This was observed in an experiment of nature occurring in fetuses with congenital high airway obstruction syndrome (CHAOS), who display impressive lung growth. Through pregnancy, fetal lungs secrete fluid during their development, which creates a positive pressure under the glottis. Fluid secretion of the lung and a cyclical pressure change are essential for development and growth of the lung [37]. Fluid secretion increases the pressure in airways but during fetal breathing movements, the pressure gradient is normalized as glottis opens. This phenomenon creates cyclical periods of tissue stretch, which are important for an optimal balance between growth and differentiation [38]. Intrauterine tracheal occlusion acts like a closed glottis trapping the fluid causing subsequently increased tissue stretch, which triggers lung growth. The tracheal occlusion decreases the number of type II alveolocytes and lowers surfactant expression in occluded lungs [39–42]. This unwanted effect may be improved by either removing the tracheal occlusion before birth and/or by antenatal steroid administration [43, 44]. Experimentally, in-utero reversal of occlusion (clinically translated as a plug-unplug sequence) achieved morphologically better lung maturation [45].

3. Conclusions

As prenatal detection of fetal CDH improved in recent years, it is important to use standardized prognosis markers around the world. Currently, available markers are not 100% accurately predictive of outcome and their use is much less accurate in the presence of chromosomal anomalies or other malformations. This shows the fact that all fetuses diagnosed with CDH should undergo an ultrasound examination by a well-trained sonographer, as well as fetal echocardiography.

Conflict of interest

No conflict of interest to declare.

Author details

Adrian Claudiu Ratiu

Address all correspondence to: ratiu.adrian@umft.ro

University of Medicine and Pharmacy "Victor Babes", Timisoara, Romania

References

[1] Gallot D, Boda C, Ughetto S, Perthus I, Robert-Gnansia E, Francannet C, Laurichesse-Delmas H, Jani J, Coste K, Deprest J, et al. Prenatal detection and outcome of congenital diaphragmatic hernia: A French registry-based study. Ultrasound in Obstetrics & Gynecology. 2007;**29**:276-283

[2] Tudorache S, Chiuţu LC, Iliescu DG, Georgescu R, Stoica GA, Simionescu CE, Georgescu EF, Nemeş RN. Prenatal diagnosis and perinatal outcome in congenital diaphragmatic hernia. Single tertiary center report. Romanian Journal of Morphology and Embryology. 2014;**55**(3):823-833

[3] Parisi MA, Zayed H, Slavotinek AM, Rutledge JC. Congenital diaphragmatic hernia and microtia in a newborn with mycophenolate mofetil (MMF) exposure: Phenocopy for Fryns syndrome or broad spectrum of teratogenic effects? American Journal of Medical Genetics: Part A. 2009;**149A**:1237-1240

[4] Pober BR, Russell MK, Ackerman KG. Congenital diaphragmatic hernia overview. In: Pagon RA, Adam MP, Ardinger HH, et al., editors. Gene Reviews. Seattle (WA): University of Washington, Seattle; 1993-2017

[5] Mehollin-Ray AR, Cassady CI, Cass DL, Olutoye O. Fetal MR imaging of congenital diaphragmatic hernia. Radiographics. 2012;**32**:1067-1084

[6] Moore KL. The Developing Human: Clinically Oriented Embryology. 3rd ed. Philadelphia: WB Saunders; 1982

[7] Yuan W, Rao Y, Babiuk RP, Greer JJ, Wu JY, Ornitz DM. A genetic model for a central (septum transversum) congenital diaphragmatic hernia in mice lacking Slit3. Proceedings of the National Academy of Sciences of the United States of America. 2003;**100**:5217-5222

[8] Birchmeier C, Brohmann H. Genes that control the development of migrating muscle precursor cells. Current Opinion in Cell Biology. 2000;**12**:725-730

[9] Babiuk RP, Zhang W, Clugston R, Allan DW, Greer JJ. Embryological origins and development of the rat diaphragm. The Journal of Comparative Neurology. 2003;**455**:477-487

[10] Hopper AF, Hart NH. Foundations of Animal Development. Oxford: Oxford University Press; 1985

[11] Spooner BS, Wessels NK. Mammalian lung development: Interactions in primordium formation and bronchial morphogenesis. The Journal of Experimental Zoology. 1970;**175**:445-454

[12] Boyden EA. Development of the human lung. In: Brenneman J, editor. Practice of Pediatrics. Hagerstown, PA: Harper & Row; 1972

[13] Keijzer R, Puri P. Congenital diaphragmatic hernia. Seminars in Pediatric Surgery. 2010; **19**:180-185

[14] Reid L. The embryology of the lung. In: de Reuck AVS, Porter R, editors. Ciba Foundation Symposium. London: J. & A. Churchill Ltd; 1967. pp. 109-130

[15] Kluth D, Keijzer R, Hertl M, Tibboel D. Embryology of congenital diaphragmatic hernia. Seminars in Pediatric Surgery. 1996;**5**:224-233

[16] Greer JJ, Allan DW, Babiuk RP, Lemke RP. Recent advances in understanding the pathogenesis of nitrofen-induced congenital diaphragmatic hernia. Pediatric Pulmonology. 2000;**29**:394-399

[17] Jesudason EC, Connell MG, Fernig DG, et al. Early lung malformations in congenital diaphragmatic hernia. Journal of Pediatric Surgery. 2000;**35**:124-127, discussion: 128

[18] Keijzer R, Liu J, Deimling J, et al. Dual-hit hypothesis explains pulmonary hypoplasia in the nitrofen model of congenital diaphragmatic hernia. The American Journal of Pathology. 2000;**156**:1299-1306

[19] Puri P, Gorman F. Lethal nonpulmonary anomalies associated with congenital diaphragmatic hernia: Implications for early intrauterine surgery. Journal of Pediatric Surgery. 1984;**19**(1):29-32

[20] Bootstaylor BS, Filly RA, Harrison MR, Adzick NS. Prenatal sonographic predictors of liver herniation in congenital diaphragmatic hernia. Journal of Ultrasound in Medicine. 1995;**14**:515-552

[21] Ruano R, Benachi A, Aubry MC, Bernard JP, Hameury F, Nihoul-Fekete C, Dumez Y. Prenatal sonographic diagnosis of congenital hiatal hernia. Prenatal Diagnosis. 2004; **24**(1):26-30

[22] Di Francesco S, Matteo Lanna M, Napolitano M, et al. A case of ultrasound diagnosis of fetal hiatal hernia in late third trimester of pregnancy. Case Reports in Obstetrics and Gynecology. 2015;**2015**. Article ID 194090, 3 pages. DOI: 10.1155/2015/194090

[23] Garne E, Quataert P, de Vigan C. Congenital diaphragmatic hernia: A European population-based study of epidemiology, prenatal diagnosis and mortality. Prenatal and Neonatal Medicine. 1999;**4**:441-447

[24] Garne E, Haeusler M, Barisic I, Gjergja R, Stoll C, Clementi M, the Euroscan Study Group. Congenital diaphragmatic hernia: Evaluation of prenatal diagnosis in 20 European regions. Ultrasound in Obstetrics & Gynecology. 2002;**19**:329-333

[25] Sebire NJ, Snijders RJM, Davenport M, Greenough A, Nicolaides KH. Fetal nuchal translucency thickness at 10-14 weeks of gestation and congenital diaphragmatic hernia. Obstetrics and Gynecology. 1997;**90**:943-947

[26] Knudtson J, Grewal H. Thoracoscopic excision of a paraesophageal bronchogenic cyst in a child. JSLS. 2004;**8**:179-182

[27] Jaggers J, Balsara K. Mediastinal masses in children. Seminars in Thoracic and Cardiovascular Surgery. 2004;**16**:201-208

[28] Ionescu C, Haradja H, Gheorghiu D, Vladescu T, Pacu I, Dimitriu M. Prenatal ultrasound diagnosis of cervical teratoma. Gineco.ro. 2011;**7**(23):25-27

[29] Metkus AP, Filly RA, Stringer MD, Harrison MR, Adzick NS. Sonographic predictors of survival in fetal diaphragmatic hernia. Journal of Pediatric Surgery. 1996;**31**:148-151

[30] Peralta CFA, Cavoretto P, Csapo B, Vandecruys H, Nicolaides KH. Assessment of lung area in normal fetuses at 12-32 weeks. Ultrasound in Obstetrics & Gynecology. 2005; **26**:718-724

[31] Jani J, Nicolaides KH, Keller RL, Benachi A, Peralta CFA, Favre R, Moreno O, Tibboel D, Lipitz S, Eggink A, Vaast P, Allegaert K, Harrison M, Deprest J. Observed to expected lung area to head circumference ratio in the prediction of survival in fetuses with isolated diaphragmatic hernia. Ultrasound in Obstetrics & Gynecology. 2007;**30**:67-71

[32] Jani JC, Peralta CFA, Nicolaides KH. Lung-to-head ratio: A need to unify the technique. Ultrasound in Obstetrics & Gynecology. 2012;**39**:2-6

[33] Deprest JA, Flemmer AW, Gratacos E, Nicolaides K. Antenatal prediction of lung volume and in-utero treatment by fetal endoscopic tracheal occlusion in severe isolated congenital diaphragmatic hernia. Seminars in Fetal & Neonatal Medicine. 2009;**14**:8-13

[34] Ionescu C, Gheorghiu D, Pacu I, Sardescu G, Ionescu V. Prognosticul fetal în hernia diafragmatică congenitală stîngă. Obstetrica si Ginecologia. 2009;**LVII**(3):183

[35] Jani JC, Cannie M, Peralta CFA, Deprest JA, Nicolaides KH, Dymarkowski S. Lung volumes in fetuses with congenital diaphragmatic hernia: Comparison of 3D US and MR imaging assessments. Radiology. 2007;**244**(2):575-582

[36] DiFiore JW, Fauza DO, Slavin R, Peters CA, Fackler JC, Wilson JM. Experimental fetal tracheal ligation reverses the structural and physiological effects of pulmonary hypoplasia in congenital diaphragmatic hernia. Journal of Pediatric Surgery. 1994;**29**:248-256

[37] Moessinger AC, Harding R, Adamson TM, Singh M, Kiu GT. Role of lung fluid volume in growth and maturation of the fetal sheep lung. The Journal of Clinical Investigation. 1990;**86**:1270-1277

[38] Nelson SM, Hajivassiliou CA, Haddock G, et al. Rescue of the hypoplastic lung by prenatal cyclical strain. American Journal of Respiratory and Critical Care Medicine. 2005;**171**:1395-1402

[39] Probyn ME, Wallace MJ, Hooper SB. Effect of increased lung expansion on lung growth and development near midgestation in fetal sheep. Pediatric Research. 2000;**47**:806-812

[40] Luks FI, Roggin KK, Wild YK, et al. Effect of lung fluid composition on type II cellular activity after tracheal occlusion in the fetal lamb. Journal of Pediatric Surgery. 2001; **36**:196-201

[41] De Paepe ME, Papadakis K, Johnson BD, Luks FI. Fate of the type II pneumocyte following tracheal occlusion in utero: A time-course study in fetal sheep. Virchows Archiv. 1998;**432**:7-16

[42] O'Toole SJ, Sharma A, Karamanoukian HL, Holm B, Azizkhan RG, Glick PL. Tracheal ligation does not correct the surfactant deficiency associated with congenital diaphragmatic hernia. Journal of Pediatric Surgery. 1996;**31**:546-550

[43] Bratu I, Flageole H, Laberge JM, et al. Surfactant levels after reversible tracheal occlusion and prenatal steroids in experimental diaphragmatic hernia. Journal of Pediatric Surgery. 2001;**36**:122-127

[44] Davey MG, Danzer E, Schwarz U, Adzick NS, Flake AW, Hedrick HL. Prenatal glucocorticoids and exogenous surfactant therapy improve respiratory function in lambs with severe diaphragmatic hernia following fetal tracheal occlusion. Pediatric Research. 2006;**60**(2):131-135

[45] Flageole H, Evrard VA, Piedboeuf B, Laberge JM, Lerut TE, Deprest JA. The plug–unplug sequence: An important step to achieve type II pneumocyte maturation in the fetal lamb model. Journal of Pediatric Surgery. 1998;**33**:299-303

2

Congenital Diaphragmatic Hernia: Part 2

Joanne Baerg, Arul Thirumoorthi and
Rajaie Hazboun

Abstract

Despite advances in neonatal and surgical care, the management of congenital diaphragmatic hernia (CDH) remains challenging with no definitive standard treatment guidelines. Several centers report mortality rates as low as 20%, but if extracorporeal membrane oxygenation (ECMO) support is required, the mortality rate rises to 50%. The disease severity is related to the degree of pulmonary hypoplasia and pulmonary hypertension that occurs with CDH. Both conditions decrease the infant's ability to ventilate and oxygenate adequately at delivery. These physiologic conditions that impair gas exchange are the important determinants of morbidity and mortality in CDH infants. Presently, delivery of infants with CDH is recommended close to term gestation. The focus of care includes gentle ventilation, hemodynamic monitoring, and treatment of pulmonary hypertension followed by surgery for the defect. Extracorporeal membrane oxygenation (ECMO) is considered after failure of conventional medical management for infants ≥ 34 weeks' gestation or with weight >2 kg and no associated major lethal anomalies. This chapter discusses long-term follow-up recommendations for survivors, which should involve a multidisciplinary approach, as there are many surgical and nonsurgical consequences to the disease process. Clinical strategies that address these multifaceted aspects of care, from prenatal to long-term follow-up, may further reduce the high mortality rate for these infants.

Keywords: respiratory failure, pulmonary hypertension, pulmonary hypoplasia, extracorporeal membrane oxygenation

1. Introduction

A congenital diaphragmatic hernia (CDH) is a developmental defect of the posterior lateral part of the diaphragm. The opening allows the abdominal organs to slide into the chest or "herniate" which may lead to underdevelopment of the lungs. The lung on the ipsilateral side of the hernia is generally smaller.

CDH is six times more common on the left than the right. The incidence is reported between one in 2200 and one in 3500 live births. Rare bilateral defects are generally fatal. The differential diagnosis includes congenital pulmonary airway malformation (CPAM), bronchogenic cyst, and eventration [1].

Despite advances in neonatal and surgical care, the management of CDH remains challenging with no definitive standard treatment guidelines. The mortality rate is high, with little change over the past few decades, and is generally reported between 30 and 45%. Several centers report mortality rates as low as 20%. If extracorporeal membrane oxygenation (ECMO) support is required, the mortality rate rises to 50% [2].

The severity of the disease is related to the degree of pulmonary hypoplasia and pulmonary hypertension that occurs with CDH. Both conditions decrease the infant's ability to ventilate and oxygenate adequately at delivery. These physiologic conditions that impair gas exchange are the important determinants of morbidity and mortality in CDH infants.

2. Embryology

Incomplete fusion of embryologic elements that give rise to the diaphragm leads to the hernia defect. CDH occurs at distinct sites. Ninety percent are a posterolateral defect (Bochdalek hernia) and 9% are an anterolateral defect (Morgagni hernia). Total agenesis may occur.

3. Inheritance patterns

Congenital diaphragmatic hernia generally presents sporadically. The CDH risk in a sibling is less than 2%, due to multifactorial patterns of inheritance [3]. There are rare incidences of dominant and X-linked recessive inheritance for isolated defects [4]. Bilateral lesions tend to familial inheritance and bilateralism, and tend to have less severe associated anomalies. Familial diaphragmatic agenesis, however, is an autosomal recessive syndrome, is a distinct syndrome with a worse prognosis than posterolateral diaphragmatic hernia [5].

There are no firmly established teratogens associated with CDH. Diaphragmatic hernia is associated with Fryn's syndrome [6], Beckwith-Wiedemann syndrome [7], and Pierre Robin syndrome [8].

4. Associated anomalies

Most fetuses with severe associated anomalies die in utero. Therefore, the incidence of prenatal abnormalities is higher than that reported in the literature by pediatric surgeons and lower than postmortem studies. In prenatal series, only about 50% of fetuses have an isolated diaphragmatic defect. In about 25% of cases, there is a chromosomal abnormality, usually Trisomy 21, trisomy 18 or 13, which is similar to omphalocele infants [9]. In another 25%, there is a major defect including cardiovascular defects atrial septal defect (ASD), ventricular septal defect (VSD), hypoplastic left heart, tetralogy of Fallot, transposition). The overall survival of infants with CDH and a chromosomal anomaly is poor.

4.1. Prenatal evaluation

Ultrasound screening examination in the prenatal period will generally diagnose a congenital diaphragmatic hernia. Prenatal evaluation of CDH is important for parental counseling, prognostication, and postnatal management. The prenatal evaluation of the postnatal prognosis of CDH is improving, but better standardization of evaluation methods is needed to compare results.

The prenatal ultrasound diagnosis is based on the following factors:

1. The presence of *abdominal organs visualized within the thoracic cavity*. Ultrasound may reveal a left-sided CDH if the stomach or loops of bowel are partially or totally within the thorax.

2. The heart position may shift, or cardiac compression may be observed, from the organs in the thoracic cavity.

3. *Polyhydramnios* is common, either due to esophageal compression or reduced absorption of fluid by the hypoplastic lungs, but it is rarely observed before 24-week gestation.

Any *mediastinal shift* or hydrothorax, abnormal position of the gallbladder, hepatic veins, or even umbilical veins should arouse suspicion of a right-sided hernia. It may be a challenging diagnosis because the lungs and liver have similar echogenicity.

At antenatal diagnosis, the following studies and consultations are recommended:

1. chromosomal analysis
2. serial prenatal ultrasound examinations
3. a fetal echocardiograph
4. pediatric surgery consultation

These investigations are relevant, even in the third trimester of pregnancy, because knowledge that the fetus is chromosomally and otherwise structurally normal allows the parents, obstetrician, pediatrician, and surgeon to discuss the mode, place, and timing of delivery.

Prognosis: The primary determinants of survival for infants with CDH are the presence of associated anomalies, pulmonary hypoplasia, and pulmonary hypertension. Prenatally discovered cases and cases diagnosed before 24-week gestation have a worse prognosis because of the early stage of the lung development when the anomaly has occurred. Mortality in this group is reported as high as 60–80% [10].

4.2. Pulmonary hypoplasia

Pulmonary hypoplasia occurs in CDH and is the main cause of mortality. Pulmonary hypoplasia is defined as incomplete development of the lungs with decreased bronchopulmonary segments and diminished alveolar septation [11]. Incomplete development results in a decreased total lung volume.

Much prenatal investigation is directed toward the accurate evaluation of pulmonary hypoplasia. Its antenatal prediction remains one of the challenges of prenatal diagnosticians. Accurate case selection identifies those cases that may benefit from prenatal surgery.

Fetuses with CDH and a "poor prognosis" with postnatal treatment have

- a low lung-to-head ratio (LHR) on ultrasound
- a diagnosis before 25-week gestation
- liver herniation on prenatal ultrasound
- a fetal magnetic resonance imaging (MRI) consistent with a low lung volume.

4.3. Lung to head ratio

The lung-head ratio (LHR) is calculated by 2D ultrasound. For accurate prognostication, the measure must be performed between 22 and 28-week gestation. The length and width of the right lung is measured and multiplied to calculate the right lung area. The right lung area is then divided by the head perimeter measure **Figure 1**.

For example:

- Right lung area: 21 mm × 10 mm = 210 mm^2
- Head perimeter: 200 mm

Lung-to-head ratio (LHR): 210/200 = 1.05

A lung-to-head ratio of 1.0 or less has a poor prognosis, despite ECMO. If the ratio is greater than 1.4, the prognosis is much better. Lung-to-head ratios between 1.0 and 1.4 have about a 38% survival rate. Most cases with an LHR in this range require ECMO. Overall, survivors have a mean lung-to-head ratio in the range of 1.4 ± 0.33 and nonsurvivors, 1.05 ± 0.3 [12].

The presence of liver in the chest on prenatal ultrasound is a poor prognosticator for survival [13, 14].

A recent meta-analysis analyzed the ability of lung-to-head ratio (LHR), observed-to-expected LHR (o/e LHR), total fetal lung volume (TFLV), o/e TFLV, percentage predicted lung volume (PPLV), and degree of liver herniation to predict neonatal morbidity and mortality in fetuses with CDH.

The primary outcome was perinatal survival and the secondary outcome was the use of extracorporeal membrane oxygenation (ECMO).

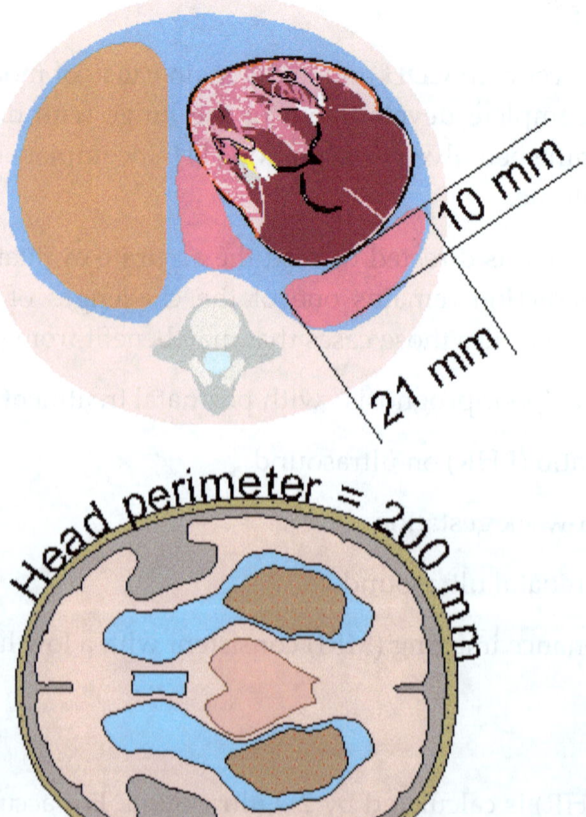

Figure 1. Calculation of lung: head ratio from 2D ultrasound. (From: 2000-05-29-17 Diaphragmatic hernia © Novakov www.thefetus.net).

Twenty-two articles published before April 2016 met the inclusion criteria.

The odds of survival with LHR <1.0 was 0.14 (CI: 0.10–0.27) and with liver herniation on ultrasound it was 0.21 (CI: 0.13–0.35).

The O/E LHR and O/E TFLV performed best in this prediction model. The most discriminatory threshold for lung volume and mortality was O/E LHR <1 and for O/E TFLV, it was 25%. LHR <1 was predictive of extracorporeal life support (ECLS) use. Overall, the O/E LHR <1, O/E TFLV (thresholds of 25%), and liver herniation are good predictors of mortality in CDH [13].

Similarly, Partridge reports that serial lung to head growth measures are a better prognosticator for lung growth and survival. Of 226 CDH infants identified over 10 years, 72 died (32%). Liver in the chest or use of patch for closure of the defect were associated with mortality. The rate of lung to head ratio increase, as measured by linear regression and slope analysis, was significantly better in survivors [15].

4.4. Fetal MRI consistent with a low lung volume

Fetal magnetic resonance imaging (MRI) has undergone major technical improvement since it was first performed over 30 years ago. It complements US studies by providing better visualization when ultrasound is limited by oligohydramnios or maternal obesity. Other advantages include a larger field of view and better tissue contrast than US. It is not limited by shadowing from osseous structures. However, the limitations include a decreased resolution compared with US, less availability, and increased cost.

Multiple MRI studies have reported normal fetal lung volumes based on gestational age. In cases of CDH, the risk for pulmonary hypoplasia can be assessed by comparing the lung volume measured by MRI with a normal value for the gestational age; however, the literature results have been inconsistent and have not reliably predicted outcome. There is a lack of standardization of MRI technique in the literature.

A curve of normal fetal lung volume values plotted against gestational age has been established and validated for fetal MRI [16]. The observed/expected total fetal lung volume (O/E-TFLV) ratio is calculated by dividing the measured fetal lung volume by the expected mean fetal lung volume for a given gestational age [16].

The fetal MRI planimetric measurements of ipsilateral, contralateral, and total fetal lung volume (TFLV) are performed with T(2)-haste sequences in transverse, coronal, and sagittal planes. All values are expressed as a ratio of what was observed over what is expected for a gestation age matched normal fetus.

One study reports the measurement of O/E LHR on ultrasound allowing a reasonable estimation and correlation of O/E contralateral FLV as well as TFLV as measured by MRI [17]. Additional parameters such as gestational age, liver position, and side of defect improved the estimation of TFLV.

Others report that lung size and liver herniation predict the need for ECMO but do not predict pulmonary hypertension [18].

A review of articles that provided normal fetal lung volumes for gestational age revealed much variability in absolute lung volume within each individual study. Each study had a solitary reporter. The best-fit curves ranged from 20 to 35 ml at 25 weeks' gestation and 58 to 95 ml at 35 weeks' gestation [19]. The study by Rypens et al. included the largest number of fetuses and, in contrast, included measurements by several observers at different institutions [16]. The ability of MRI to predict prognosis and survival for CDH is inconsistent, although multiple studies have shown a correlation between fetal lung volume in CDH and postnatal outcomes of neonatal survival and ECMO.

Infants with CDH generally have O/E-TFLV measurements ranging from 25 to 45% or lower. They require more pulmonary support than omphalocele and congenital lung malformation infants. Clinical-radiologic correlation studies support the use of prenatal MRI to predict perinatal and postnatal outcomes. The measurements may guide fetal therapy with improved postnatal results. An O/E TFLV below 35% is associated with increased ECMO use and a higher mortality [20].

One review of articles encompassing 269 fetuses with congenital diaphragmatic hernia reported areas under the receiver operating characteristic (ROC) curves ranging from 0.786 to 0.900 in the prediction of survival. Two others involving MRI-measured fetal lung volume reported the area under the ROC curves to range from 0.653 to 0.770 in the prediction of extracorporeal membrane oxygenation requirement. All of the above studies utilized MR measurements of fetal lung volume compared with normal lung volume data from either the Rypens et al. study or formulas based on gestational age or biometric parameters [19].

Further studies are needed to assess and develop the full potential of MRI measurement of fetal lung volume in predicting neonatal prognosis.

4.5. Prenatal surgery

If LHR is <1, LHR 0/E is less than 25%, or liver is in the thorax, survival for CDH infants is less than 25%. In these fetuses, in utero treatments are sometimes offered such as fetal endotracheal occlusion (FETO) [10, 21].

Many experimental models of in utero surgery for CDH exist. Prenatal treatment of the fetus has been proposed to avoid pulmonary hypoplasia. However, a hysterotomy is required. The subsequent caesarian section on an otherwise healthy mother has significant morbidity and risk of premature labor.

Open fetal surgery, while feasible, does not improve survival over standard postnatal treatment in the subgroup of congenital diaphragmatic hernia fetuses without liver herniation. The data from this randomized trial suggest that fetuses with a prenatally diagnosed CDH without evidence of liver herniation should be treated postnatally [10].

Fetal endotracheal occlusion (FETO) is thought to prevent outward movement of pulmonary fluid. The retention of lung fluid may improve lung expansion and even possibly promote reduction of the viscera into the peritoneal cavity [21]. The placement of a "tracheal clip" may accelerate lung growth and avoid the development of fatal pulmonary hypoplasia [22]. Endoscopic techniques decrease the risk of preterm labor and other complications of open fetal surgery.

The best candidates for this procedure are fetuses with a left CDH, liver herniation, and a low lung-to-head ratio that are at high risk of neonatal demise [23]. A minimally invasive intraluminal tracheal occlusion technique, which avoids laparotomy, hysterotomy, and fetal neck dissection, has been recently accomplished. This technique may change the surgical approach to the fetus with severe CDH [24].

In 2017, 20 fetuses with CDH, an LHR<1 and liver herniation were reviewed [24]. Nine were managed without tracheal balloon occlusion; tracheal occlusion was offered in 11 and in 10, it was successful. The mean gestational age at FETO was 27.9 (1.1) weeks. The occlusion was reversed at 34 weeks and the infants were delivered at 35 weeks. One required an EXIT procedure to remove the balloon. All underwent postnatal repair of CDH with patch. The 6-month, 1-year, and 2-year survival were significantly higher in the treated than nontreated cohort. They concluded that FETO is feasible and associated with improved postnatal outcomes in severe Left CDH infants. A large multicenter randomized trial is still needed to demonstrate the real benefits of FETO [25].

5. Pulmonary hypertension

The developing lung is subject to genetic, pathological, and environmental influences that affect lung adaptation, development, and growth.

Neonates with CDH are primarily classified as having vascular hypoplasia, yet lung histology of fatal cases typically shows marked muscularization of pulmonary arteries, and clinically, these patients frequently respond to vasodilator therapy.

An early developmental arrest in the normal pattern of airway branching in both lungs, resulting in reduced lung volume and impaired alveolarization, will present as a severely symptomatic CDH after birth [26].

This arrest may occur in pulmonary arterial branching and result in a reduced cross-sectional area of the vascular bed, thickened media, and adventitia of small arterioles, and abnormal medial muscular hypertrophy that extends distally to the acinar arterioles. Although in utero lung compression by herniated viscera may be the primary mechanism of the lung abnormalities of CDH, decreased pulmonary blood flow alone may cause lung hypoplasia [27].

After birth, pulmonary vascular resistance (PVR) often remains at suprasystemic levels. This increased pulmonary right-to-left shunting across the foramen ovale and ductus arteriosus manifests in the infant as profound hypoxemia. High PVR is related to multiple factors, including the small cross-sectional area of pulmonary arteries, structural vascular remodeling, vasoconstriction with altered reactivity, and left ventricular dysfunction. The mediators of altered pulmonary vascular reactivity in CDH are not well understood, although much evidence points to disruptions in nitric oxide (NO), cyclic guanosine monophosphate (GMP) and endothelin signaling [28].

The pathophysiology of hypoxemia in CDH is also related to abnormalities of cardiac development and function. The left ventricle, left atrium, and intraventricular septum are hypoplastic in infants that die of CDH relative to age-matched controls, perhaps from low fetal and postnatal pulmonary blood flow and/or compression by the dilated right ventricle [28].

CDH is also associated with increased resistance of the pulmonary vasculature. Pulmonary hypertension (PHN) is characterized by elevated pulmonary vascular resistance, resulting in right to left shunting and hypoxemia. Differential hypoxemia is observed between the preductal- and postductal saturation monitors. Pulmonary hypertension is confirmed and monitored by serial echocardiography. Studies that aim to diagnose impaired vascular development are needed.

Yamoto et al. investigated the prenatal echocardiography factors that relate to outcomes in left-sided CDH [29]. Data were collected between 2006 and 2010. Severe cardiac anomalies and chromosomal anomalies were excluded. Of 84 patients, 8 died before 90 days (9.5%). Initial analysis revealed that the postnatal echo predictors of poor outcome were continuous right to left shunting, left pulmonary artery diameter of <2.7 mm, a right pulmonary artery diameter of <3.3 mm, and a left ventricular diameter of <10.8 mm. Logistic regression analysis found a small right pulmonary diameter and a smaller left ventricular diastolic diameter that were independently associated with poor outcomes. However, the postnatal echo was sometimes performed within 24 hours after birth, during the time of transitional circulation, and is a limitation of this study.

The optimal management of the structural and functional changes in the heart, pulmonary vasculature, airways, and lung parenchyma is challenging. The treatment of PHN in infants with CDH evolves and changes as the underlying pathophysiology evolve in the days and weeks after birth. Unlike other diseases resulting in persistent pulmonary hypertension of the newborn, infants with CDH are often refractory to inhaled nitric oxide (iNO). Nitric oxide mediates pulmonary vasodilatation at birth in part via cyclic GMP production. Evidence suggests several disorders exist in CDH infants (e.g., surfactant deficiency, decreased antioxidant activity, increased vascular reactivity with decreased nitric oxide and increased endothelin 1 activity, and left heart hypoplasia) which may be associated with impaired lung development. It is unclear at present how nitric oxide, sildenafil, and bosentan will modulate pulmonary hypertension in CDH infants. Chronic pulmonary hypertension can persist into childhood and may contribute to late mortality [26].

6. Postnatal management

It is recommended that CDH infants are delivered as close to 39 weeks as possible. Neuromuscular blockade is avoided in the delivery room. The preductal saturation is kept between 80 and 95%, and the postductal at greater than 70%. The target pCO_2 is 50–70 mmHg on conventional ventilation. Intravenous sildenafil should be administered in the presence of severe pulmonary hypertension.

6.1. Immediate postnatal resuscitation and medical management

In fetuses known antenatal to have CDH, the aim of resuscitation at birth is to obtain cardiopulmonary stability, and interrupt the progression to hypercapnia, hypoxemia, acidosis, and worsening PHN. Infants are intubated, and mechanically ventilated. The initial ventilation mode is conventional mandatory ventilation (CMV). High frequency oscillatory ventilation (HFOV) is initiated when criteria for transition from conventional to HFOV are met. HFOV offers more invasive ventilation support, while minimizing barotrauma to the lungs. Cardiovascular support to avert PHN is needed. ECMO is reserved for patients with severe pulmonary or cardiac compromise refractory to medical management.

Carbon dioxide level and subsequent management can provide predictive information regarding the outcome of CDH. The initial CO_2 is significantly higher and PaO_2 is lower in 30-day mortalities than in survivors. Infants who remain hypercarbic after resuscitation also have a worse prognosis. $PaCO_2$ levels are a biomarker of successful management. The best oxygen index on the first day of life has been shown to predict outcome. Park et al. reported the PaO_2 and $PaCO_2$ from the first blood gas after birth predicted the need for ECMO and mortality [30].

Initial management includes nasogastric decompression, central venous access, total parenteral nutrition, and careful fluid management to optimize cardiopulmonary stability. Frequent echocardiography is required to identify structural cardiac anomalies and assess function and response to therapy [31].

6.2. Score for neonatal acute physiology (SNAP score)

Predictive outcome models are essential for outcome analysis of CDH. The ideal equation should generalize across CDH datasets. Existing mortality-predictive models include those of the CDH study group (CDHSG) based on birth weight and 5-minute Apgar score, the score for Neonatal Acute Physiology version II, and the Wilford Hall/Santa Rosa clinical prediction formula (WHSR(PF)) derived from blood gas measurements. The score for neonatal acute physiology (SNAP 2) score is one of the most applicable scoring systems for CDH infants.

The CDH EURO consortium expanded the implications of the SNAP score first published by Skarsgard et al. [32]. A prospective randomized study of 11 centers that participate in the CDH EURO consortium was undertaken [33]. Data were collected between 2008 and 2013 (SNAP 2). High volume centers were included and were defined as centers that treat at least 10 CDH infants per year. Infants with prematurity below 34 weeks were excluded, so those with premature lung physiology would not influence results.

The exclusion criteria were gestation below 34 weeks, severe chromosomal anomalies, severe cardiac anomalies with need for operation within 60 days, renal anomalies associated with oligohydramnios, and severe orthopedic, skeletal, and central nervous system (CNS) anomalies. All infants were inborn. The out-born infants were excluded because out-born survivors tend to have less severe disease and therefore contribute bias to the results.

The aims of the SNAP 2 study were to prospectively evaluate whether SNAP 2 predicted mortality, the need for ECMO or bronchopulmonary dysplasia (BPD) development.

All infants were randomized to a standard protocol of CMV or HFOV.

The SNAP 2 was collected in the first 12 hours of life and included the worst score of each of the following data points: mean blood pressure, temperature, PaO_2, inspired oxygen concentration (fi02), serum pH, the presence of multiple seizures, and the lowest urine output.

Infants met the criteria for ECMO if they met the following failure criteria for 3 hours: inability to maintain a preductal saturation above 85%, or a postductal saturation above 70%, an increase in CO_2 of greater than 65 mmHg, a peak inspiratory pressure of greater than 28 cm of H_2O, inadequate O_2 delivery with metabolic acidosis defined as pH < 7.2 or an oxygen index consistently greater than 40.

Of 171 infants, 46 died (27.0%). Of 108 treated at ECMO centers, 40 received ECMO (37.0%) and 27 died (25%). Of those treated in 63 centers without ECMO, 19 died (30.0%). The difference in mortality rate between ECMO and nonECMO centers was not significant ($p = 0.46$). Of 125 survivors, 39 developed BDP (31.2%).

In nonsurvivors, the median SNAP 2 was 42.5, and in survivors it was 16.5, a significant difference ($p < 0.001$). Of 108 born in ECMO centers, the median SNAP 2 was 35 in those treated with ECMO and 16 in those that did not undergo ECMO, also a significant difference ($p < 0.001$). The median SNAP 2 was also significantly different for ECMO survivors and nonsurvivors: 32 vs. 40, $p = 0.04$. Logistic regression and ROC analysis showed the SNAP 2 was significantly associated with mortality, need for ECMO and BPD.

This large study of prenatally detected CDH infants concluded that the SNAP 2 calculated in the first 12 hours of life reliably predicts survival outcomes and the need for ECMO in inborn infants with CDH with gestational age > 34 weeks. The SNAP takes only 2–4 minutes to calculate. The SNAP 2 score is considered independent of initial ventilation strategy [34].

Some now report the use of the SNAP 2 score with perinatal extension—the SNAPPE. This score includes APGARS, birth weight and gestational age, but it is time consuming to calculate. The report also includes out-born infants which is a confounder [35].

Implementation of the SNAP 2 score will provide insight into prognosis and can be used to compare severity of illness and evaluate differences in outcomes between centers.

6.3. Permissive hypercapnia and avoidance of lung injury

In the 1990s, the realization that aggressive overventilation causes barotrauma and a worse outcome leads to the introduction of minimal ventilation and permissive hypercapnia. This approach involves decreased airway pressures to reduce barotrauma, spontaneous respiration where possible, and acceptance of higher $PaCO_2$ and lower pH than previously accepted. The introduction of this strategy had the most significant influence on mortality reduction for CDH infants over the past three decades [36].

Barotrauma is commonly attributed as the principal cause of death in autopsy studies of CDH infants [37].

Complications such as pneumothorax have a detrimental effect on CDH infants. In more than one study, all infants with pneumothorax died [38].

The usual limit of permissive hypercapnia in many studies are a $PaCO_2$ within the 40s and pH of 7.2. The oxygen saturation is kept at 90–95%. Postductal oxygen saturation is correlated to other measures of adequate perfusion including lactate, blood pressure, and urine output, while maintaining acceptable ventilator parameters.

The next step in management is the introduction of HFOV. Pressure limits range from 12 to 15 cm H_2O. The benefit of HFOV has not been completely established. It is often used with other management strategies. A trial comparing CMV and HFOV is presently underway [39].

7. Management of PHN

Ensuring good oxygenation is the first step in preventing or treating PHN. The institution of effective ventilation is critical. Fluids and inotropes maintain perfusion and should be guided by serial echocardiography. When PHN worsens, a cycle of worsening hypoxia and hypercapnia from right to left shunting at both the preductal and postductal levels occurs and sets off a vicious cycle of deterioration.

Inhaled nitric oxide (iNO) is a direct pulmonary vasodilator. The inhalation dose ranges between 5 and 20 ppm. Although it may reduce the need for ECMO in other newborns without

CDH, it has not been shown to reduce the need for ECMO in CDH. Response to NO should be confirmed by echocardiography [40].

Sildenafil is a selective cGMP phosphodiesterase inhibitor that can be administered intravenously or as an oral medication. It may enhance inhaled NO-mediated vasodilation. Sildenafil Infusion has been shown to be associated with improved oxygenation in CDH. Overall, its use is increasing. Presently, conflicting reports exist as to whether it improves outcome or not [41].

Milrinone is a phosphodiesterase 3-inhibitor and acts to decrease pulmonary vascular resistance and improve cardiac function. There are few case reports of its efficacy in neonates. Although it is widely used, there is no literature that documents an advantageous effect in CDH [42, 43].

7.1. ECMO

The most severe CDH cohort fails conventional management and utilizes ECMO for support. Infants that undergo ECMO are typically profoundly hypoxemic and acidotic prior to and during ECMO cannulation. ECMO benefits infants with reversible lung disease, however infants with reversible versus irreversible lung disease can be challenging to identify. Infants with reversible lung disease, without CDH, have better documented outcomes. The advantage of ECMO in CDH infants requires continuous evaluation to resolve the issue of whether ECMO actually provides benefit.

A Cochrane review into the randomized controlled trials that investigated the benefits of ECMO in neonates concluded the benefit in CDH infants is unclear. The morbidity in those that do survive is high and can be costly from complications such as intracranial hemorrhage (ICH), bleeding, seizures, or infection. One fifth of infants with CDH that undergo ECMO have severe neurodevelopmental problems [42, 43]

The introduction of gentle ventilation strategies, permissive hypercapnia and spontaneous respiration had a more significant effect on survival than HFOV or ECMO as rescue therapy [35, 39]. These strategies increased survival from 50 to nearly 75% for CDH. Standardized postnatal treatment protocols at ECMO centers is associated with significantly improved survival [44].

7.2. Selection criteria

ECMO is useful if lung disease is reversible. Careful infant selection is critical. Due to the fact that the identification of specific CDH infants that will benefit from ECMO is not clear, some advocate that all infants with respiratory failure should get ECMO as many with poor prognosticators have been shown to survive. It is difficult to identify the influence of inadequate lung volume (pulmonary hypoplasia) versus reversible pulmonary hypertension in CDH infants and the overlap of the two entities. Many infants with CDH will have a honeymoon phase where they demonstrate sufficient lung parenchyma for gas exchange prior to clinical deterioration secondary to pulmonary hypertension. Some authors advocate utilizing clinical parameters and offering ECMO to any patient who can sustain a preductal oxygen saturation ≥90% for at least 1 hour, a PaO_2 of 100 on FiO_2 1.0 and at least one recorded $PaCO_2 < 50$ mmHg [45]. CDH infants with progressive hypoxemia who meet these initial criteria supported with ECMO have 85% survival to discharge [46].

7.3. Factors associated with survival

A retrospective review of the CDH Study Group database found that the overall survival for CDH infants was 67% and for those requiring ECMO, it was 61%. Of the infants that required ECMO and underwent surgical repair, survivors had greater gestational age (>38 weeks), greater birth weight (>3 kg), were less likely to be prenatally diagnosed, less likely to have Apgar <7 at 5 minutes, less likely to have a patch repair and had shorter ECMO runs of median 9 +/- 5 days [47].

7.4. Oxygen index and alveolar-arterial oxygen gradient ($AaDO_2$)

Objective criteria for ECMO patient selection have been suggested in the literature. The two most commonly utilized measures are oxygenation index (OI) and alveolar-arterial oxygen gradient ($AaDO_2$).

The mortality risk in neonatal respiratory failure can be measured by an OI which is based on Pao_2, and mean airway pressure (MAP).

It is computed by:

$$OI = MAP \times FiO_2 \times 100/PaO_2. \quad (1)$$

In early ECLS studies, OI >40 in three of five postductal arterial blood gas measures 30–60 minutes apart, a mortality rate > 80% (8, 9) was predicated. Some advance initiation of ECLS based on an OI of 25 or greater which has a mortality of 50%. ECMO is considered when respiratory failure exists and the OI is calculated at between 25 and 40 [39].

Alternatively, $AaDO_2$ has also been shown to be sensitive for predicting mortality [48].

$$AaDO_2 = (P_{ATM} - 47)\left(FiO_2\right) - \left[\left(PaCO_2\right)/0.8\right] - PaO_2 \quad (2)$$

When the OI ≥ 40 or $AaDO_2$ > 625 mmHg for 4 hours (or >600 mmHg for 12 hours), ECMO is considered mandatory.

7.4.1. Contraindications to ECMO

In addition to unique clinical parameters to assess pulmonary hypoplasia in CDH, there are generalized contraindications to neonatal ECMO that correspond to high mortality:

- Prematurity: gestational age <34 weeks (high risk of intracranial hemorrhage) [49]
- A known pre-ECMO IVH greater than grade 2 [50]
- Weight <2 kg (technical limitation due to cannula size)
- Mechanical ventilation >7–14 days due to risk of fibroproliferative pulmonary disease [51]

- Hypoxic ischemic encephalopathy [52]
- Chromosomal abnormalities (other than trisomy 21) [53].

7.4.2. Relative contraindications

- Multisystem organ failure or irreversible critical illness [54]
- Evidence of bleeding diathesis/disseminated intravascular coagulation (DIC) (correct prior to ECMO) [55]
- Immune compromise [56]
- Seizures prior to ECMO [57]
- Cardiac arrest was previously considered a contraindication but now survival of up to 40% after cardiac arrest is reported. The causes of the arrest are variable and the identification and treatment of the underlying cause will influence outcome [58]. Of those who survive, at least 60% have a reasonable neurologic outcome.

7.4.3. ECMO complications

Complications during ECMO support are associated with worse outcomes. Complications increase with prolonged ECMO support.

7.4.3.1. Bleeding:

Bleeding is associated with heparinization. It is the most common complication, occurs in 10–30% of ECMO runs, and can be devastating [59].

- Intracranial hemorrhage (ICH): ICH is the most common cause of death in newborns on ECMO. The etiology is multifactorial. After heparinization, platelet function remains disrupted for 48 hours after ECMO is discontinued [60]. This effect is increased in infants below 37 weeks' gestational age.
- Bleeding at extracranial sites, e.g., gastrointestinal (GI) hemorrhage
- The incidence of bleeding attributed to technical failure is between 2 and 5%. Cannula site bleeding may be as high as 6%. Cardiac patients requiring ECMO have a higher incidence of bleeding.

In order to decrease the risk of bleeding, the platelet count is kept above 100,000 mm^{-3}. The ACT is maintained between 180 and 240 seconds [61]. The occasional discontinuation of heparin may be needed.

7.4.3.2. Neurologic

The most serious post-ECMO morbidities are neurologic. Morbidity and mortality increase with greater prematurity. This implies that factors present prior to ECMO are related to neurologic outcomes. By 2.5–3 years, infants with CDH requiring ECMO had worse neurologic outcomes than nonCDH ECMO survivors [62, 63].

Neonatal seizures are associated with long-term morbidity and poor outcome including cerebral palsy and epilepsy [42, 43]. Clinical seizures occur in 5–10% of ECMO neonates [64, 65]. Abnormal electroencephalogram (EEGs) are predictive of developmental delay. Only 18% of ECMO infants with normal EEGs have developmental delays; 35% with one abnormal EEG, and 58% with two or more abnormal EEGs [66].

Sensorineural hearing loss occurs in 5% of ECMO survivors, though this rate is comparable to nonECMO PPHN infants [67].

7.4.3.3. *Pneumothorax*

Boloker et al. reported 120 consecutive inborn infants managed with a care strategy based on permissive hypercapnia, spontaneous respiration, and elective repair [39]. The overall survival rate was 75.8%, but, excluding 18 of 120 not treated for lethal anomalies, overwhelming pulmonary hypoplasia, or prerepair ECMO-related neurocomplications, 84.4% survived to discharge. In this series with excellent outcomes, the need for tube thoracostomy was rare, however, every inborn patient ($n = 11$) requiring a chest tube for pneumothorax died. Generally, the incidence of pneumothorax is reported between 4 and 14% and carries a grave prognosis.

7.4.3.4. *Mechanical failure*

Mechanical failure of the ECMO circuit can occur [65]. Examples included: thrombus in the circuit (65%), cannula problems (12%), failure of the oxygenator (6%), pump malfunction (2%), and air in circuit (5%). The effect of technical complications on survival is not as great as other physiologic complications.

7.4.3.5. *Timing of operation*

Although surgical management was historically an emergency for infants with CDH, this is no longer the approach. Previously, CDH was associated with a poor prognosis and a survival rate of approximately 50% with significant morbidity. The aim of medical management in infants with CDH is to stabilize for operation. The results of several studies suggest that delayed repair of CDH after prolonged stabilization has a beneficial effect on the survival rate. Other authors report conflicting results. The optimal time for surgical repair remains controversial and is not completely established.

The primary goal of preoperative stabilization is resolution of pulmonary hypertension. However, complete resolution of PHN can be challenging. Preliminary experience with the use of nitric oxide in infants with CDH has suggested that most infants with hypoxic respiratory failure did not show a sustained response.

Almost 500 infants undergoing early (<48 hours) versus delayed (>48 hours) were recently compared. The primary outcome was 90-day survival, and treatment duration (ventilation, oxygen, and hospitalization) was the secondary outcome. To adjust for disease severity, infants were stratified into three severity groups by Apgar score at 1 minutes ("mild" had an Apgar of 8–10, "moderate" 4–7, and :severe" 0–3). Outcomes were compared between early repair and delayed repair within each severity group [68].

Although 90-day survival was significantly different among the three severities ("mild" 97%, "moderate" 89%, and "severe" 76%, $p = 0.002$), there were no differences in 90-day survival between delayed repair and early repair in each group. In "mild," there were no differences in treatment duration between early and delayed repair. In "moderate," treatment duration was shorter in the early repair group (ventilation 11 vs. 16 days, oxygen 15 vs. 20 days, and hospitalization 34 vs. 48 days). In the "severe" group, treatment duration was shorter in the early repair group.

The timing of CDH repair appeared to have no influence on 90-day survival regardless of disease severity. Infants in the moderately severe category may benefit from the early repair by reducing treatment duration.

Some reports suggest that early repair on ECMO was associated with a decreased time on ECMO, decreased complications, and increased survival [69]. Others refute this and report increased survival if repair can be delayed until the infant is discontinued from ECMO [70].

Over about one decade (1992–2000), a single institution challenged conventional CDH management in the context of a clinical care strategy based on permissive hypercapnia and gentle ventilation. All infants underwent a respiratory care strategy based on permissive hypercapnia and spontaneous respiration, combined with elective repair. Arterial blood gas values and concomitant ventilator support were recorded.

All CDH infants and the following criteria were retrospectively reviewed: (1) respiratory distress requiring mechanical ventilation, (2) in-born infants, or (3) infants transferred preoperatively within hours of birth. Outcome markers such as the need for ECMO, time to discharge to home, need for supplemental oxygen at discharge, and the influence of nonECMO ancillary therapies (surfactant, nitric oxide, and high-frequency oscillatory ventilation) were examined.

For 120 consecutive infants with CDH, the overall survival rate was 75.8%. When 18 of 120 that were not treated were excluded (6 lethal anomalies, 10 overwhelming pulmonary hypoplasia, 3 prerepair ECMO-related neurocomplications), 84.4% survived to discharge. A total of 67/120 were inborn (55.8%). NonECMO ancillary treatments, such as iNO, HFOV, or surfactant, had no impact on the survival rate. ECMO was used in 13.3%. Surgery was transabdominal in all and 7% required a patch. Tube thoracostomy was rarely required, but every inborn patient ($n = 11$) who required a chest tube for pneumothorax died. The overall mean settings for respiratory support before surgery in survivors were: PIP: 22, FiO_2: 43%, PaO_2: 66 Torr, $PaCO_2$: 41 Torr and Ph: 7.32. Two infants that were successfully discharged on oxygen died at 4 and 7 months, respectively and the cause of death was not recorded.

The majority of infants with life-threatening CDH treated with a care strategy of permissive hypercapnia, spontaneous respiration, and elective surgery survive to discharge with minimal pulmonary morbidity [42, 43].

Overall, the approach of delayed surgery after stabilization is based on clinical evaluation, best practices, and retrospective evidence. Delay of operation while waiting for physiologic stabilization may shift mortality from post-op to pre-op in infants that do not survive. The delayed operation approach favors better resource utilization and physiologic stress reduction during hemodynamic instability and pulmonary hypertension. The delayed approach also favors infant self-selection as they demonstrate that they can stabilize during the waiting period.

8. Low risk CDH infants

There are few data in lower risk infants to support specific timing of repair of elective CDH after hemodynamic stability is achieved. The CDH study group data for low risk CDH infants were analyzed. The aim of the analysis was to understand the effect of timing of repair on survival in patients who did not require ECMO. Delayed repair did not appear to improve survival and if surgery is significantly delayed, there is an incidence of bowel obstruction and even volvulus in CDH infants [70].

8.1. Right-sided CDH

Previously, right-sided CDH was considered a subgroup of CDH infants with a poor prognosis. Twenty-seven cases of right CDH that presented for prenatal evaluation (MR or fetal echo) or postnatal treatment between 1995 and 2002 were retrospectively reviewed. In all cases, the fetal liver was herniated into the right chest [71].

The mean gestational age at evaluation was 26.1 weeks. The lung area to head circumference ratio (LHR) ranged from 0.32 to 2.5. Associated anomalies were common. There were four terminations. Fifty percent of continuing pregnancies had polyhydramnios, premature rupture of membranes, or preterm labor. The mean gestational age at birth was 36.8 weeks. One patient underwent tracheal occlusion at 27 weeks and two died before postnatal repair. The overall survival rate was 70% and the postnatal survival rate was 83%. A patch was utilized in 67% of neonates undergoing surgery. Fifty percent required ECMO with a 75% survival rate. Significant morbidity occurred in 53% of survivors and included neurologic sequelae in 32%.

MRI was considered helpful in the determination of liver position and confirmation of the diagnosis. This subgroup has a high incidence of preterm complications, comorbidities, and a frequent need for ECMO. Close prenatal surveillance and delivery at a tertiary care center with ECMO capability is recommended.

In contrast, a more recent series found right CDH was not associated with increased mortality, but it was associated with increased requirement for pulmonary vasodilatory therapy and requirement for tracheostomy [72]. However, the conclusion was similar in that the high incidence of pulmonary complications indicates an increased severity of pulmonary hypoplasia in right CDH and supports a role for delivery in tertiary centers with expertise in CDH management.

9. Repair on ECMO

In contrast to some that recommend delayed operation, others report that, if data are unadjusted for severity of disease, delaying CDH repair is associated with increased mortality [70].

One multivariate analysis of early versus late repair reports that timing of repair confers no difference in outcomes [73]. Most recommend CDH repair should be based on the optimization of clinical parameters as opposed to a specific time period to improve outcome.

Others report that surgical repair on ECMO may confer a slight survival advantage and the complications from bleeding may be lessened by the use of tranexamic acid [74]. Others contradict this recommendation [75]. Similarly, there are significant differences between repaired and nonrepaired CDH infants and significant center variation in the rate of nonrepair exists. Aggressive surgical management, leading to a low rate of nonrepair, is associated with improved risk-adjusted mortality [76].

An increase in survival to surgery does not always equate to increased survival overall. Some authors suggest that if the liver is down, the PHN is less severe, the defect tends to be smaller, and the recommended approach is stabilization and delayed repair [76]. For those with the liver up, the PHN tends to have increased severity with a larger defect and those may benefit from repair on ECMO, but more investigation is needed [77].

9.1. Care strategy for repair of CDH

It is recommended that the operation is delayed until $FIO_2 < 50\%$, PIP < 25 cm H_2O, MAP < 12, with resolution of pulmonary hypertension by clinical criteria and echo. The infant should have a normal acid base balance, stable blood pressure, resolution of anasarca, and almost meet parameters for ECMO discontinuation or have undergone decannulation.

If the infant is on ECMO, consider the use of an AMICAR infusion @20 mg/kg/hour, following a loading dose of 100 mg/kg. One must prepare for the large transfusion protocol, and blood products should be prepared to allow rapid infusion if needed during operation. The infant must have access from anesthesia and surgery and adequate venous and arterial access for administration of blood products, medications, and monitoring. Both preductal and postductal saturation monitors must be in full view. Blood gases will be monitored at baseline and then approximately every 30 minutes during the operation. Extensive team communication between anesthesia, surgery, and neonatology is imperative during the CDH repair operation.

9.2. Outcomes and long-term follow-up

The improvement in ventilation and resuscitation modalities in recent years has improved survival in CDH infants. The increased survival led to an increase in the long-term morbidity burden. As more survivors are advancing in years, our understanding of the complexity of the CDH pathology has improved [78, 79].

The CDH patient is a complicated patient with an intricate disease course. Follow-up should be composed of a multifaceted approach as there are surgical and nonsurgical consequences to the disease process.

9.3. Hernia recurrence

Recurrence of the diaphragmatic hernia has been reported in 8–50% of CDH survivors. The size and the type of repair (patch vs. primary closure and thoracoscopic vs. open repair) appear to be the most commonly reported factors affecting recurrence [80–84]. Survivors with large defects or who underwent patch or laparoscopic repair tend to be more prone to have a recurrence. Recurrence can occur months to years from the initial repair. Recurrences can present with a spectrum of findings from the asymptomatic patient to a patient with bowel obstruction.

9.4. Thoracoscopic versus open repair

Conflicting studies exist regarding the hernia recurrence rate after thoracoscopic or open repair for infants with CDH. Many studies report an increased incidence of recurrence after thoracoscopic repair. In general, these are poorly controlled, retrospective studies. It has been difficult to determine if the increased recurrence is secondary to patient selection, technical variations in repair, experience of the surgeon, or a combination of all of the above. The International Pediatric Endoscopic Group (IPEG) reported one of the first multiinstitutional studies across seven tertiary care pediatric hospitals and attempted to address these questions. IPEG attempted to specifically evaluate the technical variations of thoracoscopic repair of CDH to identify if certain methods are associated with recurrence [85].

They compared primary versus patch repair, type of patch and suture utilized, technique of patch application, and use of extracorporeal/rib fixation sutures. The study concluded there was no statistically significant technical factor related to recurrence to currently recommend a standardized surgical approach to thoracoscopic repair [85].

9.5. Pulmonary outcomes

CDH survivors are more prone to experience a pulmonary morbidity. Around 25% of CDH survivors develop an obstructive airways disease [86, 87]. An estimated 55% of survivors develop recurrent respiratory infections regardless of their chronic pulmonary or airway morbidity [88]. Pulmonary hypertension can also persist and correlates with early mortality [89].

9.5.1. Neurological and developmental outcome

Longitudinal neurodevelopmental and neuroimaging studies of CDH survivors have demonstrated the survivors' susceptibility to neurodevelopmental delay. Magnetic resonance studies revealed anatomic abnormalities in 17% of CDH patients [90]. Delayed brain maturation appears to be prevalent, especially in infants with severe CDH [91]. Such findings correlate with future cognitive impairment. The findings correlated with ECMO treatment, right-sided CDH, intrathoracic liver, patch repair, and prolonged oxygen use after multivariate analysis [67].

Sensorineural hearing loss, independent of ECMO use, has been described in CDH survivors [92, 93] and is believed to stem in part as a side effect of treatment. Approximately 35% of survivors will require hearing aids [94, 95].

9.5.2. Nutritional, growth, and gastrointestinal outcomes

Failure to thrive has been well documented in CDH survivors, with estimates of between 20 and 50% of survivors experienced growth retardation and remains in the lower percentiles on the growth chart [96, 97] and it is believe to be a result of complex processes including oral aversion, GERD, increased metabolic stress due to ingoing morbidity. Around 33% of survivors require some form of tube feeding [80, 98].

Gastroesophageal dysmotility and regurgitation has been found to be prevalent in CDH survivors with a prevalence of between 45 and 90% reported [97–101]. The tendency to GERD may contribute to the survivor's failure to thrive. However, at present, there is no evidence that routine fundoplication is needed.

9.5.3. Musculoskeletal outcomes

Chest wall deformities and scoliosis have been reported in CDH survivors. The literature estimates the prevalence of chest wall deformities to be approximately 16–48% [86, 102–105]. While thoracic scoliosis has been reported in 10–27% of survivors [82, 105]. Though prevalent, not all deformities will require intervention. The prevalence of scoliosis has been found to be more prevalent in survivors with big defects who underwent patch repairs [84, 105].

9.5.4. Other outcomes

In addition to the above-mentioned long-term morbidities, associated congenital defects have been reported in around 33–40% of CDH infants [106–112]. Associated congenital anomalies such as cardiac defects, genitourinary abnormalities, and neurological anomalies should be taken into consideration when planning long-term follow-up.

9.5.5. Follow-up

The complexity of the CDH patient mandates a structured multidisciplinary follow-up. In 2008, the American Academy of Pediatrics published an outline for the follow up of the patient with CDH [107]. This was done to identify and treat morbidities to prevent any further disability. The outline is summarized in **Table 1** [107].

	Before discharge	**1–3 months after birth**	**4–6 months after birth**	**9–12 months after birth**	**15–18 months after birth**	**Annual through 16 years**
Weight, length, occipital-frontal circumference	X	X	X	X	X	X
Chest radiograph	X	If patched	If patched	If patched	If patched	If patched
Pulmonary function testing			If indicated		If indicated	If indicated
Childhood immunizations	As indicated throughout childhood	X	X	X	X	X

	Before discharge	1–3 months after birth	4–6 months after birth	9–12 months after birth	15–18 months after birth	Annual through 16 years
RSV prophylaxis	RSV season during first 2 years after birth (if evidence of chronic lung disease)	X	X	X	X	X
Echocardiogram and cardiology follow-up	X	If previously abnormal or if on supplemental oxygen	If previously abnormal or if on supplemental oxygen	If previously abnormal or if on supplemental oxygen	If previously abnormal or if on supplemental oxygen	If previously abnormal or if on supplemental oxygen
Head computed tomography or MRI	If (1) abnormal finding on head ultrasound; (2) seizures/ abnormal neurologic findings[a]; or (3) ECMO or patch repair	As indicated	As indicated	As indicated	As indicated	As indicated
Hearing evaluation 44	Auditory brainstem evoked response or otoacoustic emissions screen	X	X	X	X	Every 6 months to age 3 years, then annually to age 5 years
Developmental screening evaluation	X	X	X	X		Annually to age 5 years
Neurodevelopmental evaluation	X			X		Annually to age 5 years
Assessment for oral feeding problems	X	X	If oral feeding problems	If oral feeding problems	If oral feeding problems	If oral feeding problems
Upper gastrointestinal study, pH probe, and/or gastric scintiscan	Consider for all patients	If symptoms	If symptoms	Consider for all patients	If symptoms	If symptoms
Esophagoscopy		If symptoms	If symptoms	If symptoms or if abnormal gastrointestinal evaluations	If symptoms	If symptoms

	Before discharge	1–3 months after birth	4–6 months after birth	9–12 months after birth	15–18 months after birth	Annual through 16 years
Scoliosis and chest wall deformity screening (physical examination, chest radiograph, and/or computed tomography of the chest)				X		X

Notes: The neurosensory tests performed and frequency of surveillance may differ among infants with CDH because of variability in neurologic, developmental, and physiologic impairments. Follow-up should be tailored to each infant. RSV indicates respiratory syncytial virus.

[a] Muscle weakness, hypotonia, hypertonia, or other abnormal neurologic sign or symptom.

Table 1. Recommended schedule of follow-up for infants with CDH [107].

10. Conclusions

The management of congenital diaphragmatic hernia remains a challenge. Mortality is dependent on associated malformations, the severity of pulmonary hypoplasia, pulmonary hypertension, and iatrogenic lung injury associated with aggressive mechanical ventilation. A comparison of the mortality rate of CDH infants in a single center between 1995 and 2005 versus 2006 and 2016 revealed that the mortality rate significantly decreased in the later time period, 17.9 compared to 4.4%. Prenatal diagnosis, intrathoracic liver, low Apgar score, and low birth weight were defined as independent risk factors for mortality. The mortality in ECMO-treated patients was 50% in both time periods [113]. Despite no significant differences in the incidence of independent risk factors and the use of ECMO between the two time periods, mortality decreased over time.

Therefore, there are many important factors involved in a successful outcome after CDH repair. Large multicenter studies are necessary to define those critical factors and to determine optimal treatment strategies.

Infants with CDH should be delivered as close to term as possible. At birth, management includes bowel decompression, avoidance of mask ventilation, and endotracheal tube placement if required. The care strategy includes gentle ventilation, hemodynamic monitoring, and treatment of pulmonary hypertension followed by surgery. Although inhaled nitric oxide is not Food and Drug Administration (FDA) approved for the treatment of pulmonary hypertension in CDH infants, it is commonly used. Extracorporeal membrane oxygenation (ECMO) is considered if conventional medical management fails for infants ≥ 34 weeks' gestation or with weight >2 kg and no associated major lethal anomalies. With advances in CDH management, the overall survival has improved and has been reported between 70 and 90% in non-ECMO infants and up to 50% in infants who undergo ECMO.

There are many important areas of research that may promote better understanding of the development of CDH. Fujinaga et al. reported that cord blood endothelial progenitor cells are altered in CDH infants, but the mechanism is unknown [114]. Russo et al. reported the use of transplacental sildenafil rescues lung abnormalities in a rabbit model of CDH, improves vascular branching, and reduces pulmonary vascular resistance [115]. This promising research may further alter and improve outcomes for infants with CDH.

Author details

Joanne Baerg*, Arul Thirumoorthi and Rajaie Hazboun

*Address all correspondence to: jbaerg@llu.edu

Loma Linda University Children's Hospital, Loma Linda, CA, USA

References

[1] Baird R, Puligandla PS, Laberge JM. Congenital lung malformations: Informing best practice. Seminars in Pediatric Surgery. 2014;**23**:270-277

[2] Downard CD, Jaksic T, Garza JJ, Dzakovic A, Nemes L, Jennings RW, Wilson JM. Analysis of an improved survival rate for congenital diaphragmatic hernia. Journal of Pediatric Surgery. 2003;**38**(5):729-732

[3] Crane JP. Familial congenital diaphragmatic hernia: Prenatal diagnostic approach and analysis of twelve families. Clinical Genetics. 1979;**16**:244

[4] Romero R, Pilu G, Ghidini A, Hobbins JC, editors. Prenatal Diagnosis of Congenital Anomalies. Connecticut/California: Appleton and Lange; 1988. p. 219

[5] Gibbs DL, Rice HE, Farrell JA, Adzick NS, Harrison MR. Familial diaphragmatic agenesis: An autosomal-recessive syndrome with a poor prognosis. Journal of Pediatric Surgery. 1997;**32**:366-368

[6] Lubinski M, Severn C, Rapaport JM. Fryns syndrome: A new variable multiple congenital anomaly (MCA syndrome). American Journal of Medical Genetics. 1983;**14**:461

[7] Thornburn MJ, Wright ES, Miller CG. Exomphalosmacro-glossia-gigantism syndrome in Jamaican infants. American Journal of Diseases of Children. 1970;**119**:316

[8] Evans JNG, MacLachlan RF. Choanal atresia. Journal of Laryngology. 1971;**85**:903

[9] Gibbin C, Touch S, Groth R, Berghella V. Abdominal wall defects and congenital heart disease. Ultrasound in Obstetrics & Gynecology. 2003;**21**:334-337

[10] Harrison MR, Adzick NS, Bullard KM, Farrell JA, Howell LJ, Rosen MA, Sola A, Goldberg JD, Filly RA. Correction of congenital diaphragmatic hernia in utero VII: A prospective trial. Journal of Pediatric Surgery. 1997;**32**:1637-1642

[11] De Paepe ME, Shapiro S, Hansen K, Gündoğan F. Postmortem lung volume/body weight standards for term and preterm infants. Pediatric Pulmonology. 2014;**49**:60-66. DOI: 10.1002/ppul.22818. Epub 2013 Aug 29

[12] Alfaraj MA, Shah PS, Bohn D, et al. Congenital diaphragmatic hernia: Lung to head ratio and lung volume for prediction of outcome. American Journal of Obstetrics and Gynecology. 2011;**205**:43.e1-43.e8

[13] Kitano Y, Nakagawa S, Kuroda T, et al. Liver position in fetal congenital diaphragmatic hernia retains a prognostic value in the era of lung-protective strategy. Journal of Pediatric Surgery. 2005;**40**:1827-1832

[14] Oluyomi-Obi T, Kuret V, Puligandla P, et al. Antenatal predictors of outcome in prenatally diagnosed congenital diaphragmatic hernia (CDH). Journal of Pediatric Surgery. 2016;**21**. S0022-3468(16)30647-9

[15] Partridge EA, Peranteau WH, Herkert L, et al. Rate of increase of lung-to-head ratio over the course of gestation is predictive of survival in left-sided congenital diaphragmatic hernia. Journal of Pediatric Surgery. 2016;**51**:703-705

[16] Rypens F, Metens T, Rocourt N, et al. Fetal lung volume: Estimation at MR imaging—initial results. Radiology. 2001;**219**:236-241

[17] Sandaite I, Claus F, De Keyzer, et al. Examining the relationship between the lung-to-head ratio measured on ultrasound and lung volumetry by magnetic resonance in fetuses with isolated congenital diaphragmatic hernia. Fetal Diagnosis and Therapy. 2011;**29**:80-87

[18] Russo FM, Eastwood MP, Keijzer R, et al. Lung size and liver herniation predict the need for extra corporeal membrane oxygenation but not pulmonary hypertension in isolated congenital diaphragmatic hernia: A systematic review and meta-analysis. Ultrasound in Obstetrics & Gynecology. 2016;**17**

[19] Deshmukh S, Rubsova E, Barth R. MR assessment of normal fetal lung volumes: A literature review. American Journal of Roentgenology. 2010;**194**:212-217

[20] Akinkuotu A, Cruz S, Abbas P, et al. Risk stratification for infants with CDH: Prenatal vs. postnatal predictors of outcome. Journal of Pediatric Surgery. 2016;**51**:44-48

[21] VanderWall KJ, Skarsgard ED, Filly RA, et al. Fetendo-clip: A fetal endoscopic tracheal clip procedure in a human fetus. Journal of Pediatric Surgery. 1997;**32**:970-972

[22] VanderWall KJ, Bruch SW, Meuli M, et al. Fetal endoscopic ('Fetendo') tracheal clip. Journal of Pediatric Surgery. 1996;**31**:1101-1103. discussion 1103-4

[23] Harrison MR, Mychaliska GB, Albanese CT, et al. Correction of congenital diaphragmatic hernia in utero IX: Fetuses with poor prognosis (liver herniation and low lung-to-head ratio) can be saved by fetoscopic temporary tracheal occlusion. Journal of Pediatric Surgery. 1998;**33**:1017-1022. discussion 1022-3

[24] Belfort MA, Olutoye OO, Cass DL, et al. Feasibility and outcomes of fetoscopic tracheal occlusion for severe left diaphragmatic hernia. Obstetrics & Gynecology. 2017;**129**:20-29

[25] Ruano R, Ali RA, Patel P, et al. Fetal endoscopic tracheal occlusion for congenital diaphragmatic hernia: Indications, outcomes, and future directions. Obstetrical & Gynecological Survey. 2014;**69**(3):147-158

[26] Gien J, Kinsella JP. Management of pulmonary hypertension in infants with congenital diaphragmatic hernia. Journal of Perinatology. 2016;**36**(Suppl 2):S28-S31

[27] Abman S, Baker C, Gien J, et al. The Robyn Barst memorial lecture: Differences between fetal, newborn, and adult pulmonary circulations: Relevance for age-specific therapies. Pulmonary Circulation. 2014;**4**:424-440

[28] Akeson AL, Cameron JE, Le Cras TD, Whitsett JA, Greenberg JM. Vascular endothelial growth factor-A induces prenatal neovascularization and alters bronchial development in mice. Pediatric Research. 2005;**57**:82-88

[29] Yamoto M, Inamura N, Terui K, et al. Echocardiographic predictors of poor prognosis in congenital diaphragmatic hernia. Journal of Pediatric Surgery. 2016;**51**(12):1926-1930

[30] Park HW, Lee BS, Lim G, et al. A simplified formula using early blood gas analysis can predict survival outcomes and the requirements for extracorporeal membrane oxygenation in congenital diaphragmatic hernia. Journal of Korean Medical Science. 2013;**28**(6):924-928

[31] Reiss I, Schaible T, van den Hout L, Capolupo I, Allegaert K, van Heijst A, Gorett Silva M, Greenough A, Tibboel D, CDH EURO Consortium. Standardized postnatal management of infants with congenital diaphragmatic hernia in Europe: The CDH EURO Consortium consensus. Neonatology. 2010;**98**:354-364

[32] Skarsgard ED, MacNab YC, Qiu Z, Little R, Lee SK, Canadian Neonatal Network. SNAP-II predicts mortality among infants with congenital diaphragmatic hernia. Journal of Perinatology. 2005;**25**:315-319

[33] Snoek KG, Capolupo I, Morini F, van Rosmalen J, Greenough A, van Heijst A, Reiss IK, IJsselstijn H, Tibboel D, Congenital Diaphragmatic Hernia EURO Consortium. Score for neonatal acute Physiology-II predicts outcome in congenital diaphragmatic hernia patients. Pediatric Critical Care Medicine. 2016;**17**:540-546

[34] Snoek KG, Capolupo I, van Rosmalen J, Hout Lde J, Vijfhuize S, Greenough A, Wijnen RM, Tibboel D, Reiss IK, CDH EURO Consortium. Conventional mechanical ventilation versus High-frequency oscillatory ventilation for congenital diaphragmatic hernia: A randomized clinical trial (The VICI-trial). Annals of Surgery. 2016;**263**(5):867-874

[35] Chiu LW, Desai J, Shanti C, et al. SNAPPE II score as a predictor of survival in neonates with congenital diaphragmatic hernia: A single center experience. European Journal of Pediatric Surgery. 2016;**26**:316-321

[36] Wung JT, Sahni R, Moffitt ST, et al. Congenital diaphragmatic hernia: Survival treated with very delayed surgery, spontaneous respiration, and no chest tube. Journal of Pediatric Surgery. 1995;**30**:406-409

[37] Wilson JM, Lund DP, Lillehei CW, Vacanti JP. Congenital diaphragmatic hernia--a tale of two cities: The Boston experience. Journal of Pediatric Surgery. 1997;**32**:401-405

[38] Boloker J, Bateman DA, Wung JT, Stolar CJ. Congenital diaphragmatic hernia in 120 infants treated consecutively with permissive hypercapnea/spontaneous respiration/ elective repair. Journal of Pediatric Surgery. 2002;**37**:357-366

[39] van den Hout L, Tibboel D, Vijfhuize S, te Beest H, Hop W, Reiss I, CDH-EURO Consortium. The VICI-trial: High frequency oscillation versus conventional mechanical ventilation in newborns with congenital diaphragmatic hernia: An international multicenter randomized controlled trial. BMC Pediatric. 2011;**11**:98

[40] Oliveira CA, Troster EJ, Pereira CR. Inhaled nitric oxide in the management of persistent pulmonary hypertension of the newborn: A meta-analysis. Revista do Hospital das Clínicas. 2000;**55**:145-154

[41] Bialkowski A, Moenkemeyer F, Patel N. Intravenous sildenafil in the management of pulmonary hypertension associated with congenital diaphragmatic hernia. European Journal of Pediatric Surgery. 2015;**25**:171-176

[42] Bassler D, Kreutzer K, McNamara P, Kirpalani H. Milrinone for persistent pulmonary hypertension of the newborn. The Cochrane Database of Systematic Reviews. 2010;(11): CD007802

[43] Mehta A, Ibsen LM. Neurologic complications and neurodevelopmental outcome with extracorporeal life support. World Journal of Critical Care Medicine. 2013;**2**(4):40-47

[44] van den Hout L, Schaible T, Cohen-Overbeek TE, Hop W, Siemer J, van de Ven K, et al. Actual outcome in infants with congenital diaphragmatic hernia: The role of a standardized postnatal treatment protocol. Fetal Diagnosis and Therapy. 2011;**29**(1):55-63

[45] Ashcraft KW, Holcomb GW, Murphy JP, Ostlie DJ. Ashcraft's Pediatric Surgery. 6th ed. London, New York: Saunders/Elsevier; 2014

[46] Stolar C, Dillon P, Reyes C. Selective use of extracorporeal membrane oxygenation in the management of congenital diaphragmatic hernia. Journal of Pediatric Surgery. 1988;**23**(3):207-211

[47] Seetharamaiah R, Younger JG, Bartlett RH, Hirschl RB, Congenital Diaphragmatic Hernia Study G. Factors associated with survival in infants with congenital diaphragmatic hernia requiring extracorporeal membrane oxygenation: A report from the Congenital Diaphragmatic Hernia Study Group. Journal of Pediatric Surgery. 2009;**44**(7):1315-1321

[48] Group UCET. UK collaborative randomised trial of neonatal extracorporeal membrane oxygenation. UK Collaborative ECMO Trail Group. Lancet. 1996;**348**(9020):75-82

[49] Rivera RA, Butt W, Shann F. Predictors of mortality in children with respiratory failure: Possible indications for ECMO. Anaesthesia and Intensive Care. 1990;**18**(3):385-389

[50] Krummel TM, Greenfield LJ, Kirkpatrick BV, Mueller DG, Kerkering KW, Ormazabal M, et al. Alveolar-arterial oxygen gradients versus the Neonatal Pulmonary Insufficiency Index for prediction of mortality in ECMO candidates. Journal of Pediatric Surgery. 1984;**19**(4):380-384

[51] Cilley RE, Zwischenberger JB, Andrews AF, Bowerman RA, Roloff DW, Bartlett RH. Intracranial hemorrhage during extracorporeal membrane oxygenation in neonates. Pediatrics. 1986;**78**(4):699-704

[52] Kim ES, Stolar CJ. ECMO in the newborn. American Journal of Perinatology. 2000;**17**(7): 345-356

[53] Kornhauser MS, Cullen JA, Baumgart S, McKee LJ, Gross GW, Spitzer AR. Risk factors for bronchopulmonary dysplasia after extracorporeal membrane oxygenation. Archives of Pediatrics and Adolescent Medicine. 1994;**148**(8):820-825

[54] von Allmen D, Babcock D, Matsumoto J, Flake A, Warner BW, Stevenson RJ, et al. The predictive value of head ultrasound in the ECMO candidate. Journal of Pediatric Surgery. 1992;**27**(1):36-39

[55] Gaffney AM, Wildhirt SM, Griffin MJ, Annich GM, Radomski MW. Extracorporeal life support. British Medical Journal. 2010;**341**:c5317

[56] Sell LL, Cullen ML, Whittlesey GC, Yedlin ST, Philippart AI, Bedard MP, et al. Hemorrhagic complications during extracorporeal membrane oxygenation: Prevention and treatment. Journal of Pediatric Surgery. 1986;**21**(12):1087-1091

[57] Gupta M, Shanley TP, Moler FW. Extracorporeal life support for severe respiratory failure in children with immune compromised conditions. Pediatric Critical Care Medicine. 2008;**9**(4):380-385

[58] Parish AP, Bunyapen C, Cohen MJ, Garrison T, Bhatia J. Seizures as a predictor of long-term neurodevelopmental outcome in survivors of neonatal extracorporeal membrane oxygenation (ECMO). Journal of Child Neurology. 2004;**19**(12):930-934

[59] Fiser RT, Morris MC. Extracorporeal cardiopulmonary resuscitation in refractory pediatric cardiac arrest. Pediatric Clinics of North America. 2008;**55**(4):929-941. x

[60] Bartlett RH, Gattinoni L. Current status of extracorporeal life support (ECMO) for cardiopulmonary failure. Minerva Anestesiologica. 2010;**76**(7):534-540

[61] Raithel SC, Pennington DG, Boegner E, Fiore A, Weber TR. Extracorporeal membrane oxygenation in children after cardiac surgery. Circulation. 1992;**86**(5 Suppl):II305-II310

[62] ELSO Anticoagulation Guidelines 2014. Ann Arbor, MI: Extracorporeal Life Support Organization

[63] Stolar CJ, Crisafi MA, Driscoll YT. Neurocognitive outcome for neonates treated with extracorporeal membrane oxygenation: Are infants with congenital diaphragmatic hernia different? Journal of Pediatric Surgery. 1995;**30**(2):366-371; discussion 71-72

[64] Danzer E, Gerdes M, Bernbaum J, D'Agostino J, Bebbington MW, Siegle J, et al. Neurodevelopmental outcome of infants with congenital diaphragmatic hernia prospectively enrolled in an interdisciplinary follow-up program. Journal of Pediatric Surgery. 2010;**45**(9):1759-1766

[65] ECLS Registry Report International Summary. Extracorporeal Life Support Organisation. 2016

[66] Graziani LJ, Streletz LJ, Baumgart S, Cullen J, McKee LM. Predictive value of neonatal electroencephalograms before and during extracorporeal membrane oxygenation. Journal of Pediatrics. 1994;**125**(6 Pt 1):969-975

[67] Schumacher RE, Palmer TW, Roloff DW, LaClaire PA, Bartlett RH. Follow-up of infants treated with extracorporeal membrane oxygenation for newborn respiratory failure. Pediatrics. 1991;**87**(4):451-457

[68] Okuyama H, Usui N, Hayakawa M, Taguchi T, Japanese CDH study group. Appropriate timing of surgery for neonates with congenital diaphragmatic hernia: Early or delayed repair? Pediatric Surgery International. 2017;**33**(2):133-138

[69] Fallon SC, Cass DL, Olutoye OO, et al. Repair of congenital diaphragmatic hernias on Extracorporeal Membrane Oxygenation (ECMO): Does early repair improve patient survival? Journal of Pediatric Surgery. 2013;**48**:1172-1176

[70] Hollinger LE, Lally PA, Tsao K, et al. Congenital Diaphragmatic Hernia Study Group. A risk-stratified analysis of delayed congenital diaphragmatic hernia repair: Does timing of operation matter? Surgery. 2014;**156**:475-482

[71] Hedrick HL, Crombleholme TM, Flake AW, et al. Right congenital diaphragmatic hernia: Prenatal assessment and outcome. Journal of Pediatric Surgery. 2004;**39**:319-323. discussion 319-323

[72] Partridge EA, Peranteau WH, Herkert L, et al. Right- versus left-sided congenital diaphragmatic hernia: A comparative outcomes analysis. Journal of Pediatric Surgery. 2016;**51**:900-902

[73] Rozmiarek AJ, Qureshi FG, Cassidy L, et al. Factors influencing survival in newborns with congenital diaphragmatic hernia: The relative role of timing of surgery. Journal of Pediatric Surgery. 2004;**39**:821-824. discussion 821-824. Review

[74] Desai AA, Ostlie DJ, Juang D. Optimal timing of congenital diaphragmatic hernia repair in infants on extracorporeal membrane oxygenation. Seminars in Pediatric Surgery. 2015;**24**:17-19

[75] Partridge EA, Peranteau WH, Rintoul NE, et al. Timing of repair of congenital diaphragmatic hernia in patients supported by extracorporeal membrane oxygenation (ECMO). Journal of Pediatric Surgery. 2015;**50**:260-262

[76] Harting MT, Hollinger L, Tsao K, Putnam LR, Wilson JM, Hirschl RB, Skarsgard ED, Tibboel D, Brindle ME, Lally PA, Miller CC, Lally KP, Congenital Diaphragmatic Hernia Study Group. Aggressive surgical management of congenital diaphragmatic hernia: Worth the effort? A multicenter, prospective, cohort study. Annals of Surgery. 2017;**27**

[77] Morini F, Goldman A, Pierro A. Extracorporeal membrane oxygenation in infants with congenital diaphragmatic hernia: A systematic review of the evidence. European Journal of Pediatric Surgery. 2006;**16**:385-391

[78] Chiu PP, Ijsselstijn H. Morbidity and long-term follow-up in CDH patients. European Journal of Pediatric Surgery. 2012;**22**(5):384-392

[79] Chiu PP, et al. The price of success in the management of congenital diaphragmatic hernia: Is improved survival accompanied by an increase in long-term morbidity? Journal of Pediatric Surgery. 2006;**41**(5):888-892

[80] Van Meurs KP, et al. Congenital diaphragmatic hernia: Long-term outcome in neonates treated with extracorporeal membrane oxygenation. Journal of Pediatric. 1993;**122**(6):893-899

[81] Ssemakula N, et al. Survival of patients with congenital diaphragmatic hernia during the ECMO era: An 11-year experience. Journal of Pediatric Surgery, 1997;**32**(12):1683-1689

[82] Lally KP, et al. Congenital diaphragmatic hernia. Stabilization and repair on ECMO. Annals of Surgery. 1992;**216**(5):569-573

[83] Moss RL, Chen CM, Harrison MR. Prosthetic patch durability in congenital diaphragmatic hernia: A long-term follow-up study. Journal of Pediatric Surgery. 2001;**36**(1):152-154

[84] Jancelewicz T, et al. Late surgical outcomes among congenital diaphragmatic hernia (CDH) patients: Why long-term follow-up with surgeons is recommended. Journal of Pediatric Surgery. 2013;**48**(5):935-941

[85] Weaver KL, Baerg JE, Okawada M, et al. A multi-institutional review of thoracoscopic congenital diaphragmatic hernia repair. Journal of Laparoendoscopic & Advanced Surgical Techniques. Part A. 2016;**26**:825-830

[86] Bagolan P, et al. Impact of a current treatment protocol on outcome of high-risk congenital diaphragmatic hernia. Journal of Pediatric Surgery. 2004;**39**(3):313-318. discussion 313-318

[87] Wischermann A, Holschneider AM, Hubner U. Long-term follow-up of children with diaphragmatic hernia. European Journal of Pediatric Surgery. 1995;**5**(1):13-18

[88] Gischler SJ, et al. A prospective comparative evaluation of persistent respiratory morbidity in esophageal atresia and congenital diaphragmatic hernia survivors. Journal of Pediatric Surgery. 2009;**44**(9):1683-1690

[89] Dillon PW, et al. The relationship of pulmonary artery pressure and survival in congenital diaphragmatic hernia. Journal of Pediatric Surgery. 2004;**39**(3):307-312. discussion 307-312

[90] Tracy S, et al. Abnormal neuroimaging and neurodevelopmental findings in a cohort of antenatally diagnosed congenital diaphragmatic hernia survivors. Journal of Pediatric Surgery. 2010;**45**(5):958-965

[91] Danzer E, et al. Abnormal brain development and maturation on magnetic resonance imaging in survivors of severe congenital diaphragmatic hernia. Journal of Pediatric Surgery. 2012;**47**(3):453-461

[92] Nobuhara KK, et al. Long-term outlook for survivors of congenital diaphragmatic hernia. Clinics in Perinatology. 1996;**23**(4):873-887

[93] Rasheed A, et al. Neurodevelopmental outcome after congenital diaphragmatic hernia: Extracorporeal membrane oxygenation before and after surgery. Journal of Pediatric Surgery. 2001;**36**(4):539-544

[94] Walton JP, Hendricks-Munoz K. Profile and stability of sensorineural hearing loss in persistent pulmonary hypertension of the newborn. Journal of Speech and Hearing Research. 1991;**34**(6):1362-1370

[95] Hendricks-Munoz KD, Walton JP. Hearing loss in infants with persistent fetal circulation. Pediatrics. 1988;**81**(5):650-656

[96] Jaillard SM, et al. Outcome at 2 years of infants with congenital diaphragmatic hernia: A population-based study. Annals of Thoracic Surgery. 2003;**75**(1):250-256

[97] Muratore CS, et al. Nutritional morbidity in survivors of congenital diaphragmatic hernia. Journal of Pediatric Surgery. 2001;**36**(8):1171-1176

[98] Stolar CJ, et al. Anatomic and functional abnormalities of the esophagus in infants surviving congenital diaphragmatic hernia. American Journal of Surgery. 1990;**159**(2):204-207

[99] Fasching G, et al. Gastroesophageal reflux and diaphragmatic motility after repair of congenital diaphragmatic hernia. European Journal of Pediatric Surgery. 2000;**10**(6):360-364

[100] Koot VC, et al. Incidence and management of gastroesophageal reflux after repair of congenital diaphragmatic hernia. Journal of Pediatric Surgery. 1993;**28**(1):48-52

[101] Kieffer J, et al. Gastroesophageal reflux after repair of congenital diaphragmatic hernia. Journal of Pediatric Surgery. 1995;**30**(9):1330-1333

[102] Di Pace MR, et al. Evaluation of esophageal motility and reflux in children treated for congenital diaphragmatic hernia with the use of combined multichannel intraluminal impedance and pH monitoring. Journal of Pediatric Surgery. 2011;**46**(10):1881-1886

[103] Lund DP, et al. Congenital diaphragmatic hernia: The hidden morbidity. Journal of Pediatric Surgery, 1994;**29**(2):258-262; discussion 262-264

[104] Arena F, et al. Mid- and long-term effects on pulmonary perfusion, anatomy and diaphragmatic motility in survivors of congenital diaphragmatic hernia. Pediatric Surgery International. 2005;**21**(12):954-959

[105] Trachsel D, et al. Long-term pulmonary morbidity in survivors of congenital diaphragmatic hernia. Pediatric Pulmonology. 2005;**39**(5):433-439

[106] Vanamo K, et al. Long-term gastrointestinal morbidity in patients with congenital diaphragmatic defects. Journal of Pediatric Surgery. 1996;**31**(4):551-554

[107] American Academy of Pediatrics Section on S, et al. Postdischarge follow-up of infants with congenital diaphragmatic hernia. Pediatrics. 2008;**121**(3):627-632

[108] Cohen MS, et al. Influence of congenital heart disease on survival in children with congenital diaphragmatic hernia. Journal of Pediatric. 2002;**141**(1):25-30

[109] Fauza DO, Wilson JM. Congenital diaphragmatic hernia and associated anomalies: Their incidence, identification, and impact on prognosis. Journal of Pediatric Surgery. 1994;**29**(8):1113-1137

[110] Colvin J, et al. Outcomes of congenital diaphragmatic hernia: A population-based study in Western Australia. Pediatrics. 2005;**116**(3):e356-e363

[111] Vanamo K. A 45-year perspective of congenital diaphragmatic hernia. British Journal of Surgery. 1996;**83**(12):1758-1762

[112] Huddy CL, et al. Congenital diaphragmatic hernia: Prenatal diagnosis, outcome and continuing morbidity in survivors. British Journal of Obstetrics and Gynaecology. 1999;**106**(11):1192-1196

[113] Kadir D, Lilja HE. Risk factors for postoperative mortality in congenital diaphragmatic hernia: A single-centre observational study. Pediatric Surgery International. 2017;**33**:317-323

[114] Fujinaga H, Fujinaga H, Watanabe N, et al. Cord blood-derived endothelial colony-forming cell function is disrupted in congenital diaphragmatic hernia. American Journal of Physiology Lung Cellular and Molecular Physiology. 2016;**310**:L1143–L1154

[115] Russo FM, Toelen J, Eastwood MP, et al. Transplacental sildenafil rescues lung abnormalities in the rabbit model of diaphragmatic hernia. Thorax. 2016;**71**:517-525

3

Laparoscopic Inguinal Hernia Repair: Technical Details, Pitfalls and Current Results

Fatih Altintoprak, Emrah Akin,
Kemal Gundogdu and Enis Dikicier

Abstract

Expanding view of minimal invasive surgery horizon reveals new practice areas for surgeons and patients. Laparoscopic inguinal hernia repair is an example in progress wondered by many patients and surgeons. Advantages in laparoscopic repair motivate surgeons to discover this popular field. In addition, patients search the most convenient surgical method for themselves today. Laparoscopic approaches to inguinal hernia surgery have become popular as a result of the development of experience about different laparoscopic interventions, and these techniques are increasingly used these days. As other laparoscopic surgical methods, experience is the most important point in order to obtain good results. This chapter aims to show technical details, pitfalls and the literature results about two methods that are commonly used in laparoscopic inguinal hernia repair.

Keywords: laparoscopy, inguinal hernia, TAPP, TEP

1. Introduction

For centuries, the inguinal hernias have played an important role in the surgical literature and continue to preserve this feature today. With many procedures, inguinal hernia interventions continue to be the most common general surgery operations worldwide and approximately 2 million people are operated for inguinal hernia every year. There are many techniques described on the surgical treatment of inguinal hernias. There is no other example of disease preoccupied in the surgical literature. Existence of the postoperative complications suggests that we have not found the ideal treatment option yet because a wide variety of techniques have been described and most of the surgeons engaged in this procedure have completed learning curves a long time ago. In 1984, about hernia, Sir Astley Paston Cooper says: "No disease from the human body, belonging to the surgeon, demands in its treatment, a better mixture of precise, anatomical knowledge along with surgical skill, compared to hernia in most of its variations". In this chapter, the details and results of two laparoscopic techniques, which have become common in inguinal hernia treatment today, are evaluated in detail.

2. Incidence and general information

The incidence of inguinal hernia varies according to age and sex. There is a bi-modal distribution in males and it increases in the first year of life and in older ages. The rate of 15% in the second decade increases with age and reaches 47% in the seventh decade. In females, this rate is 3% for life. There is a significant difference between the male/female ratio and is reported as 1:15. Although the majority of the inguinal hernia patients do not face great problems in resuscitating their lives, the incidence of general incidence and emergency case incidence (incarceration-strangulation) increases with age [1].

Inguinal hernias are classified as direct or indirect inguinal hernia according to their mechanism and anatomical characteristics. Indirect inguinal hernias are the most common subtype and the risk of strangulation is much higher compared to direct hernias. In the case of strangulation, it is also necessary to mention that the femoral hernias head to this issue. Femoral hernias, which are found in 70% of women and generally settled in the principle of "should be fixed when they are detected", due to the risk of strangulation, have not been included in this section [2].

When the side is concerned, it is a fact that all inguinal hernias are seen more on the right side. One of the theories developed to explain this is that there is anatomically protective effect of the sigmoid colon present on the left side and delayed atrophy of the processus vaginalis due to the slower descent of the scrotum on the right side during embryological development.

3. History

The word "hernia" came from the Latin word "rupture" and was described as a disease in the first fifteenth century in papyrus. The idea of repairing surgery came out between fifteenth and seventeenth centuries although the inguinal region anatomy has been described in detail by Hesselbach, Cooper, Camper, Scarpa and Gimbernat during eighteenth and nineteenth centuries. In the twentieth century, "tension-free repairs" started to be proposed and in the last 25 years, parallel to technological developments, videoscopic repairs became widespread. As a result of this development, surgical procedures have now become the standard procedure for "strengthening the abdominal wall in the transverse fascia plan" and are accepted all over the world [3].

The idea of laparoscopic repair was first alleged by Ger in 1982 by the collapse of the internal loop. In 1990, Schultz used transperitoneal plugs and developed the intraperitoneal onlay mesh (IPOM) technique, which was performed in the same year by patching the Fitzgibbons peritoneum. Transabdominal preperitoneal (TAPP) patch application was first performed by Leroy in 1990. Then in 1991 Dulucq and in 1992 McKernan introduced total extraperitoneal (TEP) intervention [4].

4. Anatomy

In the inguinal region, four different types of hernia—indirect, direct, femoral and obturator—can develop. One of the most important advantages of the posterior approach is the ability to reveal the entirety of hernia types. There are median, medial and lateral ligaments in the anterior wall of the abdomen after fetal period, followed by urachus obliteration, umbilical artery obliteration and inferior epigastric vessels, respectively. In addition, there are iliopubic tractus, pectineal ligament (Cooper) and lacunar ligament in pubic region, pubic tubercule, spina iliaca anterior superior (SIAS) and superior pubic ramus bones [5].

There are two potential gaps in the preperitoneum. The "Bogros gap" is located between the transverse fascia and the peritoneum. Preperitoneal fatty tissue and porous connective tissue fill this area. The medial part of the preperitoneal cavity on the bladder is known as the "Retzius cavity". The posterior view angle allows examination of the myofektineal orifice, which is a relatively weak part of the abdominal wall and is divided by the inguinal ligament [6].

The external iliac vessels are anastomosed with the inferior epigastric vessels and the superior epigastric vessels. They supply the abdominal wall and penetrate the rectus abdominus through the cranial route within the vagina musculature rectus. Posteriorly inspected anulus inguinalis profundus will reveal the deep location of inferior epigastric vessels. In addition, the aberrant obturator arteries formed by the anastomosis of the pubic ramus of the epigastric artery with the obturator artery, known as "Corona Mortis", constitute the basis of the death triangle. The medial side of this triangle is vas deferens, the lateral side is the spermatic cord and the posterior border is the peritoneal margin.

The inferolateral border of the iliopubic tract, the superomedial border of the gonadal vessels and the lateral border of the peritoneal catheter is defined as the area of the pain triangle and the intermediate cutaneous branches of the lateral femoral cutaneous nerve, the femoral branch of the genitofemoral nerve and the anterior branch of the femoral nerve contain posterior anatomical approach.

5. Material and methods

We performed laparoscopic inguinal hernia surgery in 163 patients between January 2017 and 2018 in our clinic. Laparoscopic hernia repair was recommended to patients who are suitable for general anesthesia, had no previous abdominal surgery or incarceration or strangulated hernia or without acute mechanical intestinal obstruction. In terms of learning curve, TAPP was performed on first 50 cases and TEP on the following cases. A total of 155 (95%) patients were male and 8 (5%) were female. A total of 51 patients received TAPP (31.2%) and 112 patients (68.7%) received TEP. Eight patients who underwent TAPP (15.6%) were operated for recurrence. Thirteen patients (25.4%) underwent bilateral repair while three (5.8%) patients underwent the same session umbilical hernia repair. The groups were evaluated in terms of operation time, pain scores, recurrence rates, duration of hospitalization and return to daily activity and complication rates. TAPP average operation time is 58 min while in bilateral cases this duration is 72 min. The duration of operation of recurrent cases was 59 min average and there was no significant difference between these patients and the primary cases. A total of 112 patients were treated with TEP technique. Nineteen patients (16.9%) were operated for recurrent hernia, and 14 patients (12.5%) underwent bilateral repair. In three patients (2.6%), the same session umbilical hernia repair was also performed. Average duration of TEP is 47 min while in bilateral cases this duration is observed as elongated, 56 min. The duration of operation in recurrent cases was 56 min and there was no significant difference between these patients and the primary cases. The hospital stay was measured as 1.2 days for TAPP and 1.1 days for TEP, and no significant difference was found between the groups. It was also found that the pain scores between the two groups were similar as 3.2 and 2.9 for TAPP and TEP, respectively. The time to return to the daily activity for TAPP was 5.6 days and for TEP was 5.3 days and no significant difference was found between the two groups. As a complication, seroma in four patients (2.4%), recurrent hernia in two patients (1.2%) and chronic persistent pain in six patients (3.6%) occurred. Patients with recurrence were reoperated. Five patients with chronic persistent pain were treated with medical therapy within 6 months, and one patient with osteitis pubis was detected and curettage was performed by orthopedics clinic. In our study, no significant difference in recurrence, return duration to work, pain score, duration of hospitalization and postoperative complication were detected between the groups.

6. Technical points

The use of laparoscopic methods for inguinal hernia surgery is advanced minimal invasive surgery with less tissue trauma, less postoperative pain, lower postoperative infection risk and faster postoperative recovery. It is possible to combine positive effects such as faster return to work and better cosmetic results. As with all surgical techniques, minimally invasive techniques also have advantages. Compared to open surgery, some disadvantages of inguinal hernia surgery are the initial operation time and the long learning curve. Also, the cost is relatively high. In addition, unlike open surgery, the lack of sense of depth in the image, that is, the operation with the 2D image requires the surgeon to dominate the inguinal region anatomy at a high level. Instead of cost problem, by time, the integration of the learning curve and the increase in the experience reduce most of the problems.

There are two main techniques when laparoscopic inguinal hernia repair is concerned. These are defined as transabdominal preperitoneal approach (TAPP) and total extraperitoneal approach (TEP). According to the International Endohernia Group's 2011 Guidelines, revised in 2015, TAPP and TEP have become the preferred repair techniques for the Lichtenstein technique, especially after hernia recurs by open pre-repair [7].

7. Laparoscopic transabdominal preperitoneal approach

It is stated that TAPP is the first method to be learned because it is applicable in all inguinal region hernia types. As an advantage of the intraabdominal approach, the posterior wall anatomy can be better dominated, so proper and adequate parietalization can be made more comfortable. Compared to TEP, the cost is lower and the learning curve is shorter. TAPP is a highly successful method for both incarcerated and scrotal hernias. Due to intraabdominal vision, providing a wide field of view study is one of its greatest advantages and is a method that can be used in laparoscopically repaired recurrent hernias.

8. Technical details

8.1. Operating room layout

The opposite side of the surgical field and both legs are in closed position. In bilateral hernia repair, both arms are in closed position. The videomonitor laparoscopy tower is placed on the patient's foot, on the side to be operated. The operator can be placed on the opposite side of the area to be operated and the camera assistant can be placed on the same side or opposite side of the surgeon depending on the experience and habits of the team. We prefer the camera assistant to sit on the same side of the surgeon (**Figure 1**).

8.2. Surgical instruments

- Standard laparoscopic equipment consisting of camera, monitor, light and bag
- 10 mm diameter and 30° angle camera
- One 10 mm and two 5 mm in diameter totally 3 trocars
- Veress needle
- Endoinstruments (Atraumatic pens, dissector, scissors, hook, acutenaculum, aspirator)
- 5 mm diameter vessel sealing device
- 15 × 15 cm polypropylene or polyester special shaped patch
- Fixing material for mesh detection and peritoneal closure (mechanical stapler, tissue adhesive or non-absorbable suture material) (**Figure 2**).

8.3. Preparation of the patient and treatment of trocars

A single dose of 1 g second-generation cephalosporin as prophylactic antibiotic is injected half an hour before the onset of operation. The patient should urinate before operation and preoperative fluid resuscitation should be kept to a minimum. Before the operation, the patient

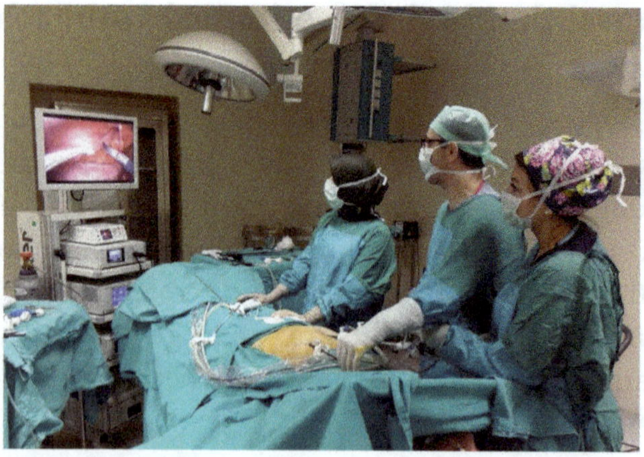

Figure 1. Operating room: The surgeon and camera assistant placed on the opposite side of the surgical area.

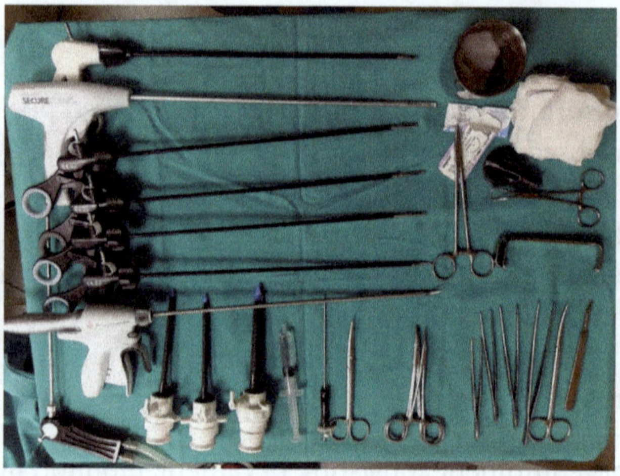

Figure 2. Surgical instruments for TAPP procedure.

is scrubbed and covered in the supine position for sterility. Under general anesthesia, by Hasson technique or with Veress needle which is placed in the infraumbilical region, produces caphno pneumoperitoneum. General intraabdominal exploration is completed with a 10 mm trocar inserted in the infraumbilical region. The operating table position is kept (30° Trendelenburg and 15°–20°opposite to the operating area). Two operating ports (5 mms) are placed on the umbilical level transverse line, with the lateral sides of both rectus muscles localized and placed under direct vision. The trocars on the operative side are placed on infraumbilical transverse line, while the opposite trocar is placed 4–5 cm caudal side on this line (**Figure 3**). In bilateral hernias, it is suggested that both trocars to be placed on the transverse line at the same level.

8.4. Intraabdominal inguinal exploration

As the trocar placements are complete, the inguinal area is examined with care. The hernia type is detected and the content—if present—of the hernia is carefully reduced to origin with atraumatic clamp. If there are elements such as intestine or omentum in the hernia sac, the vitability of intestine or omentum is checked after reducement.

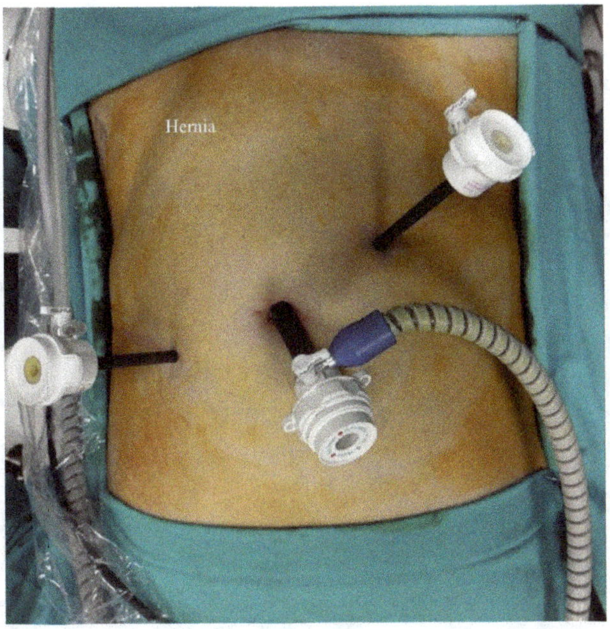

Figure 3. Trocar placement for TAPP procedure.

8.5. Peritoneal incision, dissection and preparation of preperitoneal area

The preparation of the peritoneal flap starts on approximately 5 cm above the hernia canal at the level of the anterior superior crista iliaca on the upper outer side of the annulus inguinalis. The incision is advanced to the medial side of the transverse plane through the upper 5 cm of the inguinal canal's inner ring and terminated at approximately 2 cm to median ligament.

The peritoneal incision can be done with endoscissors or hooks. Rest of the peritoneal flap on the inguinal canal inner ring can be easily disrupted with the help of intraabdominal CO_2 pressure, stretched with endograsper. Peritoneal dissection, below the inguinal canal inner ring, is a little more difficult. The lower peritoneal flap is liberated until lateral visualization of the iliopubic tract, and medial visualization of the Cooper ligament. The hernia sac is carefully dissected from the spermatic cord and elements that are attached through the lower peritoneal membrane (**Figure 4**). The peritoneal upper and lower flaps are dissected in each direction to provide large parietalization and vision of myopectineal orifice. Thus, enough space is available to lay a mesh on probable direct, indirect and femoral herniation defect sources. If bilateral hernias are present, the peritoneal incision can be extended from one side of the crista iliaca to the other side of the crista iliaca, but in the literature it is suggested that a single incision should be made and a peritoneal bridge could be released in the midline.

8.6. Preparation, placement and detection of the mesh patch

Special shaped polypropylene or polyester patches prepared in size appropriate to the anatomical characteristics of the hernia of the patient are used. The patch is rolled from the outside to the inside and from top to bottom in the form of a roll with limb or without limb (**Figure 5**). It is placed into the abdomen through a 10 mm trocar. With the help of two endograspers, placed in the working ports, the roll is unfolded in the opposite direction and is laid to cover

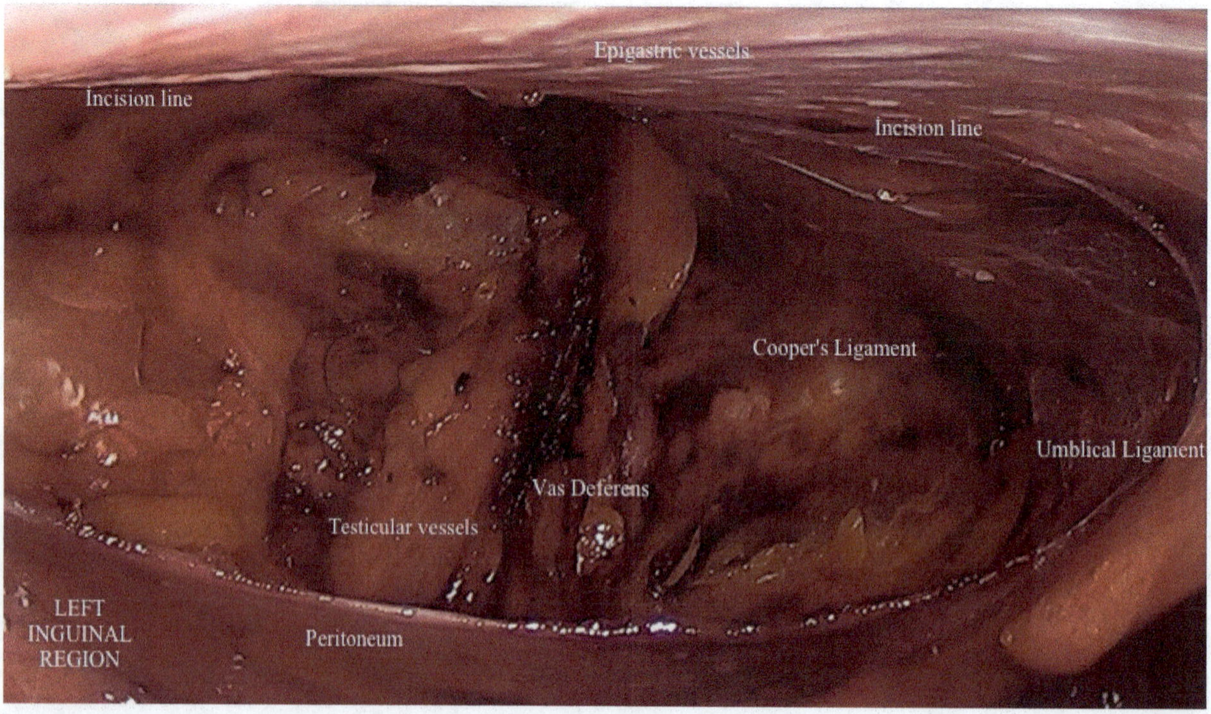

Figure 4. Anatomic details of left inguinal region after peritoneal flap preparation.

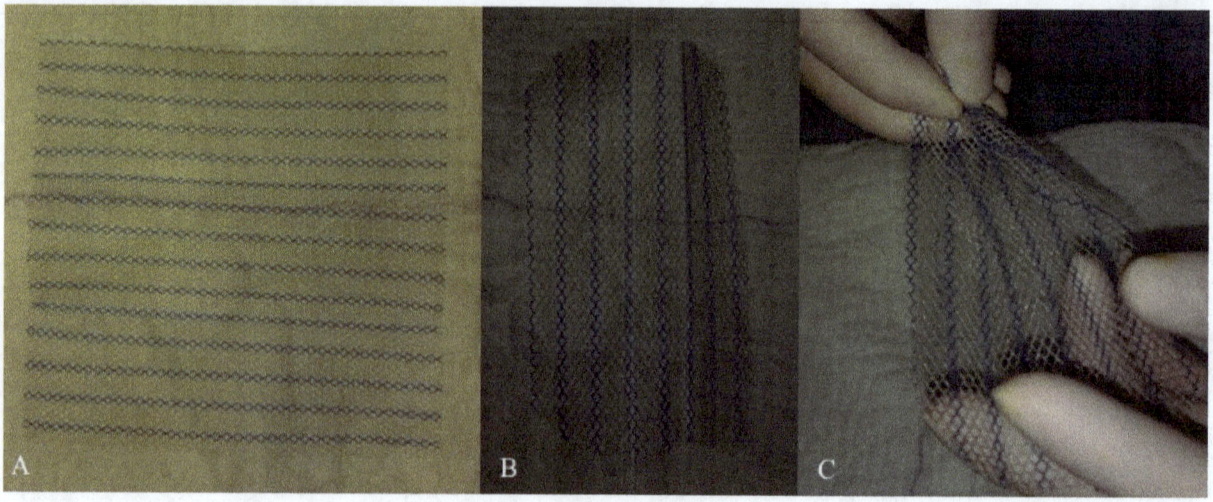

Figure 5. Mesh preparation.

the existing hernia defect and potential hernia sources. Also, it must be ensured that the patch is placed with a proper tension. When a limb patch is applied the lower limb is passed under the spermatic cord and it is wrapped in a tie and is joined laterally with the upper limb again. The location and number of staples is very important for the immobilization of the mesh patch. The basic rule—with different suggestions about this—is that the staples must be placed on the ileo-pubic tract. We prefer to fix it with two absorbable staples totally, one medially to the Cooper ligament and one to the back of the transverse fascia (**Figure 6**). Tissue adhesives or absorbable suture materials may also be used for detection.

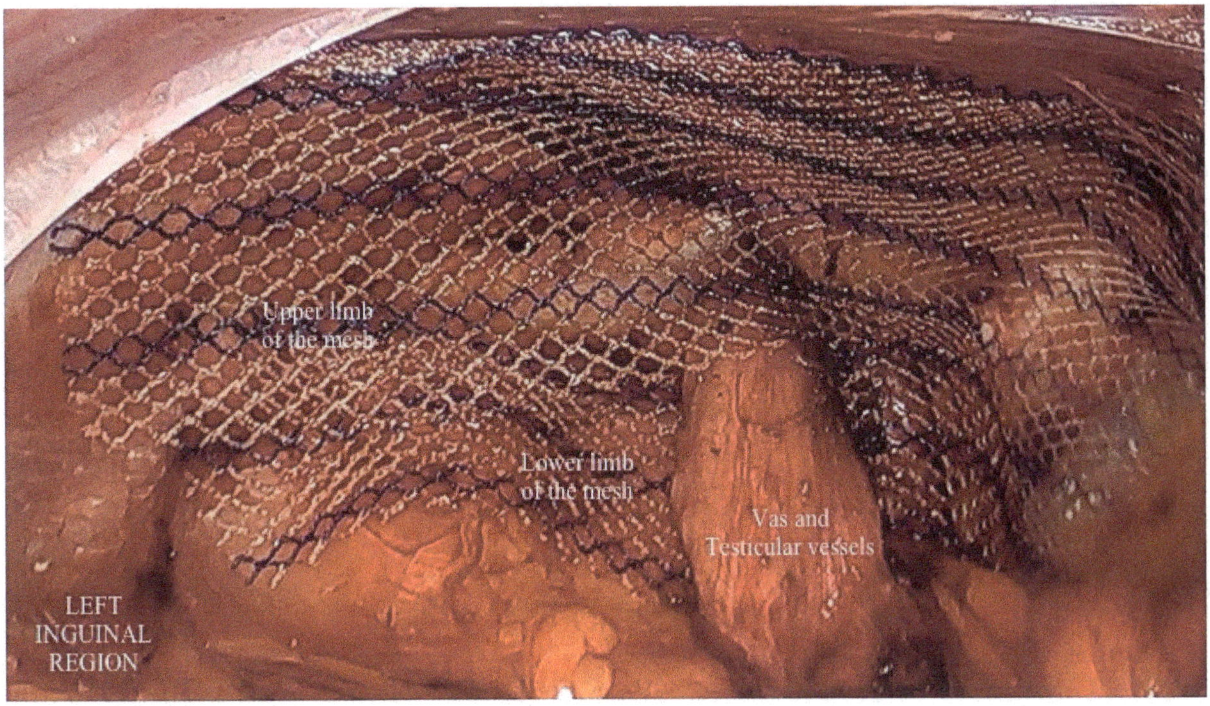

Figure 6. After mesh fixation in TAPP procedure.

8.7. Closure of peritoneum over mesh

After the integration of fixation, the upper and lower leaves of the peritoneum are covered on the patch and the opposite edges are closed with either continuous stitches or with clips. Closing the peritoneum with stitches is more convenient but requires more time and experience. The hernia sac, which is usually left in the lower peritoneal sheet and reduced into the peritoneum, can be left if it is small, also the larger sacs can be partially resected before closing the peritoneal leaves. According to experience and preference, a drain can be placed behind the peritoneal flap. After the peritoneum is closed, 5 mm ports are removed under direct vision and the operation is terminated.

8.8. Postoperative care

Oral intake can be started a few hours after surgery and the patient is mobilized the same evening. The following day the patient can be discharged by removal of the drain. There is no need to regulate postoperative medical treatment other than oral analgesics.

9. Laparoscopic total extraperitonal approach

Despite discussions about the use of laparoscopy in the repair of primary unilateral groin hernias, the superiority of TEP in bilateral or recurrent hernias is accepted. The major advantages of this method are that it is extraperitoneal and there is no break in peritoneum. The dominance of the anatomy of the posterior wall is not as good as TAPP, but sufficient parietalization is possible with TEP. Nowadays it becomes the first choice especially for athletes both men and women.

9.1. Operating room layout

The opposite side of the surgical field and both legs are in closed position. In bilateral hernia repair, both arms are in closed position. The videomonitor laparoscopy tower is placed on the patient's foot, on the side to be operated. The operator can be placed on the opposite side of the area to be operated and the camera assistant can be placed on the same side or opposite side of the surgeon depending on the experience and habits of the team. We prefer the camera assistant to sit on the same side of the surgeon.

9.2. Surgical supplies

Standard laparoscopic equipment consisting of a camera, a monitor, a light and an insuflator

- 10 mm diameter balloon trocar
- Laparoscope with a diameter of 10 mm and a 30° angle
- A 10 mm, two 5 mm diameter, totally 3 trocars
- Atraumatic clamps, endodissectors, endoscissors, endohooks, endoclapms, endoaspirators
- 5 mm diameter vessel sealing device
- 15 × 15 cm polypropylene or polyester special shaped patch
- Fixation material (mechanical staple or tissue adhesive)

9.3. Preparation of the patient, application of extraperitoneal trocars

A single dose of 1 g second-generation cephalosporin as prophylactic antibiotic is injected half an hour before the onset of operation. The patient should urinate before operation and pre-operatory fluid resuscitation should be kept to a minimum. With general anesthesia, the operation starts in supine position. In method of TEP, the patient should be wider painted than the TAPP technique, from the nipple to the perineum. Infraumbilical, slightly lateralized incision is made on the hernia side and then the rectus sheath is opened by transverse incision. Rectus fibers are removed with Farabeuf retractor and blunt dissection is performed to reach the Bogros area. A tunnel is made between umbilicus to pubis. In front of this tunnel, there is a parietal peritoneum from the back of the rectus muscle and from the end of this fascia to the transverse course of the linea semilunaris. After blunt dissection and cannula is completely inserted from the preperitoneal tunnel to the pubis, it is removed from the trocar cannula and replaced with a telescope, and the cannula is inflated with a balloon attached to the mandrel. Air is discharged 20–25 times with puar after waiting for 30 s and this process is repeated three times. With some balloons, it is possible to view inside with scope as it inflates. It can also be monitored whether the definite surgical area is viewed during this observation. Upper view of rectus fibrils and lower view of parietal peritoneum indicates the right position. A 10 mm trocar is placed in the infraumbilical incision to prevent gas leakage and the telescope is placed. The preperitoneal space is inflated with 10–12 mmHg CO_2. Two 5 mm ports are placed at a distance of 5 cm from the midline in direct view (**Figure 7**).

9.4. The dissection of extraperitoneal area and herniated sac

After the 30° camera is inserted, the inferior epigastric artery and vein are observed along the bottom of the rectus muscle. The parietal peritoneum is dissected in the medial and lateral directions to remain underneath. The Cooper ligament is visible in the inferomedial area and it is removed. The lateral aspect of the rectus is up to the border of the crista iliaca and the fascia transversalis is opened with blunt and sharp dissections posteriorly. The potential hernia areas are examined and the hernia type is determined (**Figure 8**). In the indirect inguinal hernia, the hernia sac is found adhered to the spermatic cord. The hernia sac should be dissected from the pubic tuberculum to the level of the external iliac vein. Large scrotal or indirect hernia may be released by Zig technique if it is confirmed that the hernia sac does not contain omentum or intestinal contents. The anatomic regions described as Femoral and Hasselbach triangles should be examined in terms of direct and femoral hernia that may be accompanied. The ililopubic tract must be detected not to injure the femoral and lateral femoral cutaneous nerves of the underlying genitofemoral nerve. The lateral dissection does not need to be as wide as the TAPP technique. The hernia sac should be gently released and reduced from the spermatic cord and cremaster fibers. If the peritoneum is wounded during the dissection procedure, the defect can be closed with a clip. If gas insufflation flows through the gap to the peritoneal defect, the enlarged abdomen will restrict the area of dissection. In order to prevent this, intraperitoneal air could be taken out from the upper left quadrant of the midclavicular line through the abdominal cavity (Palmer's point) with Veress needle. The valve is left open, the evacuation of the gas is provided and the operation can be continued.

9.5. Preparation, placement and detection of the mesh patch

Special shaped 15 × 15 cm polypropylene or polyester patch can be used according to the anatomy of the patient. The patch can be prepared with limb or without limb. It is rolled up

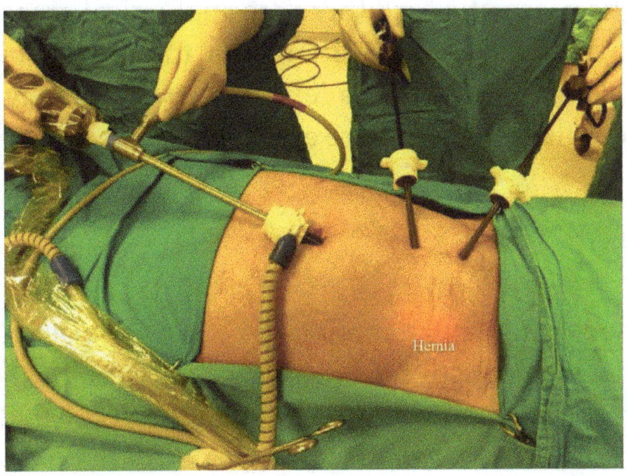

Figure 7. Trocar placement for TEP procedure.

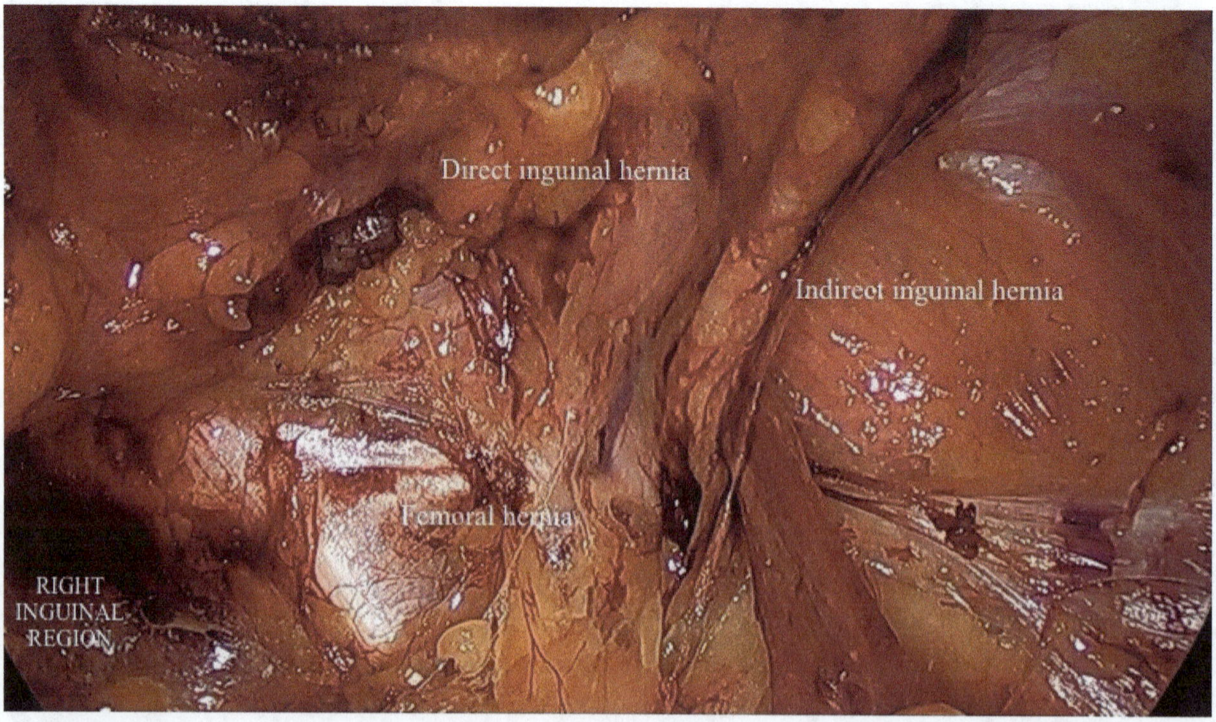

Figure 8. Potential hernia areas for TEP procedure.

from the top and laid to the extraperitoneal space by the 10 mm camera trocars. With the help of two endograspers placed in the working ports, the patch is unfolded in the opposite direction and is laid to cover the existing hernia defect and potential hernia areas. It should be ensured that the area where the patch is applied covers it with a proper tension. When a limb patch is applied, the lower limb is passed under the spermatic cord and it is wrapped in a tie and is laterally joined to the lower limb (**Figure 9**). The lower edge of the patch is placed so that it remains at least 2 cm above the released hernia sheath. The locations and numbers are very important if the absorbable staple is preferred for the detection of the mesh. The basic rule, with different suggestions about this, is that the mesh must be placed on the ileo-pubic tract. We prefer to fix it with a total of two absorptive staples, one medially to the Cooper ligament and one to the back of the transverse fascia laterally. On the lateral edge of the spermatic cord there are anatomical areas defined as the triangle of pain mentioned above and the death triangle at the medial border. Staples must be avoided in these areas. Tissue adhesives have also been used today as fixing material. The use of drains varies according to experience and habits. We routinely use aspirative drain after TEP.

9.6. Postoperative care

Oral intake can be started a few hours after surgery and the patient is mobilized the same evening. The following day the patient can be discharged by removal of the drain. There is no need to regulate postoperative medical treatment other than oral analgesics.

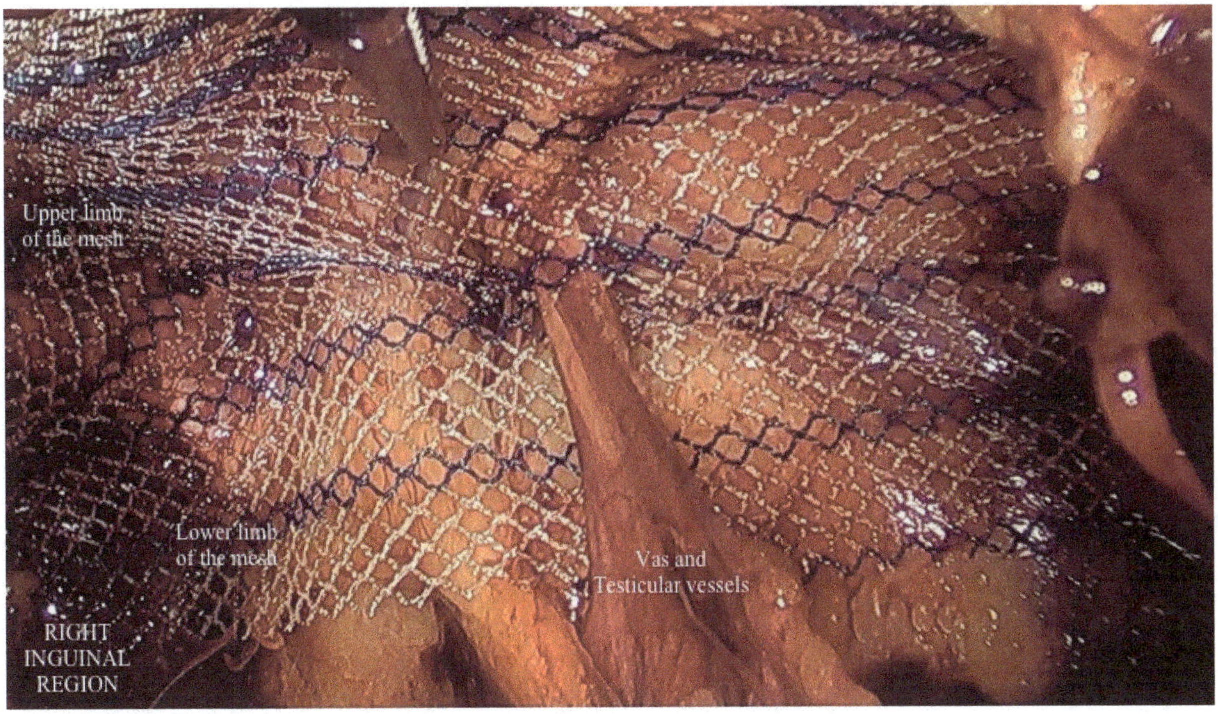

Figure 9. After mesh fixation.

10. Pitfalls

In this chapter, details take place as noted; details in current practice are given while applying the laparoscopic hernia repair. The points to be considered are evaluated for both techniques. In addition, the difficulties faced by the surgeon are itemized.

10.1. TAPP

- As all laparoscopic operations, the first point to note in laparoscopic hernia surgery is trocar entry sites. Correct positioning of the appropriate points will prevent intestinal injuries that may occur at the time of first entry and bleeding which may be caused by the injury of the abdominal wall, especially the epigastric vessels.
- A complete exploration should be done in terms of hernia type, size, presence of accompanying incarceration and other pathologies in intraabdominal exploration.
- Taking enough width for dissection during the preparation of the peritoneal flap will ensure that the exploration area is convenient. Working on a sufficient width of dissection will facilitate the spread of the patch, the adequate closure of the hernia defect and the operator's work during the detection of the patch.
- A very careful dissection should be performed in order to avoid damage to the spermatic cord structures, especially in the presence of indirect hernia, when the hernia incision is

dissected, as interference with the anatomical planes may result in attempts made for recurrent hernia.

- Should be very careful not to hold Vas Deferens by endo-devices so as to not disturb.
- The dissection should be performed at an adequate width of the myopectinale opening, but should be avoided from the extreme dissection in front of the psoas site in the lateral direction. There is an anatomic area defined as triangular pain in this region and it should be especially noted that the cutaneous femoral lateralis and femoral branches of genitofemoral nerves are not damaged. Postoperative chronic pain syndromes can be encountered in the event of a possible nerve injury.
- Death triangle is defined as the anastomotic area between the external iliac vein and the obturator vein and should be avoided from the extreme dissection. Because, in the event of a possible vascular injury in this region, catastrophic consequences may be encountered.
- The staples used for patch detection due to the same reasons should never be used under the iliopubic tract.
- Should be sure to place the staples on the medial side, especially on the Cooper ligament, so that postoperative osteitis pubis is avoided.
- It is generally advised to use the least amount of other materials that can be used for stapling or patch fixation.
- Wide laying of the mesh will reduce the recurrence rate by covering the three hernia areas.
- Reducing the intraabdominal CO_2 pressure during the peritoneal flap closure and correcting the patient's position will facilitate closure because it will reduce tension. The effective closing of the flap is important to prevent postoperative intestinal adhesions.

10.2. TEP

- The infraumbilical incision should be made from slightly left or right lateral. What should be noted here is to be on the rectus front sheath. If the linea alba is opened by mistake, the gas will flow to the intraabdominal region and strengthen the technique at the start.
- It is important to notice the bright white color of the rectus posterior sheath, and it is important that the balloon is inflated by advancing the balloon trocar in this space. The balloon dissection between the fibers of the rectus will cause bleeding between the muscle fibers, disturbing the dissection plans and preventing the vision.
- If gas flows into the abdomen during possible peritoneal injuries in the TEP technique, as mentioned in the techniques section, the gas must be evacuated with the Veress needle, which will be entered from the Palmer point.
- Large peritoneal defects may cause postoperative patchy contact with the intestines and lead to postoperative intestinal adhesion development. For this reason, large peritoneal defects should be closed with endoclips.

11. Complications and management

In this section, complications related to laparoscopic inguinal hernia surgery, literature information about management of these complications and suggestions based on our own experience are included.

11.1. Local complications

The most common complications are serous fluid deposits (seroma) and bleeding(hematoma) which may develop during operation. Patients should be informed in the preoperative period about these complications. Postoperative seromas usually resorb spontaneously within 2 weeks and do not require treatment. Therapeutic drainage needs arise in the presence of seroma persistent for longer than 6–8 weeks or in the presence of seroma causing clinical symptoms. The use of peroperative aspirative drains in risky patients of who may be predicted seroma and hematoma development may prevent the development of these complications. Scrotal elevation is recommended in the postoperative period. If abdominal wall ecchymosis occur, mechanical compression, cold application and medical treatment can be tried. Subcutaneous emphysema is often untreated and spontaneous. In rare occasional hydrocele cases, it will be more appropriate to consult with a urologist.

11.2. Neurological complications

The treatment of chronic pain syndromes after laparoscopic hernia surgery is often long and difficult. Chronic postoperative pain has been reported in up to 63% of all groin repairs and significantly affects clinical outcomes. The pain following laparoscopic surgery is usually neuropathic pain. The cause is usually the damage or trapping of the lateral femoral cutaneous or femoral branch of the genitofemoral nerve. Clinically it occurs as acute burning and/or crushing pain in a particular dermatome. Mareljia parestetika is the name of a pain clinic that develops after a lateral femoral cutaneous nerve injury and persistent paresthesia lateral of the femoral area. It is recommended to apply corticosteroids or anesthetic injections which can be applied at rest, cold application, NSAIDs, physical therapy, locally. Osteitis pubis is; the name of the pain clinic that occurs due to public inflammation and arises especially on the middle of the groin or on the pubis, especially with femoral adduction. Diagnosis can be made by excluding recurrent hernia diagnosis radiographically and performing bone imaging. The treatment approach is the same as neuropathic pain. Often, 6 months are required to respond to treatment. However, if the cure is not available, the orthopedic consultation may be needed to consider possible bone resection or curettage options.

11.3. Cord and testicular injury

Ischemic orchitis should be considered in the complaints of hardened, enlarged and painful testicles that appear about 10 days after the repair of the inguinal hernia. It is often self-limiting. It is usually the result of a possible damage to the pampiniform plexus, not the testicular artery. Ultrasound can distinguish necrosis or ischemia. If testicular necrosis is detected, urgent orchiectomy may be necessary. Treatment includes IV hydration and NSAIDs. If testicular artery is damaged, it can be caused testicular atrophy after long periods of operation. Vas deferens may not be manipulated during surgery and maximum effort to avoid disturbing their nutrition may help to avoid these complications.

11.4. Recurrents

Postoperative pain, swelling and the presence of a mass in the inguinal region should be considered. Diagnosis can be made by radiological examinations. Technical factors that play a role in the development of recurrence include inappropriate patch size, inadequate patch, stress or inaccurate detection, lack of experience, tissue ischemia and infections. Factors related to the patient include malnutrition, obesity, wound healing disorders and uncontrolled diabetes mellitus. Surgical intervention should be considered in the treatment.

Other complications include urinary retention, which can be prevented by the patient's urination before surgery or by peroperative urinary catheterization. Paralytic ileus, visceral injuries, vascular injuries, intestinal obstruction, hypercapnia, pneumothorax and gas embolism are also uncommon complications.

12. Literature review

The results of laparoscopic and open inguinal hernia surgeries are now being compared very much. Postoperative pain complications, recurrence rates, patient satisfaction, cost analysis are frequently discussed. Papachariston and colleagues in their postoperative evaluation of pain study [8], even though it was reported to require more analgesic in the first 6 h in the TAPP group, pain was reported in 2–11% of the open surgery group and reported as 1–4.2% in the laparoscopic group. In the same study, persistent pain lasting from seventh day to 1 year in the open surgical group was associated with postoperative fibrosis, while point pain in the laparoscopic group was associated with scar tissue rupture. In a meta-analysis evaluating persistent pain [9], patch repair has been shown to reduce persistent pain as opposed to pain relief, and it has also been found that chronic pain is less in the laparoscopic method.

In a study in which approximately 10,000 patient outcomes were assessed in the United States and patients were followed for 3 years [10], the recurrence rate of the laparoscopic method was found to be 0.4%, and it was emphasized that the most important difference between open and laparoscopic operations was the achievement of sufficient experimentation, the number of operations performed. According to this recommendation, a randomized controlled trial conducted by the Veterans Affairs Cooperative Study and reporting of 2-year follow-ups [11], recurrence rates were reported as 10% for laparoscopic repair and 5% for open repair, but after 250 laparoscopic cases techniques, results were improved. In a more recent study, Lal et al. [12] has shown that surgeons have reduced recurrence rates from 9 to 2.9% after 100 operations. In different studies, it has been reported that the laparoscopic techniques are spreading and the time to assess the competence of the surgeons is between 50 and

100 cases. A meta-analysis by Köckerling et al. [13] evaluating the relationship between patch fixation and recurrence, cases that patch fixation was performed and in cases not performed, there was no difference in the duration of operation, patch-related complications, recurrence and duration of hospital stay.

In a randomized controlled meta-analysis in which Wei and colleagues evaluated the outcomes of 1000 patients published in 2015, there was no difference between the two surgeries, pain score, operation time, return to daily activity, hospitalization time, complication and cost between the two surgeries. In conclusion, TEP was found to be more complicated than TAPP and advised to start laparoscopic surgery with TAPP to inexperienced surgeons [14]. In a study published by Köckerling et al. [15] there was no difference between two surgeries in terms of intraoperative complications and reoperation rates. However, after TAPP surgery, complication rates were found to be higher due to possible large complications, more scrotal hernia, elderly patient selection.

In a study conducted by Payne et al. [16] to measure postoperative quality of life, it has been shown that patients' compliance with straight leg exercises is better after laparoscopic surgery. Designed in the same way and studied by Lawrence et al. [17], this difference was more evident in bilateral hernia repair.

The problem of cost is still an important problem, with the fact that it has been removed from the big picture compared to the past. In the study conducted by Stylopoulos et al. [18] in 2003 and the results of 1.5 million patients evaluated, laparoscopic operations have been claimed to reduce costs compared to long-term open surgery when salary, health insurance costs, reduced job quality, delayed work shifts and the salary of the worker looking after the patient are taken into consideration. Farinas et al. [19] showed that 60% reduction in indirect costs could be achieved despite the 40% increase in the direct costs of using non-disposable devices and shortening of the operation time.

When TEP and TAPP were compared, there was no difference between the two techniques in terms of hospitalization time, recovery time and short term recurrence rates. The duration of the TEP technique is shorter than that of the TAPP technique [20]. However, according to the International Endohernia Association, it has been suggested that surgeons should apply the TEP technique after learning the TAPP technique and acquiring a certain experience in the learning curve [21].

In our study, we have found that there is only a minimal difference between TAPP and TEP techniques, in terms of operative time. There was no difference in both techniques when recurrence, return to work, pain score, duration of hospitalization and complications were evaluated. Particularly, we observed that bilateral and recurrent hernia had high patient satisfaction. Also we observed that TAPP surgery in the early stages of surgery, shortened the learning curve.

In conclusion, laparoscopic inguinal hernia surgery takes place in daily practice as an increasingly widespread up-to-date treatment method in which training and experience gained over time and patient satisfaction of clinical outcomes are very good.

Conflict of interest

The authors declare that they have no conflict of interest.

Author details

Fatih Altintoprak[1]*, Emrah Akin[2], Kemal Gundogdu[2] and Enis Dikicier[1]

*Address all correspondence to: fatihaltintoprak@yahoo.com

1 Istinye University Faculty of Medicine, Department of General Surgery, Istanbul, Turkey

2 Sakarya University Research and Educational Hospital, Department of General Surgery, Sakarya, Turkey

References

[1] Wagner JP, Brunicardi CF, Amid PK. İnguinal Hernias Schwartz's Princeples of Surgery. 10th ed. In: Brunicardi CF, editor. New York: In chief. McGraw Hill publishing; 2016. pp. 1510-1517

[2] Mark A, Malangomi and Michael J. Dosen Hernias Sabiston Textbook of Surgery: The biological basis of modern surgical practice 19th ed. In: Townsend CM, Beauchamp RD, Evers BM, Matteox KL, editors. London: Saunders publishing; 2012. pp. 1114-1141

[3] Van Hee R. History of inguinal hernia repair. Turnalul de Chirurgie. 2011;**73**:301-314

[4] Sachs M, Damm M, Enche A. Historical evaluation of inguinal hernia repair. World Journal of Surgery. 1997;**21**(2):218-223

[5] Bianutto SN, Repetto E, Aliendo MM, Borginho VW. İnguinal canal development: The muscular wall and the role of the gubernaculum. Clinical Anatomy. 2009;**22**(5):614-618. DOI: 10.1002/ca.20820

[6] Rosenberger RT, Loewneck H, Meyer G. The cutaneous nerves encountered during laparoscopic repair of inguinal hernia: New anatomical findings for the surgeon. Surgical Endoscopy. 2000;**14**(8):731-735

[7] Brittner R, Montgomery MA, Arregui, et al. Erratum to: Update of guidelines on laparoscopic(TAPP) and endoscopic (TEP) treatment of inguinal hernia (İnternational Endehernia society). Surgical Endoscopy. 2015;**29**(6):1655-1656. DOI: 10.1007/s00464-015-4156-3

[8] Papachariston EA, Mitselou MF, Finokaliotis ND. Surgical outcome and hospital cost analysis of laparoscopic and open tension free hernia repair hernia. 2002;**6**(2):68-72. PMID:12152642

[9] EU Hernia trialists Colloboration. Repair of groin hernia with synthetic mesh: Meta analysis of randomized controlled trials. Annals of Surgery. 2002;**235**(3):322-332.PMID:11882753

[10] Felix EL, Harbestson N, Vartanian S. Laparoscopic hernioplasty; significant complications. Surgical Endoscopy. 1998 Apr;**13**(4):328-331. PMID:10094740

[11] Neumayer L, Giobbie-Hurder A, Jonasson A, et al. Veterans cooperative studies program 456 investigators. Open mesh versus laparoscopic mesh repair of inguinal hernia. The New England Journal of Medicine. 2004;**350**(18):1819-1827. DOI: 10.1056/NEJMoa040093

[12] Lal P, Kajla RK, Chander J, et al. Laparoscopic total extraperitoneal (TEP) inguinal hernia repair: Overcoming the learning curve. Surgical Endoscopy. 2004;**18**(4):642-645. Epub 2004. DOI: 10.1007/s00464-002-8649-5

[13] Köckerling F, Jacob DA, Chowbey P, et al. A meta-anlysis examining the use of tucker fixation versus no-fixation of mesh in laparoscopic inguinal hernia repair. International Journal of Surgery. 2012;**10**(6):325. DOI: 10.1016/J.ijsu. 2012.04.014

[14] Fx W, Zhang YC, Han W, et al. Transabdominal preperitoneal (TAPP) versus totally extraperitoneal (TEP) for laparoscopic hernia repair: A meta-analysis. Surgical Laparoscopy, Endoscopy and Percutaneous Techniques. 2015;**25**(5):375-383. DOI: 10.1097/SLE.0000000000000123

[15] Köckerling F, Bittner R, Jacob DA. TEP versus TAPP: Comparision of the perioperative outcome in 17.587 patients with a primary inguinal hernia. Surgical Endoscopy. 2015;**39**(12):3750-3760. DOI: 10.1007/s00464-015-4150-9

[16] Payne JH, Grininger LM, Izawa WT, et al. Laparoscopic or open inguinal hernioraphy? A randomized prospective trial. Archives of Surgery. 1994;**129**(9):973-979. PMID:8080380

[17] Lawrence K, Mc Whinnie D, Goodwin A, et al. Randomized controlled trial of laparoscopic versus open repair of inguinal hernia: Early results, BMJ. 1995;**311**(701):981-985. PMID:7583639

[18] Stylopoulos N, Gazelle GS, Rattner DW, et al. A cost-utility analysis of treatment options for inguinal hernia in 1,513,008 adult patients, Surgical Endoscopy. 2003;**17**:180-189. DOI: 10.1007/900464-002-8849-z

[19] Farinas LP, Griffin FD. Cost containment and totally extraperitoneal laparoscopic herniorraphy. Surgical Endoscopy. 2000;**14**(1):37-40. PMID:10653233

[20] Qıu K, Ma J. Comments on TAPP versus TEP for laparoscopic hernia repair: A meta-analysis. Surgical Laparoscopy Endoscopy and Percutaneous Techniques. 2016;**26**(2):171. DOI: 10.1097/SLE.0000000000000251

[21] Bittner R, Köckerling F. Endorsement of the hernia surgical guidelines by the International Endohernia Society. Hernia. 2018;**22**(1):179. DOI: 10.1007/s10029-017-1674-z

4

Inguinal Hernia in Infants and Children

Ahmed Abdelghaffar Helal

Abstract

Congenital inguinal hernia is a very important subject for both general and pediatric surgeons, and many issues related to the inguinal hernia in infants and children are still confusing. Herein, the subject of congenital inguinal hernia, including the relevant embryology, related anatomy, the symptoms and signs essential for diagnosis, and the needed examination tests and investigations, is presented in a systematic manner. Also, the updated treatment options were discussed including both open and laparoscopic approaches with spotlight on the very recent single incision laparoscopic inguinal hernia repair in children. Finally, at the end of the chapter, there are many valuable references for more details.

Keywords: congenital inguinal hernia, inguinal canal, infants, children, laparoscopic hernia repair

1. Introduction

Congenital inguinal hernia in infants and children is a common surgical problem. Numerous issues, including the rational and timing of the repair, the need to explore the contralateral side, the use of laparoscopy, and anesthetic precautions, remain unsettled. Moreover, inguinal hernias in both full-term and preterm infants are commonly repaired shortly after diagnosis to avoid incarceration of the hernia, may be due to the lack of definitive data regarding optimal timing for repair of inguinal hernias in infants. In this chapter, the reader will be able to know and understand:

- the embryology and anatomy of pediatric inguinal hernia,
- the different clinical presentations of pediatric inguinal hernia,

- the differential diagnosis of inguinal hernia in infants and children,
- the treatment options for pediatric inguinal hernia, and
- the common open and laparoscopic approaches to pediatric inguinal hernias.

2. Embryology

Inguinal hernia in children represents arrest of development rather than acquired weakness. It is directly related to the descent of the developing gonads. The testes are preceded in their descent to the scrotum by a "finger" of peritoneum, the processus vaginalis (PV), which is first seen around the 12th week of gestation, and it is usually closed between the 36th and 40th weeks of gestation, except for the part that becomes the tunica vaginalis. In many newborns, this process is incomplete, leaving a patent processus vaginalis (PPV).Usually, the closure of PV is completed at birth; however, it may be delayed to postnatal period. Approximately 40% of PPV will close during the first months of life and an additional 20% close by 1 year of age. The closure of the PV on the left side precedes closure on the right; therefore, it is not surprising that 60% of congenital inguinal hernia occurs on the right side. The assumption that PPV is the same as an inguinal hernia is not true. The presence of PPV is necessary but not sufficient to develop a congenital inguinal hernia. In other words, all congenital inguinal hernias are preceded by PPV, but not all PPV go on to become inguinal hernia. About 12–14% of boys with PPV will develop inguinal hernia in their life time. The exact cause of the obliteration of the PPV is unknown. When PPV fails to close, a sac is present through which abdominal contents can be herniated via the inguinal canal. However, sometimes the entrance may be adequately covered by the internal oblique and transverses abdominal muscles, preventing escape of abdominal contents for many years, or allowing only fluid to pass through it forming a communicating hydrocele. If closure occurs proximally while fluid is trapped within the tunica distally, a non-communicating hydrocele is the result [1, 2].

3. Anatomy

3.1. Open anatomy

The inguinal canal is an oblique inter-muscular passage that extends from the deep to superficial inguinal rings and transmits the spermatic cord in males and round ligament in females. Most of the canal consists of the aponeurosis of the external oblique muscle as it curves inward to form the inguinal ligament. The roof of the canal is formed of the lower arched fibers of internal oblique and transverses abdominis muscles. The posterior wall of the canal consists of the transversalis fascia along its whole length. The inferior border of the canal is formed by the rolled fibers of inguinal ligament medially, and then the pectineus fascia and the insertion of the lacunar ligament (**Figure 1**). In neonates and infants, the inguinal canal is not well developed, and it was very short with both external and internal inguinal rings overlapping. Therefore, during open herniotomy before 1 year of age, there is no need to open the external oblique muscle [3, 4].

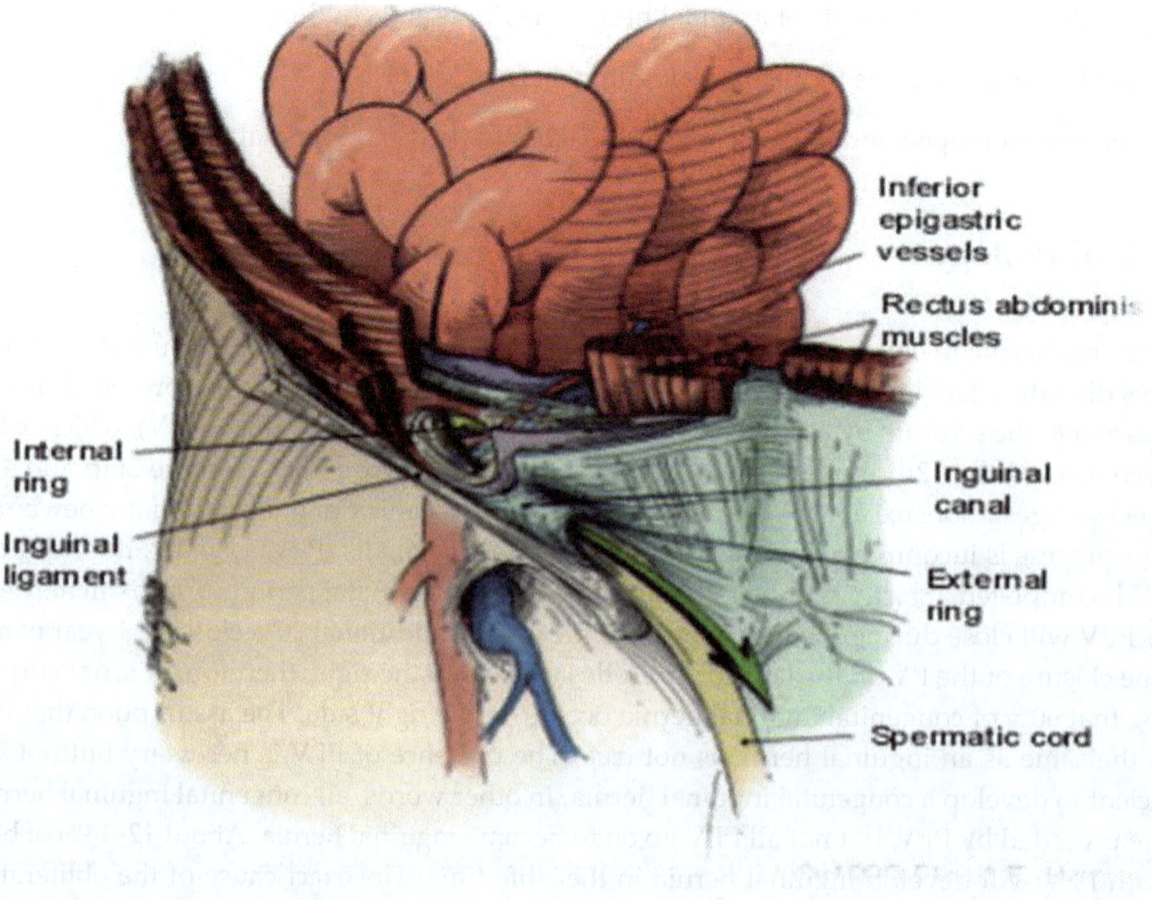

Figure 1. The open anatomy inguinal canal.

3.2. Laparoscopic anatomy

In 1945, Lytle wrote "The surgeon knows little about the anatomy of the posterior wall of the inguinal canal, as it is hidden from his view." During laparoscopic hernia repair, the hernia is no longer viewed as a protrusion from the abdominal wall, but rather as an extrusion of a viscous from the peritoneal cavity. So, the layers of the inguinal region and the abdominal wall are viewed in a reversed order or practically it is seen from an opposite view point. Therefore, during laparoscopic hernia repair, the following changes must be considered: the inguinal anatomy is visualized from inside with an optimal panoramic view of the posterior surface of the abdominal wall. Moreover, the inguinal anatomy is visualized with a paralyzed and expanded abdominal wall muscles. The pneumoperitoneum itself distorts normal anatomy, stretches ligaments, tenses parietal peritoneum, and inflates hernia sac. This laparoscopic change modifies the tension, texture, and handling characteristics of the peritoneum and the abdominal wall muscles when compared with its normal characteristics found during laparotomy (**Figure 2**) [5, 6].

Laparoscopically, the abdominal wall below the umbilicus shows five peritoneal folds, with three convergent fibrous cords in the center and two vascular bundles peripherally. In the mid-line is the median umbilical ligament, which represents the obliterated remnant of the embryonic urachus and extends from the fundus of the bladder to the umbilicus. The medial umbilical ligament consists of a peritoneal fold covering the obliterated distal portion of the

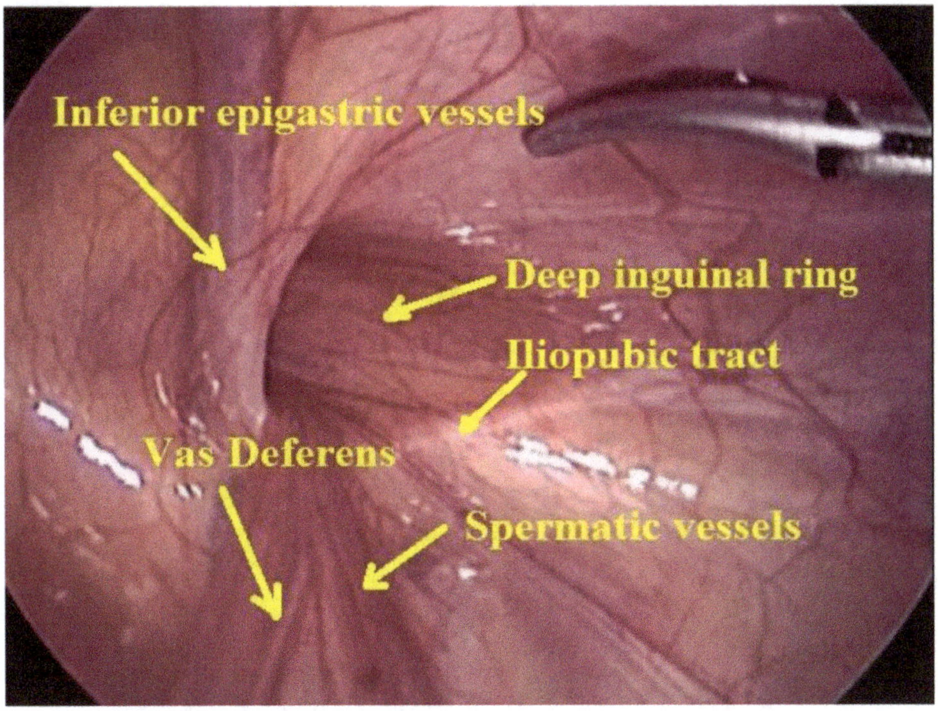

Figure 2. The laparoscopic view of inguinal anatomy.

umbilical artery. The lateral umbilical ligament consists of a fold of peritoneum around the inferior epigastric vessels together with a variable amount of fatty tissue [7, 8].

The pre-peritoneal space is important for the laparoscopic surgeon. It contains a variable amount of connective tissue, the residual of the umbilical artery, and the inferior epigastric vessels. The external iliac vessels and the inferior epigastric vessels lie free in this space and have no intimate anatomic relationship with the fascia transversalis, a fact that is important during laparoscopic hernia repair. The obturator artery originating from the inferior epigastric or external iliac vessel has been observed in approximately 30% of the patients. Damage to this artery during inguinal hernia repair may cause serious hemorrhage into the pre-peritoneal space. Finally, the laparoscopic pediatric surgeon must become familiar with the pre-peritoneal space anatomy and its vascular contents, as vascular injury during laparoscopic hernia repair is easy and usually leads to severe hematoma formation [9–11].

The vas deferens ascends from the side wall of the pelvis, curving upward around the obliterated umbilical artery, below the level of the transverse vesical fold as it passes from medial to lateral across the external iliac vessels. Then, it disappears from view as it meets with the testicular vessels immediately lateral to the base of the epigastric artery. The round ligament alone enters the deep inguinal ring. The artery to the vas or round ligament accompanies each structure, with several minor veins, often visible through the thin peritoneal covering. While the vas forms just a ridge beneath the peritoneum, the round ligament tends to lie deeper at an intra-peritoneal level. The testicular vessels usually not seen through the peritoneum disappear from laparoscopic view as they meet with the vas on its lateral aspect, and they enter together the deep ring on its posteromedial edge (**Figure 3**) [12, 13].

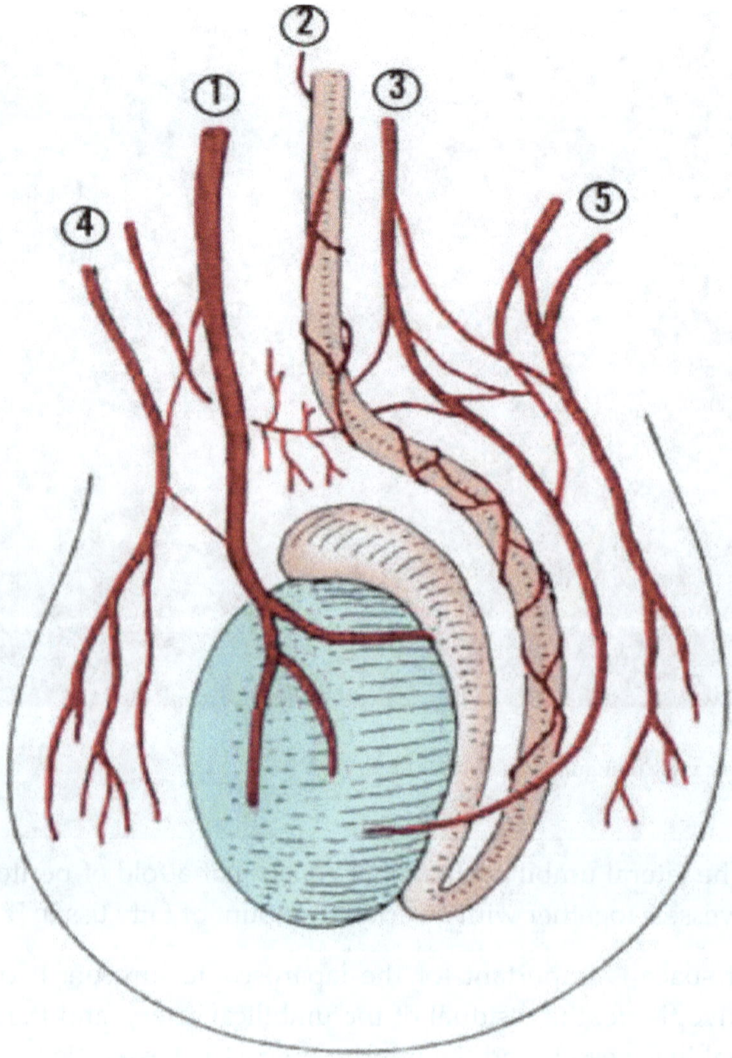

Figure 3. Arterial supply of testis and epididymis. (1) Testicular artery. (2) Deferential artery. (3) Cremasteric artery. (4) Posterior scrotal artery. (5) Anterior scrotal artery.

4. Clinical presentations

The incidence of congenital inguinal hernia in infants and children ranges from 1 to 5%. With 60% occurring on the right side, premature infants are at higher risk. The male-to-female ratio is estimated to be 6:1. Inguinal bulge with straining or crying is the most common presentation described by the parents or observed during physical examination. Classically, the diagnosis is established by history taking and clinical examination.

4.1. History taking

The parents usually described a visible, intermittent swelling or bulge in the inguino-scrotal region in boys or inguino-labial region in girls appears with crying or straining, and usually it disappeared during night while the baby is sleeping. The swelling is usually not associated with pain or discomfort. But, sometimes, the parents may perceive the bulge as being painful, which is not true as it in facts causes no discomfort to the baby except if complicated. The presence of a painful bulge should alert the pediatric surgeon to the presence of an incarcerated inguinal hernia. Most pediatric surgeons diagnose and operate child with congenital inguinal hernia depending on a classic history description by parents or a referring physician, others still insist on seeing the hernia themselves and may return the child for a second examination after 2–3 weeks [14, 15].

4.2. Clinical examination

Local examination is essential to confirm the diagnosis of congenital inguinal hernia, and it usually starts with inspection of the inguinoscrotal region to see the inguinal bulge, and if it is not obvious by inspection, holding baby legs and arms gently against the examination table will result in crying with increased intra-abdominal pressure and appearance of the inguinal bulge. For older children, blowing bubbles, or having them blow up balloons or examination gloves will increase intra-abdominal pressure and inguinal bulge may appear. The "silk purse" or "silk glove" sign is an important local physical sign. It elicited by gently rolling the cord structures across the pubic tubercle. The feeling of a sac moving on itself is considered positive finding. Published reports showed a wide variation in diagnostic accuracy of the silk purse sign, with a sensitivity of 91% and specificity of 97.3%. Currently, the most reasonable approach is to consider the silk purse sign as supporting but not conclusive evidence to confirm the diagnosis. It is essential to palpate both testicles, to rule out an undescended or retractile testicle, which can be associated with an inguinal hernia. In girls, feeling the ovary in the hernia sac is not uncommon and may be mistaken for a lymph node [16, 17].

Direct hernias through the floor of the inguinal canal due to muscular weakness are extremely rare in children. It classically presents medial to the inferior epigastric vessels. Due to the rarity of the direct hernia in children and the fact that direct hernia in children will never reach scrotum, the pediatric surgeon can easily diagnose that an inguinal hernia in a child is of the indirect type. Femoral hernia in children can be very difficult to differentiate from an indirect inguinal hernia. It is located below the inguinal canal, through the femoral canal. The only possible differentiation is during the operative repair as the anatomy and relationship to the inguinal ligament are clearly visualized. The clinical presentations of femoral hernias in children are essentially the same as indirect inguinal hernias. In a case of incarcerated inguinal hernia, there will be tender firm mass in the inguinal region or scrotum, and the child may be fussy, unwilling to feed, and crying inconsolably. The overlying skin may be edematous, erythematous, and discolored. On the other hand, the hernia may be huge enough to be easily diagnosed as seen in (**Figure 4**) [18, 19].

The differentiation between congenital inguinal hernia and hydrocele in young children is not always straightforward. The well-known trans-illumination test is essential for distinguishing between the presence of a sac filled with fluid in the scrotum and the presence of bowel in the scrotal sac. However, in cases of incarcerated inguinal hernia, trans-illumination test may be equivocal, as distended viscera with fluid in the scrotum of a young infant will trans-illuminate. Finally, the use of inguinal ultrasound may be needed to differentiate between PPV

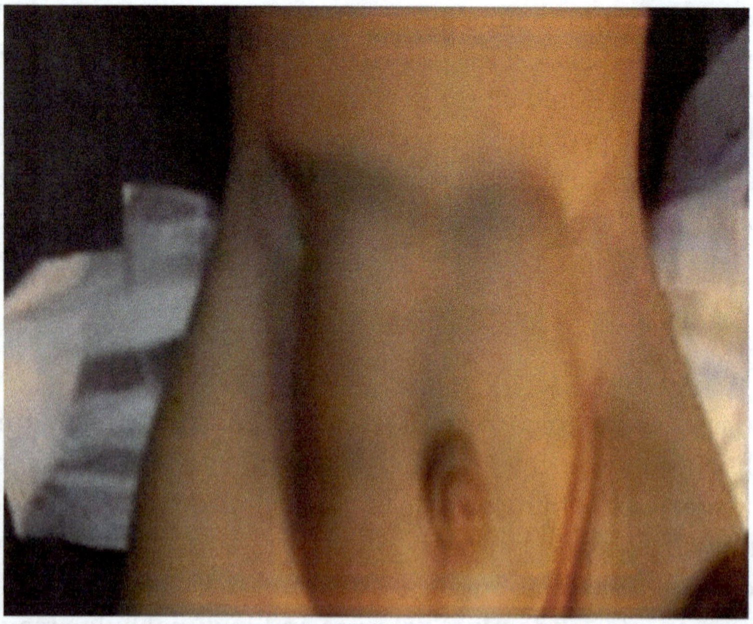

Figure 4. Bilateral huge congenital inguinal hernia.

and inguinal hernia. It can differentiate between hydrocele, incarcerated hernia, and testicular torsion. In most cases, inguinal ultrasound was used to increase the diagnostic accuracy of inguinal hernia in children from 84% on physical examination alone to 97.9% and that hypoechoic structure in the inguinal canal measuring 4–6 mm was a PPV, and greater than 6 mm was a hernia [20, 21].

5. Treatment

Congenital inguinal hernia repair is one of the most common operations performed by pediatric surgeons, and consultations for inguinal hernia are among the most frequent reasons for pediatric surgical referral. In infants and young children, the risk of incarceration of the unrepaired inguinal hernia is as high as 31% (usually in the first few months of life), posing a significant risk to the bowel and testicle. Accordingly, surgical repair of a symptomatic inguinal hernia is recommended soon after diagnosis. Parents are instructed to do gentle pressure on the inguinal bulge to prevent incarceration of the contents until the elective surgery is performed. On the other hand, in neonates, the surgical treatment of hydrocele is delayed for 12–18 months because in such case the PPV opening is very small and may have already closed or be in the process of closing. If the hydrocele persists after this observation period, operative repair is usually indicated [22, 23].

5.1. Open repair

Open hernia repair in children is usually an outpatient procedure. Surgery should be postponed in the presence of upper respiratory tract, otitis media, or significant napkin dermatitis. The basic principle of the repair includes high ligation and excision of the hernia sac with or without narrowing of the internal inguinal ring. The classical open herniotomy is performed as follows: a lower abdominal skin crease incision is made, and then both Scarp's fascia and the external oblique are opened. The cremasteric fibers are bluntly dissected until the sac can be seen. The sac is then gently separated from the cord structures, dissected to the level of the internal inguinal ring, ligated, and divided at this level. In patients with a wide internal ring, narrowing of the internal ring can be added with repair of the inguinal floor. The distal sac is either split anteriorly or excised. The excision versus splitting of the distal hernia sac continues to be controversial issue; however, it was founded that there is no difference in recurrence or hydrocele formation, suggesting that simply opening the anterior wall is sufficient in children and neonates. On the other hand, complete excision of the distal sac may increase the risk of injury to the cord structures and the testis and may cause hematoma. It is important to ensure that the testis is in the scrotum at the end of the operation to avoid iatrogenic cryptorchidism. If undescended testis is discovered during herniotomy, it must be fixed in the scrotum, even if the infant is younger than 12 months old. This avoids the possible risk of incarceration, strangulation, and testicular infarction [24, 25, 26].

Contralateral exploration for PPV in children with unilateral hernia is still debatable. Contralateral PPV was present in about 30–40% of children presenting with unilateral hernia. The introduction of the telescope through the sac of the hernia to visualize the contralateral PPV is used to avoid contralateral exploration, and recently, during laparoscopic hernia repair, contralateral PPV is easily diagnosed [27, 28].

5.2. Laparoscopic repair

Laparoscopic hernia repair recently challenged the conventional open herniotomy, with reported results that comparable to open herniotomy with nearly similar recurrence rate and superior cosmetic results. The basic principle for laparoscopic inguinal hernia repair (LIHR) in children is a high ligation of the hernia sac from inside either in continuity using complete purse string suture or after complete dissection of the peritoneum around internal inguinal ring (IIR) to separate the distal hernia sac (like open herniotomy). The most wildly used techniques for laparoscopic hernia repair are as follows: (1) Insertion of a complete purse-string suture around the internal inguinal ring with intra-corporeal knotting using either two laparoscopic instruments, or recently using only single laparoscopic instrument technique. (2) Complete separation of the peritoneum around the IIR to disconnect the distal hernia sac (dissection technique). (3) Percutaneous extra-corporeal ligation of the IIR under laparoscopic guidance [29, 30].

5.2.1. *Intra-corporeal techniques*

The first laparoscopic technique described for repair of inguinal hernia in children use three ports for the repair, two intra-peritoneal working instruments to make a complete purse string suture around the opened IIR, and a camera port. The technique started with insertion of the umbilical camera port by the open Hasson's technique. Then pneumoperitoneum was established to a pressure of 8–12 mm Hg according to age. Laparoscopic exploration of the pelvis and both internal inguinal rings were done. Then two 3-mm ports for the working instruments (two laparoscopic needle holders) were inserted at the lateral borders of the rectus muscles at the level of the umbilicus. Non-absorbable 3-0 Prolene suture was used to make a complete purse suture around the opened internal inguinal ring, with intra-corporeal knot tying. The sutures include only the peritoneum with no underlying tissues. The contralateral IIR was closed if its diameter is more than 2 mm. This technique is not cosmetically superior in children, when compared to open herniotomy, which was performed through a small lower abdominal crease incision. Recently, in 2015, Helal modified this traditional laparoscopic hernia repair technique and introduced a novel technique for laparoscopic hernia repair using only single laparoscopic instrument (laparoscopic needle holder). The principle of his repair is the closure of the IIR with complete purse string suture using single laparoscopic needle holder instrument, with intra-corporeal knotting using single instrument tie. He reported that his novel technique is feasible, simple, secure, and more cosmetic. It permits extension of benefits of minimal access surgery. Also, he reported that it reduces operative time especially in bilateral cases and allows for quick return to normal activity of children (**Figure 5**) [18, 31, 32].

5.2.2. *Percutaneous extra-corporeal technique*

This technique entails percutaneous insertion of complete purse string suture using non-absorbable sutures around the IIR under laparoscopic guidance and the suture was tightened

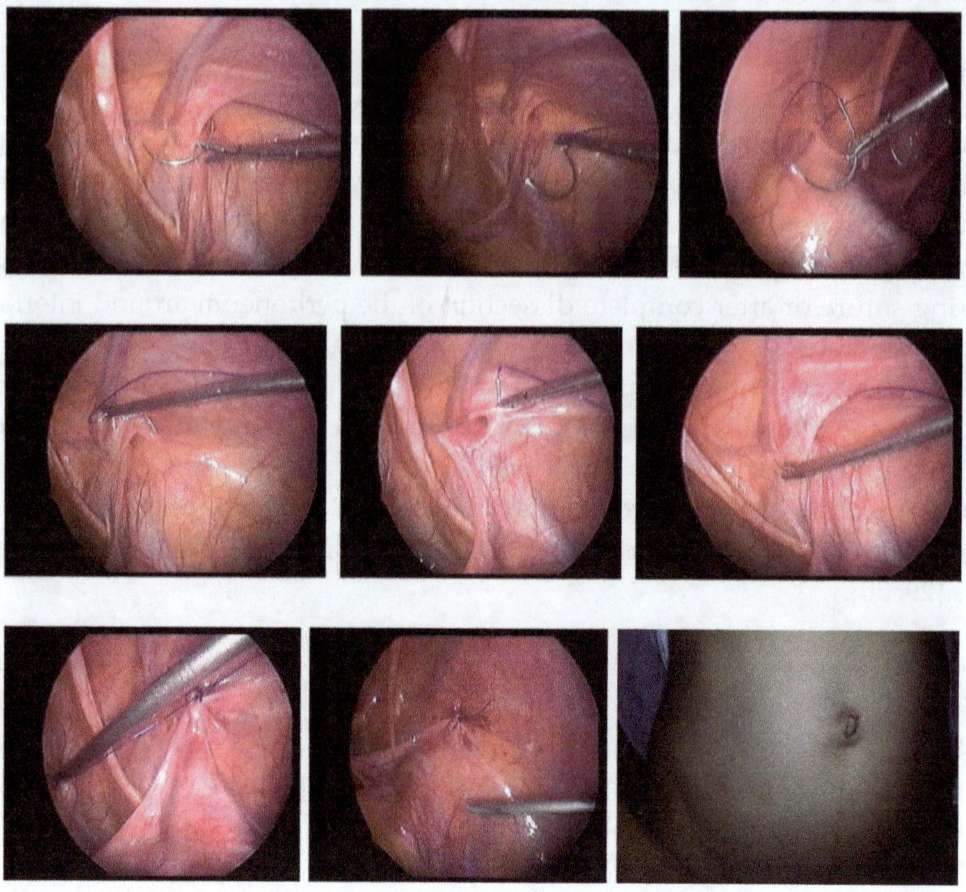

Figure 5. Steps of laparoscopic single instrument repair of inguinal hernia (Helal technique).

extra-corporeally and burred subcutaneously. The suture crosses over the spermatic duct or the gonadal vessels to avoid their injury. In girls, the round ligaments were not dissected, and it is included with the closure of the hernia sac. It is safe, effective, and reliable technique, with short operative time. It is suitable for laparoscopic surgeons that don't have a good experience in intra-corporeal laparoscopic suturing and tying techniques. However, the main concerns about this technique are the presence of the suture subcutaneously which may cause stitch granuloma or sinus formation. Also, the inclusion of the abdominal wall muscles with the suture may cause later losing of the suture or the suture may cut through the muscle which may increase the risk of hernia recurrence. The subcutaneous endoscopic assisted ligation (SEAL) technique entails percutaneous insertion of complete purse string suture around the IIR without any intra-peritoneal laparoscopic instrument. The technique was described by Ozgediz et al., and its main principles include passing a curved needle threaded with a 2/0 non-absorbable suture through the anterior abdominal wall under direct vision to surround the IIR peri-peritonealy in a U-shaped manner. The tip of the needle is grasped in a needle driver, and the heel of the needle is backed through the subcutaneous tissue to come out through the original stab incision. The suture is then secured and ligated subcutaneously. The needle may jump over the vas and vessels, and a peritoneal gap may be left untouched. This skip area is the cause of recurrence of hernia. However, if the size of the defect is extraordinarily wide, an additional instrument to assist guidance of the needle or conversion to open herniotomy is necessary. The steps of the technique are showed in **Figure 6**. The SEAL technique is then modified by injecting saline in the pre-peritoneal space for hydro-dissection to separate the peritoneum over the vas and the vessels [33, 34].

5.2.3. *Single incision laparoscopic hernia repair*

Recently, single incision laparoscopic surgery is advancing significantly, and nowadays, many laparoscopic surgeons prefer to perform most laparoscopic operations through several tiny incisions rather than one large incision, to improve the cosmetic outcome. At the

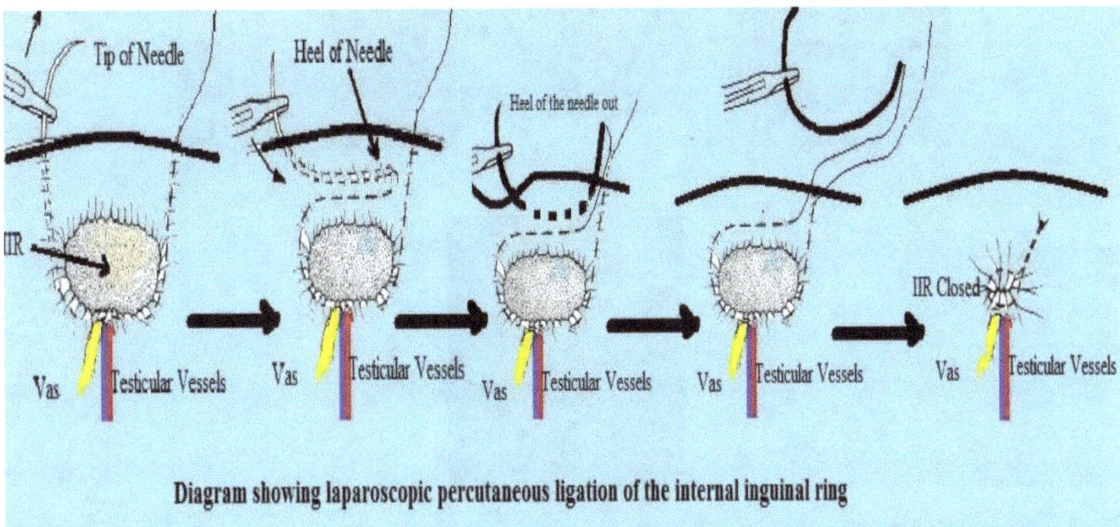

Figure 6. The steps of the subcutaneous endoscopic assisted ligation technique.

moment, single incision laparoscopic hernia repair (SILHR) has been well reported in the literature with many studies describing its feasibility and safety in children. SILHR is a newly developed technique for minimizing the post-operative pain, reducing the invasiveness of traditional laparoscopy, and reducing hospital stay with nearly scar less surgery. It is a new paradigm in minimally invasive surgery world. In our hospital, we perform laparoscopic inguinal hernia repair in children using the needlescopic assisted SILHR by using epidural needle gauge 18 to make complete purse string suture around the IIR, and we tied the suture extra-corporally using the self-sliding clinch knot (as shown in **Figure 7**) with an outstanding cosmetic results making great parent satisfaction. We think that there would be no reason to perform multiple incisions in laparoscopic hernia repair in children as SILHR is a safe and secure technique with excellent cosmetic results because it results in single umbilical wound which is already scar area in the body, the scar is hidden in the fold of the umbilicus, and the puncture wounds from the epidural needle are practically unnoticeable. Finally, SILHR in children is safe, perhaps even less technically demanded than open herniotomy [35–37].

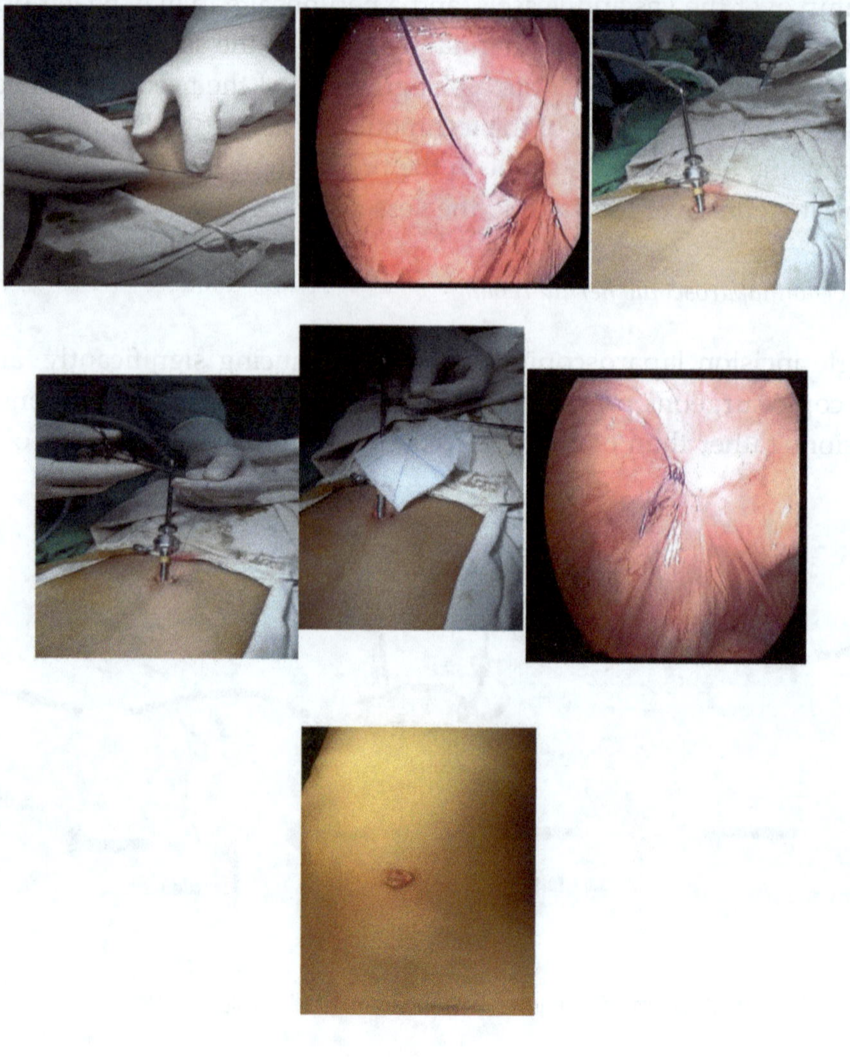

Figure 7. Single incision laparoscopic hernia repair in children with intra-corporeal knotting and finally the umbilical scar is practically unnoticeable.

6. Post-operative care

Most patients are discharged home on the same day after open or laparoscopic inguinal hernia repair. Small premature babies may need overnight observation and monitoring due to the risk of post-operative apnea. Post-operative follow-up after inguinal hernia repair requires only one clinic visit. Post-operative scrotal swelling and bruising for 1–2 weeks are very common, and they represent normal post-operative changes rather than a complication. Post-operative hydrocele (non-communicating) is not uncommon, and it usually reabsorbed spontaneously in 95% of the cases. Only major physical activity should be avoided after open or laparoscopic inguinal hernia repair in children for 1–3 weeks. Post-operatively, most children do well with acetaminophen alone, although the addition of non-steroidal anti-inflammatory drugs may be necessary for some children. The most common complications of herniotomy include injury to the vas deferens, iatrogenic cryptorchidism, and testicular atrophy. Iatrogenic cryptorchidism occurs in 0.6–2.9 %of patients. Injury to the vas deferens has been reported to occur in as many as 1.6% of patients. Testicular atrophy occurs in 1–2% and decreased testicular size in 2.7–13% of patients. Increased incidence of complications may present with inexperienced surgeons. Very rarely infertility may result from injury to both Fallopian tubes in girls subjected to bilateral herniotomy during childhood. Factors that may contribute to recurrence after congenital inguinal hernia repair include failure to ligate the sac high enough, tear in the sac or missing the posterior wall of the sac, leaving wide internal ring, and the presence of comorbid conditions (e.g., collagen disorders, severe malnutrition) [38].

7. Summary

Inguinal hernia in children can be a simple problem or a major catastrophe. True direct hernia is extremely rare in children. Recurrence of inguinal hernia in a child should be investigated for a general cause rather than a pure local reason. There is a difference between the hernia "sac" and the hernia "defect" which is actually a normal hiatus that allows passage of the cord structures or round ligament and should therefore not require repair *per se*. In fact, narrowing of a normal internal inguinal ring may cause entrapment of the cord structures. Instead, simple ligation and division of the hernia sac should allow the hiatus to close down to a normal functional size.

The open herniotomy through a lower skin crease incision is still the gold standard for inguinal hernia repair in children. It is very safe, well-tolerated, with low recurrence rate, leaving early invisible scar. On the other hand, at the moment the great advancement in laparoscopic techniques for inguinal hernia repair challenged this traditional operation, because of short operative time after learning curve, the untouched cord structure with increased fertility later on also allows it to rule out a contralateral PPV, finally the outstanding cosmetic results especially in female children, with great parent's satisfaction. I hope to someday be proven that laparoscopic hernia repair in children will be a gold standard like laparoscopic cholecystectomy.

Incarcerated inguinal hernia is defined as obstruction to the blood supply of the hernia contents, and if not corrected within reasonable time (from 4 to 6 hours), gangrene will occur. Therefore, repair of inguinal hernia in children should be undertaken as soon as possible after diagnosis.

In case of incarcerated hernia if a trial of manual reduction is to be performed, the following precautions must be considered, the use of sedation is mandatory even anesthetic consultation may be needed in very irritable child, gradually increasing pressure for 2–3 min with short periods of rest for 1 min in between. Don't forget that during reduction of the incarcerated hernia, two edematous surfaces are being rubbed together (similar to that of two pickles). Tense hydrocele may be confused with an incarcerated hernia, and in such situation, urgent surgical exploration is mandatory without losing time in doing diagnostic investigations.

Laparoscopic hernia repair needs a learning curve especially in doing intra-corporeal suturing and knot tying which is the basic step in conventional laparoscopic approach; however, extra-corporeal self-sliding knot becomes a suitable solution for replacing traditional intra-corporeal suturing and knotting during laparoscopic hernia repair. It is very important for junior pediatric surgeons not to be in hurry to perform laparoscopic repair of inguinal hernia without mastering the open herniotomy and dealing with its different complications. Laparoscopic complete purse string suture around the internal inguinal ring is very sufficient for repair of inguinal hernia in children. However, laparoscopic dissection of the hernia sac is mandatory in recurrent cases and in the presence of very wide internal ring which needs repair of the muscular defect. Injection of saline will elevate the peritoneum over the vas and vessels and make a plane for the needle to pass safely. The needle sign is very important during laparoscopic repair of inguinal hernia in which the needle and the thread are clearly seen under the peritoneum. Inclusion of tissue with the suture around internal inguinal ring will cause later losing of the suture with increased recurrence rate.

Home message

- Congenital inguinal hernia is a common surgical problem in infants and children.
- More than 98% of inguinal hernias in children are indirect hernias.
- Incarcerated hernia if not managed within a reasonable time will lead to bowel necrosis and testicular atrophy.
- History is very important aspect in diagnosis of inguinal hernia in children.
- Hernias in children are usually painless, except if complicated.

Author details

Ahmed Abdelghaffar Helal

Address all correspondence to: helalhmada@yahoo.com

Department of Pediatric Surgery, Faculty of Medicine, Al-Azhar University, Cairo, Egypt

References

[1] Becmeur F, Philippe P, Lemandat SA, et al. A continuous series of 96 laparoscopic inguinal hernia repairs in children by a new technique. Surgical Endoscopy. 2004;**18**:1738-1741

[2] Bharathi RS, Arora M, Baskaran V. How we "SEAL" internal ring in pediatric inguinal hernias. Surgical Laparoscopy Endoscopy & Percutaneous Techniques. 2008;**18**:192-194

[3] Bharathi RS, Arora M, Baskaran V. Minimal access surgery of pediatric inguinal hernias. A review. Surgical Endoscopy. 2008;**22**:1751-1762

[4] Canes D, et al. Transumbilical single-port surgery: Evolution and current status. European Urology. 2008;**54**:1020-1029

[5] Chang YT, Wang JY, Lee JY. A simple single-port laparoscopic assisted technique for completely enclosing inguinal hernia in children. The American Journal of Surgery. 2009;**198**:13-16

[6] Chang YT. Technical refinements in single-port laparoscopic surgery of inguinal hernia in infants and children. Diagnostic and Therapeutic Endoscopy. 2010;1-6

[7] Chen K, Xiang G, Wang H, Xiao F. Towards a near-zero recurrence rate in laparoscopic inguinal hernia repair for pediatric patients. Journal of Laparoendoscopic & Advanced Surgical Techniques. Part A. 2011;16

[8] Chinnaswamy P, Malladi V, Jani KV, et al. Laparoscopic inguinal hernia repair in children. Journal of Second Language Studies. 2005;**9**:393-398

[9] Chow A, Purkayastha S, Paraskeva P. Appendicectomy and cholecystectomy using single-incision laparoscopic surgery (SILS): The first UK experience. Surgical Innovation. 2009;**16**:211-217.

[10] de Armas IA, Garcia I, Pimpalwar A. Laparoscopic single port surgery in children using Triport: Our early experience. Pediatric Surgery International. 2011;**27**:985-989

[11] Dorsey JH, Sharp HT, Chovan JD, et al. Laparoscopic knot strength: A comparison with conventional knots. Obstetrics & Gynecology. 1995;**86**:536-540

[12] Ein SH, Njere I, Ein A. Six thousand three hundred sixty-one pediatric inguinal hernias. A 35-year review. Journal of Pediatric Surgery. 2006;**41**:980-986

[13] El-Gohary MA. Laparoscopic ligation of inguinal of inguinal hernia in girls. Pediatric Endosurgery & Innovative Techniques. 1997;**1**:185-187

[14] Endo M, Watanabe T, Nakano M, et al. Laparoscopic completely extraperitoneal repair of inguinal hernia in children. A single-institute experience with 1257 repairs compared with cut-down herniorrhaphy. Surgical Endoscopy. 2009;**23**:1706-1712

[15] Erez I, Rathause V, Vacian I, et al. Preoperative ultrasound and intraoperative findings of inguinal hernia in children: A prospective study of 642 children. Journal of Pediatric Surgery. 2002;**37**:865-868

[16] George EK, Qudesluys MAM, Madern GC, et al. Inguinal hernia containing the uterus, fallopian tube and ovary in premature female infants. Journal of Paediatric. 2000;**136**:696-703

[17] Giseke S, Glass M, Priyanka TP, et al. True laparoscopic herniotomy in children evaluation of long-term outcome. Journal of Laparoendoscopic & Advanced Surgical Techniques Part A. 2010;**20**:191-194

[18] Helal AA. Laparoscopic single instrument closure of inguinal hernia in female children: A novel technique. Journal of Pediatric Surgery. 2015;**50**(9):1613-1616

[19] Koivusalo AI, Korpela R, Wirtavuori K, et al. A single-blinded, randomized comparison of laparoscopic versus open hernia repair in children. Pediatrics. 2009;**123**:332-337

[20] Kumar A, Ramakrishnan TS. Single port laparoscopic repair of pediatric inguinal hernias: Our experience at a secondary care centre. Journal of Minimal Access Surgery. 2013;**9**:7-12

[21] Lee DY, Baik YH, Kwak BS, et al. A purse-string suture at the level of internal inguinal ring, taking only the peritoneum leaving the distal sac: Is it enough for inguinal hernia in pediatric patients? Hernia. 2015;1348-1347

[22] Lukong CS. Surgical techniques of laparoscopic inguinal hernia repair in childhood: Critical appraisal. Journal of Surgical Technique and Case Report. 2012;**4**:1-5

[23] Luo CC, Chao HC. Prevention of unnecessary contralateral exploration using the silk glove sign (SGS) in pediatric patients with unilateral inguinal hernia. European Journal of Pediatrics. 2007;**166**:667-669

[24] Mcclain L, Streck C, Leshar A. Laparoscopic needle assisted inguinal hernia repair in 495 children. Surgical Endoscopy. 2014;**29**:781-786

[25] Cam C, Celik C, Sancak A, et al. Inguinal herniorrhaphy in childhood may result intubal damage and future infertility. Archives of Gynecology and Obstetrics. 2009;**279**:175-176

[26] Schier F. Laparoscopic inguinal hernia repair—a prospective personal series of 542 children. Journal of Pediatric Surgery. 2006;**41**:1081-1084

[27] Parelkar SV, Oak S, Gupta R, et al. Laparoscopicinguinal hernia repair in the pediatric age group; Experience with 437 children. Journal of Pediatric Surgery. 2010;**45**:789-792

[28] Patkowski D, Czernik J, Chrzan R. Percutaneous internal ring suturing: A simple minimally invasive technique for inguinal hernia repair in children. Journal of Laparoendoscopic & Advanced Surgical Techniques Part A. 2006;**16**:513-517

[29] Ponsky TA, Diluciano J, Chwals W, et al. Early experience with single-port laparoscopic surgery in children. Journal of Laparoendoscopic & Advanced Surgical Techniques Part A. 2009;**19**:551-553

[30] Rothenberg SS, Shipman K, Yoder S. Experience with modified single-port laparoscopic procedures in children. Journal of Laparoendoscopic & Advanced Surgical Techniques Part A. 2009;**19**:695-698

[31] SarangaBharathi R, Arora M, Baskaran V. Pediatric inguinal hernia: Laparoscopic versus open surgery. Journal of Second Language Studies. 2008;**12**:277-281

[32] Schier F. Laparoscopic herniorrhaphy in girls. Journal of Pediatric Surgery. 1998;**33**:1495-1497

[33] Ozgediz D, Roayaie K, Lee H, et al. Subcutaneous endoscopically assisted ligation (SEAL) of the internal ring for repair of inguinal hernias in children. Report of a new technique and early results. Surgical Endoscopy. 2007;**21**:1327-1331

[34] Turial S, Enders J, Krause K, Schier F. Laparoscopic inguinal herniorrhaphy in babies weighing 5 kg or less. Surgical Endoscopy. 2011;**25**:72-78

[35] Uchida H, Kawashima H, Goto C. Inguinal hernia repair in children using single-incision laparoscopic-assisted percutaneous extraperitoneal closure. Journal of Pediatric Surgery. 2010;**45**:2386-2389

[36] Yang C, Zhang H, Pu J, et al. Laparoscopic vs open herniorrhaphy in the management of pediatric inguinal hernia: A systemic review and meta-analysis. Journal of Pediatric Surgery. 2011;**46**:1824-1834

[37] Helal AA. Single incision laparoscopic closure of inguinal hernia in female children: a simplified technique. Mini-invasive Surg 2017 May 23.

[38] Zallen G, Glick PL. Laparoscopic inversion and ligation inguinal hernia repair in girls. Journal of Laparoendoscopic & Advanced Surgical Techniques. 2007;**17**:143-145

5

Imaging of Hernias

Mohamed Abdelmohsen Bedewi and
Mohamed El-sharkawy

Abstract

Abdominal wall hernias are usually suggested by the patient's history and confirmed by physical examination; however, the history may be not typical, especially in patients with abdominal pain, distention, and overweight patients or in patients with small hernias located in unusual sites. Although most abdominal hernias are asymptomatic, the fear of developing complications like irreducibility, incarceration, and strangulation may necessitate prophylactic surgical repair; thus, early and accurate diagnosis is important. Before 20 years, herniorrhaphy was considered for imaging of hernias; however, in recent years, computed tomography (CT) (especially multidetector CT (MDCT)), together with ultrasound represented the mainstay of the diagnosis of abdominopelvic wall hernias by imaging, and magnetic resonance imaging (MRI) could be used as a diagnostic aid in a minority of the cases. Each imaging modality has its own privilege. The main advantage of ultrasound is the dynamic ability for assessment, while the main advantage of computed tomography is the multiplanar reformatting, allowing identification and accurate diagnosis of the hernia type, its content, and also the associated complications. Radiologists should be familiar with common sites of hernias and their detailed normal anatomy in order to reach the diagnosis easily.

Keywords: hernia, ultrasound, imaging, abdominal wall, strangulation

1. Introduction

Abdominal wall hernias are mostly diagnosed by typical history and clinical examination; however, in some cases, the history is not typical, especially in patients with marked abdominal distention, and overweight patients or in cases of occult hernias. Although most abdominal hernias are asymptomatic, the fear of developing complications like irreducibility, incarceration, and strangulation may necessitate prophylactic surgical repair; thus, early and accurate diagnosis is important. Before 20 years, herniorrhaphy was considered for imaging of hernias; however, in recent years, computed tomography (CT) (especially multidetector CT (MDCT)), together with ultrasound represented the mainstay of the diagnosis of abdominopelvic wall hernias by imaging, and magnetic resonance imaging (MRI) could be used as a diagnostic aid in a minority of cases. Each imaging modality has its own privilege. The main advantage of ultrasound is the dynamic ability for assessment, while the main advantage of computed tomography is the multiplanar reformatting [1, 2, 3], allowing identification and accurate diagnosis of the hernia type, its content, and also the associated complications. MDCT technology also has the benefit of fast acquisition times, which reduces motion artifact, such as those related to bowel peristalsis and respiration. MDCT also has the postprocessing ability to manipulate the data to create three-dimensional surgical planning models [4]. Radiologists should be familiar with common sites of hernias and their detailed normal anatomy in order to reach the diagnosis easily [5] (**Figures 1, 2**).

The absence of a reducible mass or a palpable defect does not rule out the presence of hernia. The term "hidden hernia" describes the situation when physical examination fails to demonstrate a palpable defect or a reducible mass, but the hernia sac is identified on surgical exploration [6]. The role for diagnostic imaging is to support clinical suspicion. Another important issue is to distinguish other lesions mimicking hernias, like desmoid tumors in the abdominal wall, seromas, abscesses, and hematomas. In inguinal region, abscesses, lipomas, and encysted hydrocele of the spermatic cord represent the most common lesions which could be put in the differential diagnosis of masses seen in the common sites of inguinal region hernias. In the next few pages, we will discuss our experience in imaging of the common hernias which we confront in practice.

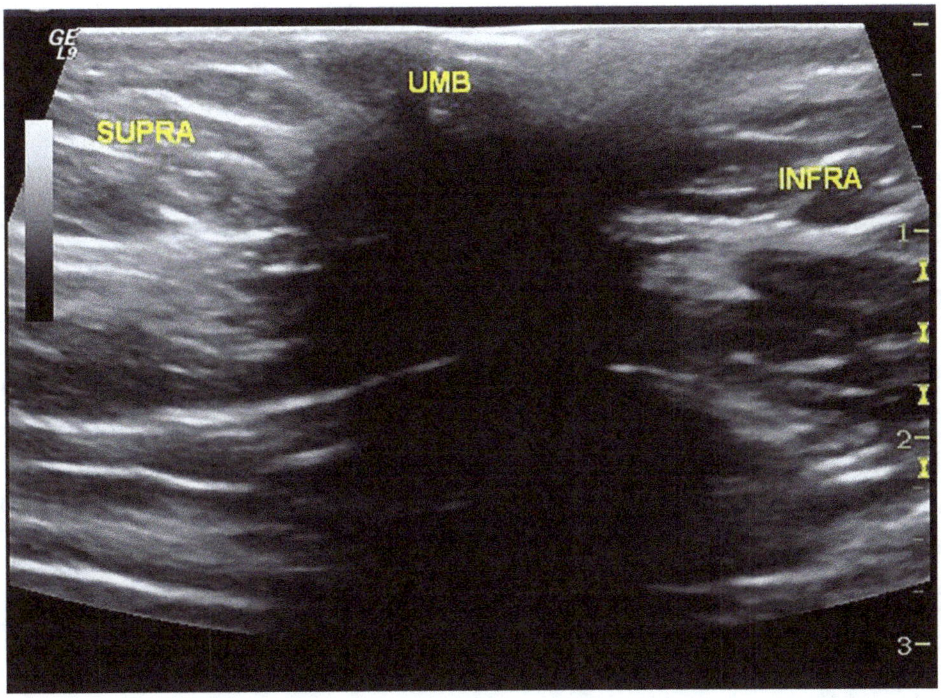

Figure 1. Normal appearance of the umbilicus by ultrasound, short axis.

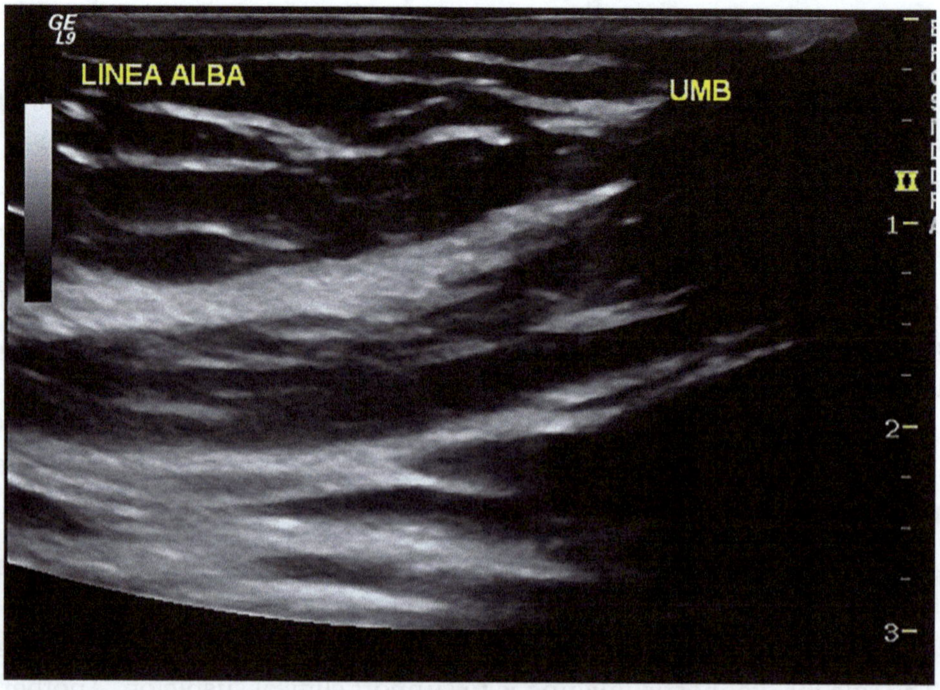

Figure 2. Normal appearance of the linea alba by ultrasound, long axis.

2. Inguinal hernia

Patients are usually diagnosed clinically, and most of the cases are operated without referral for imaging. There are two common types, direct and indirect; both are related to the inguinal ligament. By ultrasound, the inguinal ligament is seen as a dense echogenic line, and followed inferomedially, till the pubic region. The differentiation between direct and indirect inguinal hernias is by the relation of the hernia sac to the inferior epigastric artery where the more common indirect inguinal hernia lies lateral to it. The sac of the less common direct inguinal hernia lies medial to the inferior epigastric artery. The appearance of hernia sac is variable, and the defect of the hernia sac ranges from 0.2 to more than 3 cm and reaching 4 cm in some cases. The advantage of ultrasound over computed tomography lies mainly in the ability to perform a dynamic scan. A linear transducer (10–15 MHZ) is used to scan the inguinal region. If the sac is clear from the beginning of the scan, provocative tests could be excluded; otherwise, the simple use of Valsalva maneuver is recommended as a first-line dynamic maneuver, and the size of the defect is measured before and after the maneuver. The second provocative test is simple standing for 30 s, again the size of the defect is measured before and after standing (**Figure 3 (A)**, **(B)**), and the third test is to let the patient walk steadily for 2 min and then examine the patient in the standing position before lying supine (**Figure 4 (A)**, **(B)**, and **(C)**) (**Table 1**). The relatively echogenic edge of the sac is easily identified, and the content is usually fat, or omentum, less commonly bowel (**Figure 5**), or a mix of all these. The relation to spermatic cord has to be determined. Irreducibility has to be reported if present. It is always recommended to examine the asymptomatic side (**Figure 6**). The examination should extend to include the scrotal sac in male patients, to assess the extension of the sac, and to detect associated hydrocele. Color Doppler is occasionally used to see the vascularity and hence to

(a)
(b)

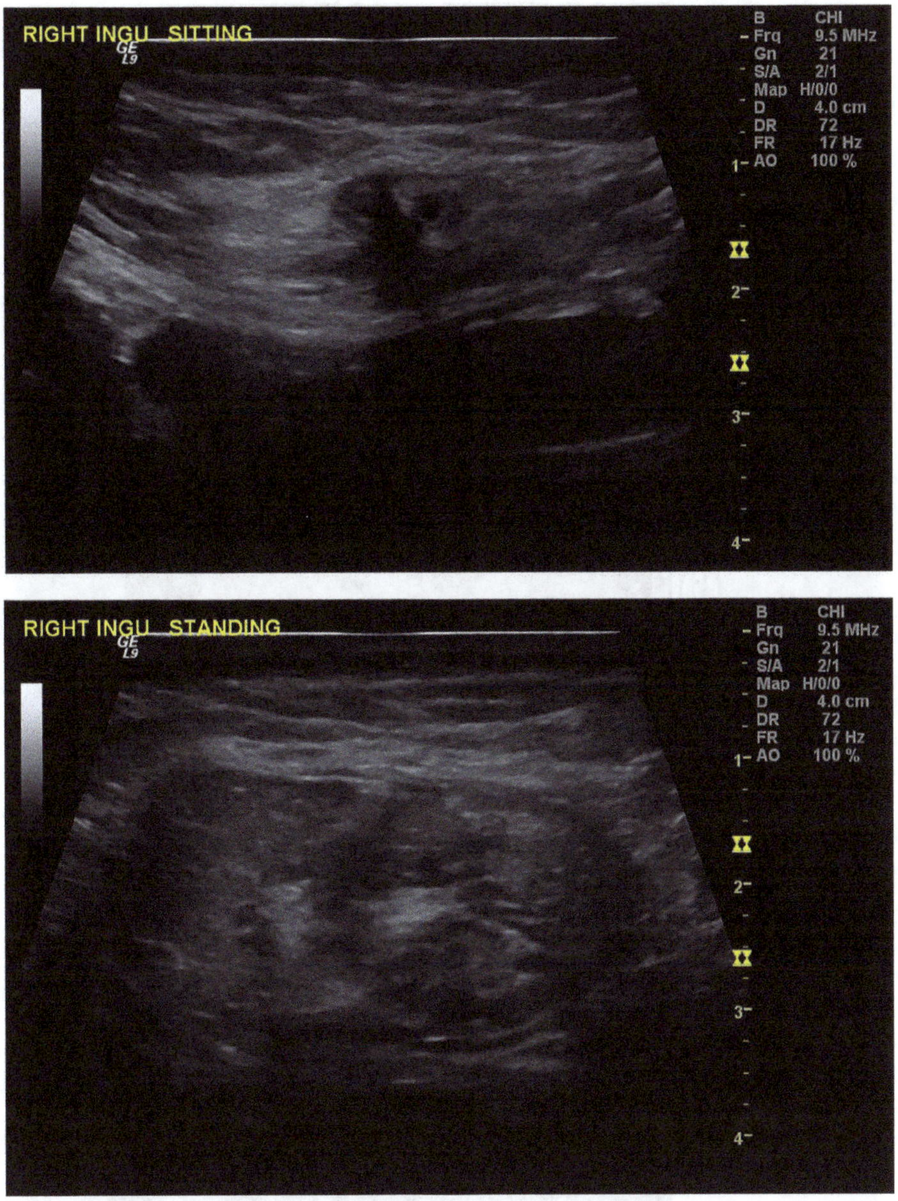

Figure 3. (A) Ultrasound right indirect inguinal hernia, sitting position. (B) Ultrasound right-sided indirect inguinal hernia standing.

indicate viability of the contents inside the sac. Care must be taken not to press too much with the transducer, because this may reduce small hernias (**Table 2**).

On computed tomography, the deep inguinal ring, is lateral to the inferior epigastric artery. The indirect inguinal hernia passes from lateral to medial, along the canal, and the neck is lateral and above the inferior epigastric vessels. The direct inguinal hernia enters the canal medial to the deep inferior epigastric artery, through Hesselbach's triangle, superior to inguinal ligament. The inferior epigastric and femoral vessels, are of key importance when diagnosing inguinal hernias as mentioned before in contrast to enhanced CT discriminating between direct and indirect hernias[4].

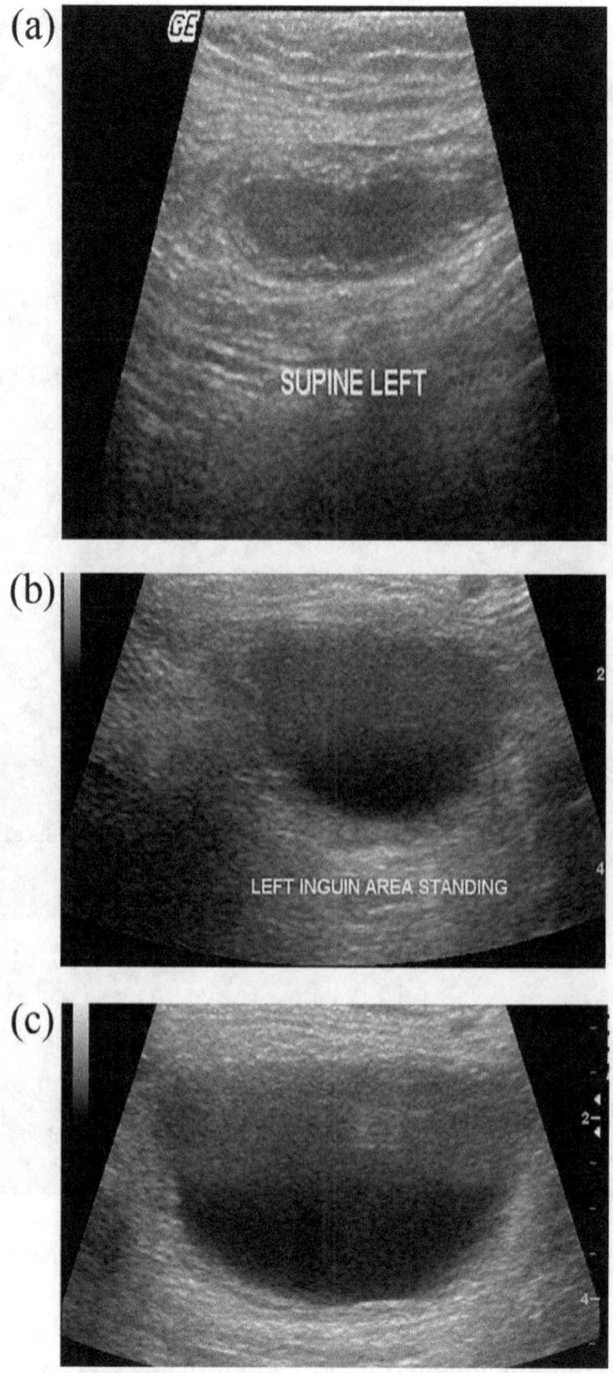

Figure 4. (A), (B), (C) inguinal hernia with provocative tests.

Dynamic maneuvers
1- Valsalva maneuver
2- Standing and supine position
3- Provocative walking

Table 1. Dynamic maneuvers used for ultrasound of the inguinal hernia.

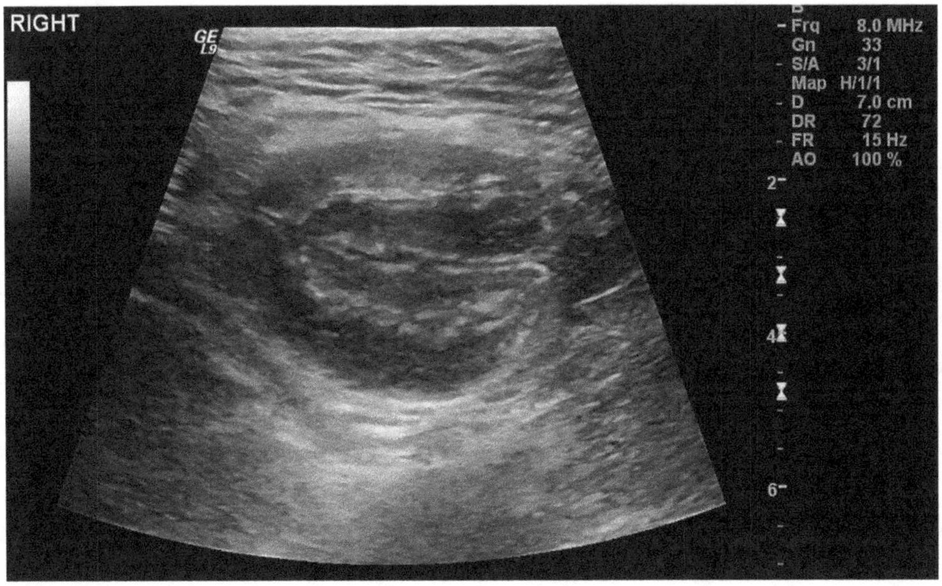

Figure 5. Right inguinal hernia with bowel content.

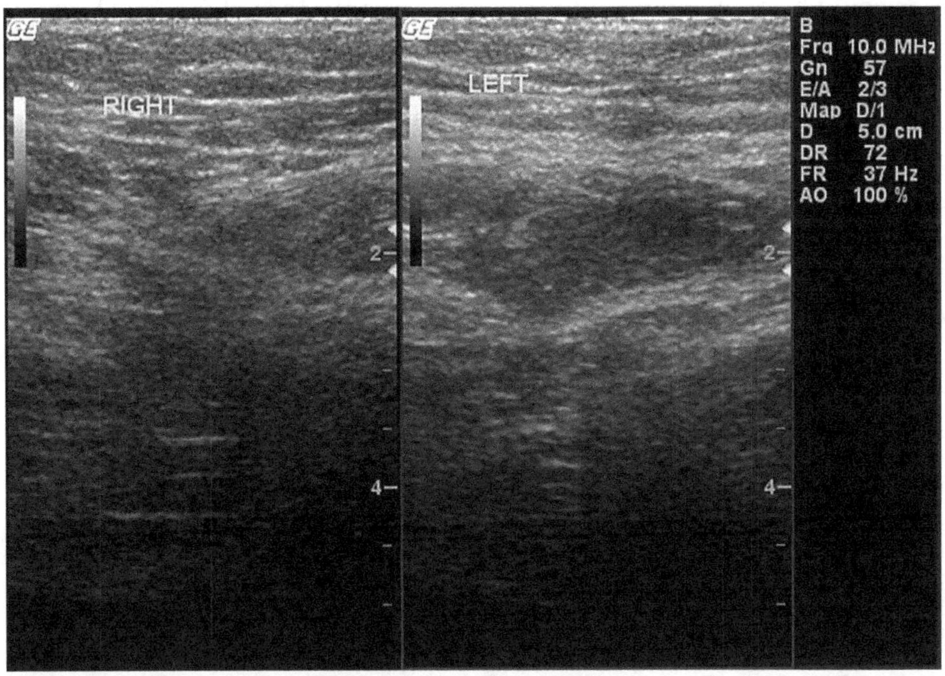

Figure 6. Comparison of the normal right inguinal hernia, to the left side of the inguinal canal with indirect inguinal hernia.

Transducer: linear, 10–15 MHZ

- Check type, and relation to the inferior epigastric vessels (direct, indirect)
- Size of the defect
- Hernia sac content
- Compare both sides

Table 2. Checklist of ultrasound exam inguinal hernias.

3. Umbilical hernia

Acquired umbilical hernia is usually associated with multiparty and increased body mass index. Commonly, the patient is referred to ultrasound if the hernia is not obvious clinically, due to its dynamic and real-time capabilities, and ability to compare both sides of the abdominal wall. It is important for the radiologist to assess the hernia orifice and size of the defect (**Figure 7**). In small-sized hernias, contents of the hernia sac are usually only omental fat (which appears slightly hyperechoic); however, intestinal loops may be present in larger size umbilical hernias, and it could be easily identified by the appearance of dirty shadowing of gas and peristaltic movement (**Figure 8**). Color and power Doppler could be used to assess its viability. The use of Valsalva maneuver has been described for both ultrasound and computed tomography [7], and in our center, this is done in the supine position. Operator dependence and long learning curve are drawbacks for ultrasound scanning. Differentiation between true hernia and other masses like desmoid tumors, or collections whether inflammatory like abscesses or noninflammatory like seromas located in the paraumbilical region, is detected by both ultrasound and computed tomography.

Small hernias could be assessed by a linear transducer 10–15 MHZ, while larger size umbilical hernias with large-sized defect should be assessed by a curvilinear transducer 7–15 MHZ. The diagnostic yield of the ultrasound decreases with large-sized hernias; hence, it is recommended in this case to refer to multidetector computed tomography, where sagittal and axial reconstruction could add some information in addition to axial sections. The presence of the surgeon or the referring physician at the time of scanning is suggested to facilitate diagnosis.

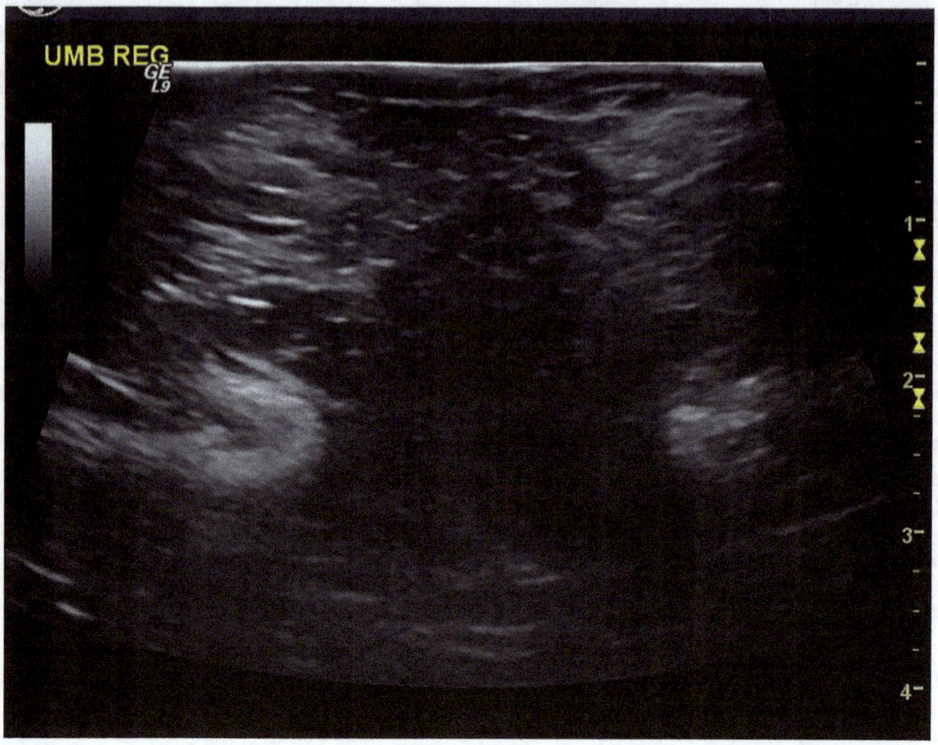

Figure 7. Clear defect of hernia orifice, umbilical hernia.

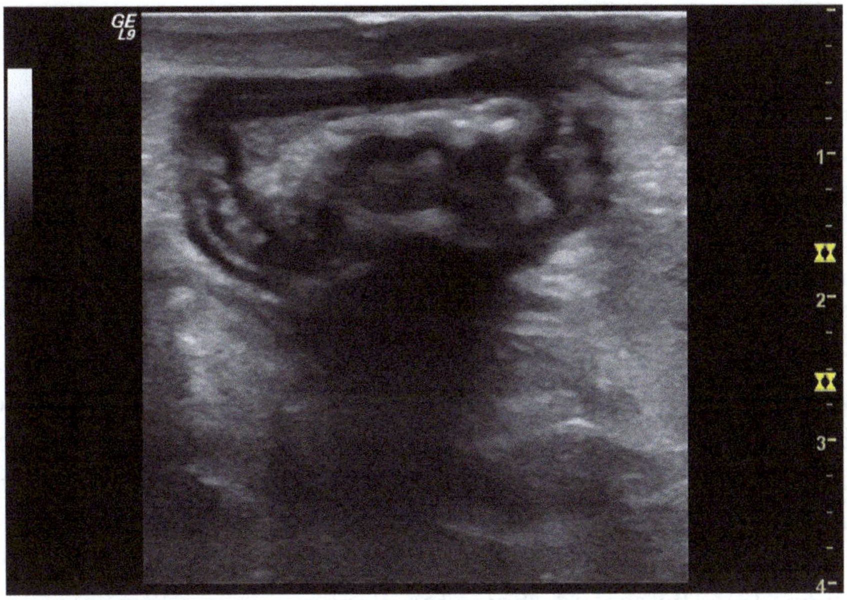

Figure 8. Umbilical hernia with intestine.

4. Epigastric hernia

It occurs in the midline above the umbilicus till the xiphisternum. Diastasis of the rectus abdominis muscle often predisposes to epigastric hernias and fatty hernia of the linea alba. Defects are usually small sized, and the content is almost always fat [8]. They have to be differentiated from other causes of epigastric pain. They could be confused with paraumbilical hernia/swelling if they are near to the umbilicus. The defect is usually small (less than 1 cm) and appears as a hypoechoic interruption of the echogenic linea alba (**Figure 9**).

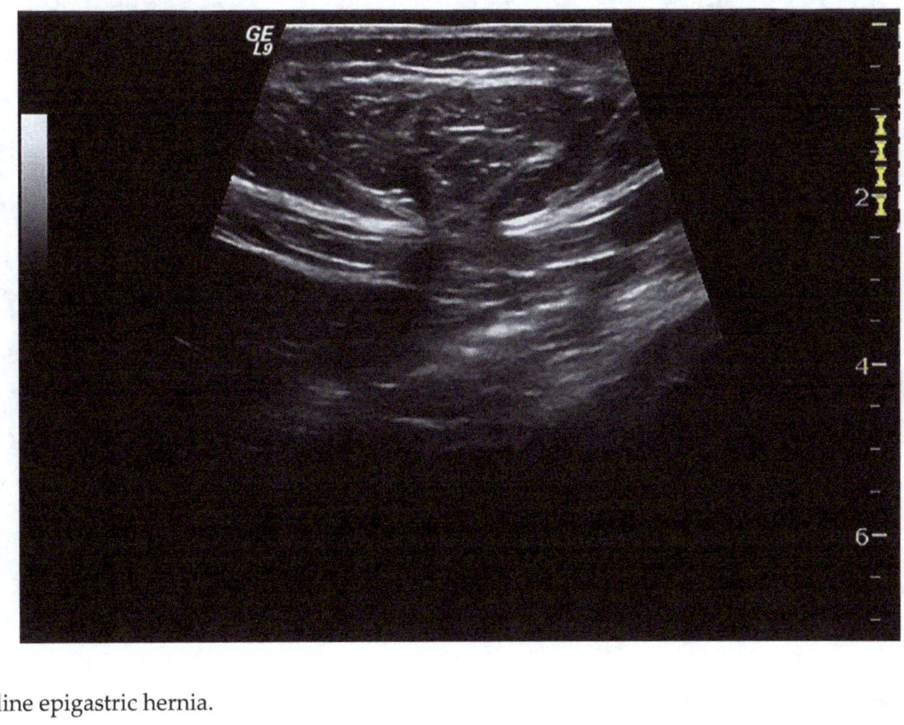

Figure 9. Midline epigastric hernia.

5. Spigelian hernia

It is named after the anatomist (Adriaan van der Spieghel) and is a rare lateral abdominal wall hernia. Most of these hernias have narrow neck and wide fundus, hence predisposing to irreducibility, incarceration, and strangulation [9] (**Figure 10**). Spigelian hernias are common in obese women, and clinical diagnosis is difficult. The hernia classically occurs caudal to the umbilicus but cranial to the junction of the linea semilunaris and the inferior epigastric vessels. Spigelian hernias traverse through the full thickness of the abdominal wall muscles [4]. Before three decades, herniorrhaphy (using contrast) was the mainstay for radiological diagnosis; however, in the last few years, the use of ultrasound has become much increased, with the capability of dynamic scanning and comparison to the asymptomatic side. A linear transducer (10–15 MHZ) is usually used for scanning; however, in obese patients, a curvilinear transducer (2–7 MHZ) is used. The use of color Doppler is helpful in the diagnosis of serious complications and incarceration and strangulation by checking the viability of the intestinal loops [8]. The second choice for diagnosis in modern imaging is computed tomography which displays excellent anatomy of the abdominal wall, especially with multidetector modern scanners; however, the risk of radiation makes it the second choice after ultrasound. An important point in either ultrasound or CT is the ability to identify the hernia orifice at the junction of the semilunar line and the semicircular line. It is important to establish a confident relationship between the radiologist and the surgeon in diagnosis of this type of hernia, as a number of cases of Spigelian hernia are falsely negative on radiologic investigation.

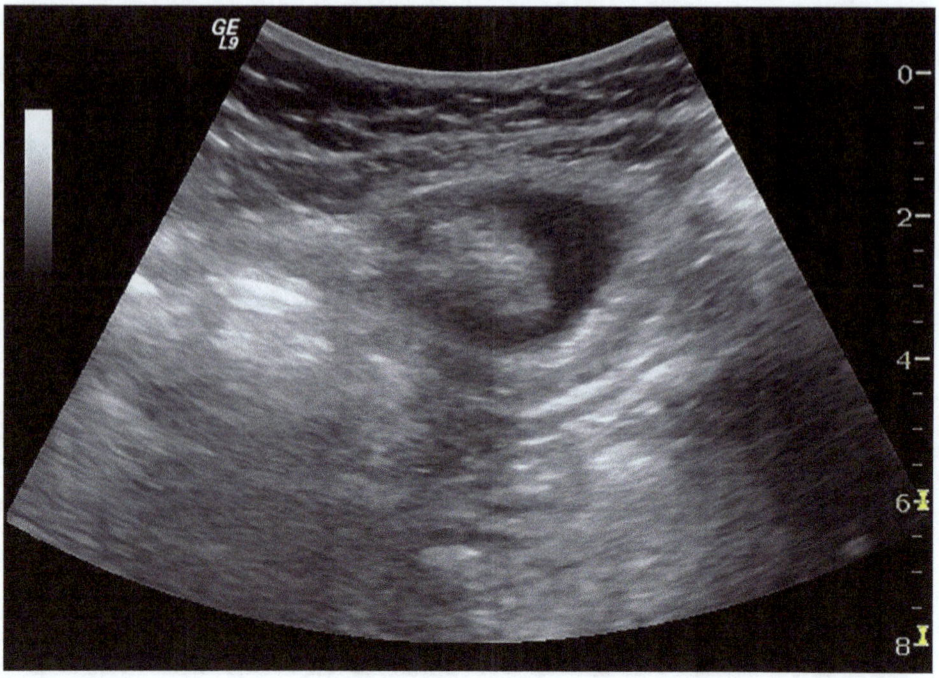

Figure 10. Ultrasound Spigelian hernia.

6. Femoral hernia

It is a rare hernia that is more common in females, likely attributed to increased intrapelvic pressure. A linear transducer of 10–15 MHZ is used, and scanning begins by identifying the echogenic inguinal ligament, then sweeping the probe inferomedially to identify the common femoral vein (**Figure 11**), where the usual site of hernia defect is medial to it. The importance of early diagnosis lies in the small size of the hernia sac of this type of hernia, making it prone to higher incidence of serious complications like strangulation. The differentiation of femoral hernia from direct and indirect inguinal hernias is not easy from the clinical point of view, and in this moment, the use of cross sectional imaging tool like CT is much more useful. On CT, the sac of an incarcerated femoral hernia lies lateral to the pubic tubercle, while the sac of the inguinal hernias is usually located medial to the pubic tubercle. Compression of the femoral vein within the canal is an important sign which could be demonstrated by both CT and ultrasound [10].

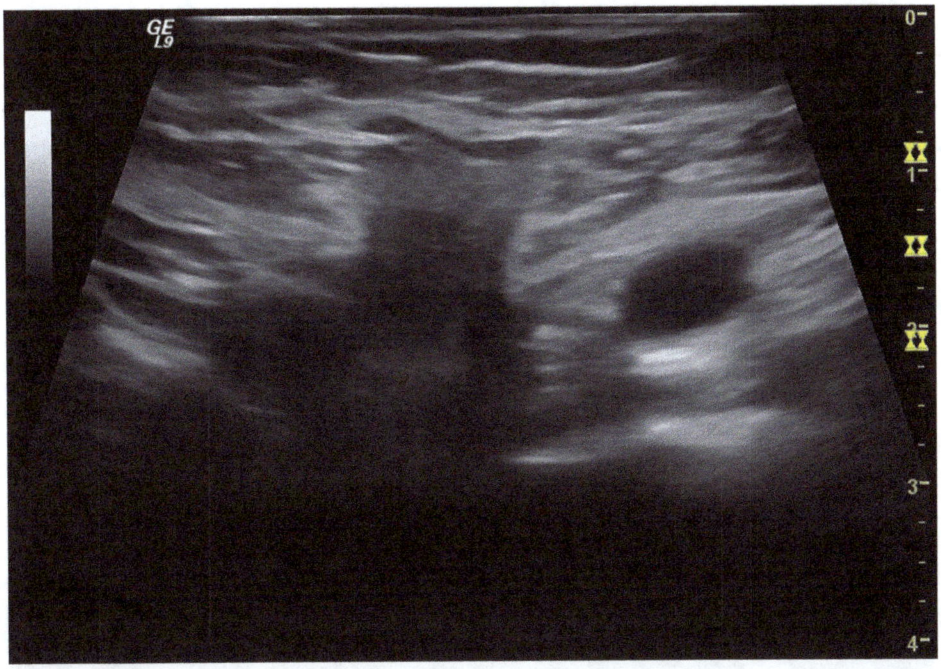

Figure 11. Left femoral hernia, note the sac is medial to left common femoral vein.

7. Obturator hernia

It is a rare type of hernia that is related to the obturator foramen and is associated with high risk of complications, hence, high morbidity. Referral for imaging is usually due to unexplained groin pain. On computed tomography, the hernia sac protrudes through the obturator foramen and lying between the obturator externus muscle from the posteromedial aspect and the pectineus muscle from the antero-lateral aspect [11].

8. Incisional and Para-stomal hernias

It is an important type of hernia that is related to the surgical incision or laparoscopy stomas. They are commonly associated with vertically oriented incisions and less frequently with transverse incisions. They could also occur with laparoscopy port sites. Para-stomal hernias are incisional hernias that occur around a stoma [4]. Incisional hernias are associated with high rate of postsurgical complications, with or without weakness of the abdominal wall muscles. The prognosis of the incisional hernia is highly related to how much of the thickness of the abdominal wall is involved by the hernia. Diagnosis could be done by ultrasound especially with the use of dynamic maneuvers; however, in cases of recurrent large incisional hernias, we recommend the use of CT as the edge of the hernia orifice may appear beyond the scope of the curvilinear abdominal low-frequency ultrasound probe. Also in cases of lateral incisional hernias (especially subcostal type), better localization of the hernia orifice is made by the modern multislice CT scanners, using the coronal and sagittal reconstruction.

9. Role of imaging in complications of hernias and postoperative period

Complications of hernias include irreducibility (**Figure 12**), obstruction, incarceration (**Figure 13 (A)** and **(B)**), and strangulation. Differentiating irreducibility from incarceration in terms of imaging is important. In our experience, simple failure of the hernia sac contents to reduce

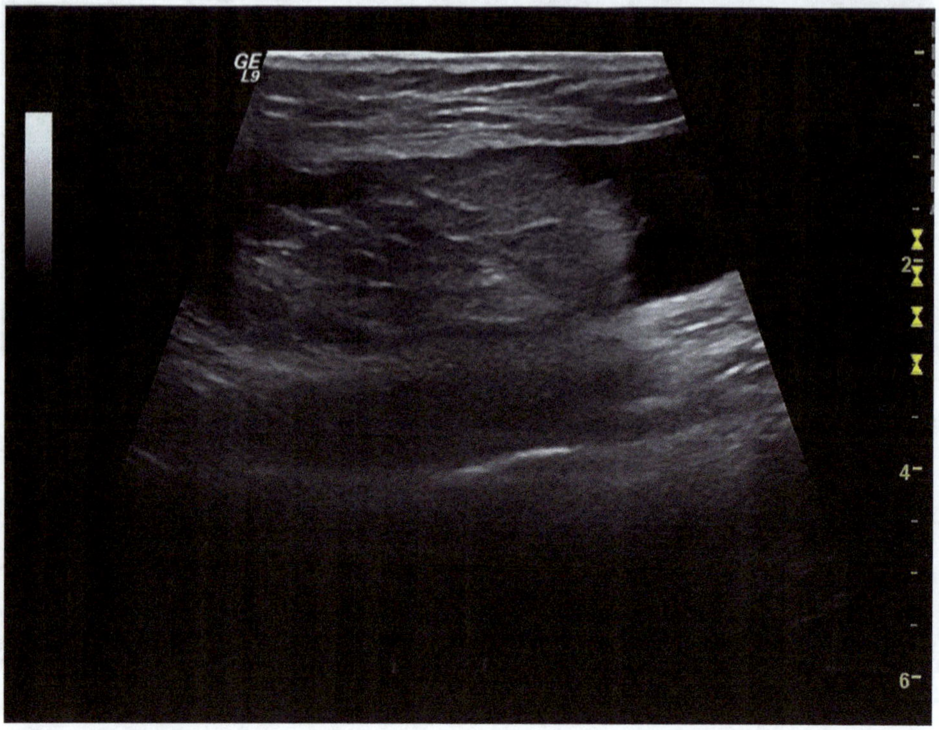

Figure 12. Irreducible umbilical hernia.

back into the sac after provocative tests should be defined as irreducibility, while presence of adhesion in addition to irreducibility signifies incarceration, and the addition of impedance of the vascular supply to the contents which are usually bowel loops signifies "strangulation." The use of color Doppler in diagnosing vascular compromise should be taken with caution, as the absence of positive vascularity may not be always associated with strangulation, and the presence of positive blood flow within the loops does not exclude strangulation. Vascular compromise is rather suggested by indirect signs of like thickening of the bowel wall, and presence of fluid inside the hernia sac.

Clinical evaluation of recurrent hernias is usually limited due to the existence of mesh (made of nonabsorbable material), and tissue fibrosis or large body habitus, contraction of the abdominal wall muscles, or any cause of distension. Under these circumstances, we usually resort to multi-detector row computed tomography for proper diagnosis. Complications after surgical hernia repair may comprise high percentage of cases, depending on surgical technique and the status of the hernia sac vasculature. Approximately one-half of these complications may require surgical re-intervention, and accurate diagnosis at multi-detector row CT is necessary for optimal patient treatment [2]. Assessment of the herniectomy site includes assessing the wound area for any collections, hematoma, seroma (**Figures 14** and **15**), stitch abscess, and recurrence. It is important to compare to the asymptomatic side and to assess the size of any collection present. Follow-up may be necessary for some complications such seroma, which have high rate of recurrence even after ultrasound-guided aspiration. The assessment of inserted mesh includes assessment of the edge and competence of the mesh, detecting any

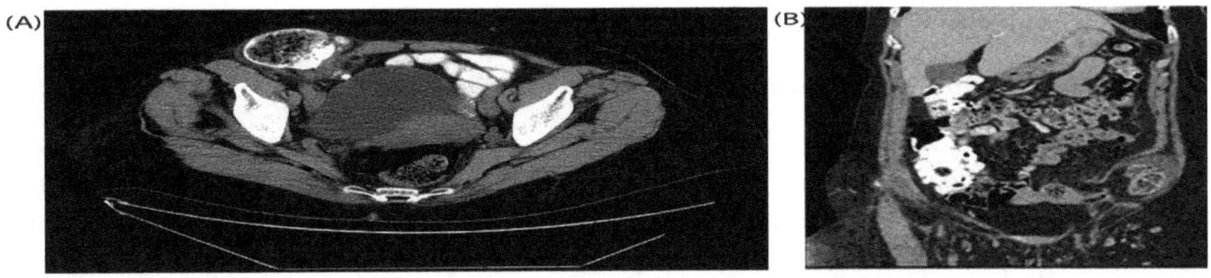

Figure 13. (A) CT incarcerated Spigelian hernia, axial. (B) CT incarcerated Spigelian hernia, coronal reconstruction.

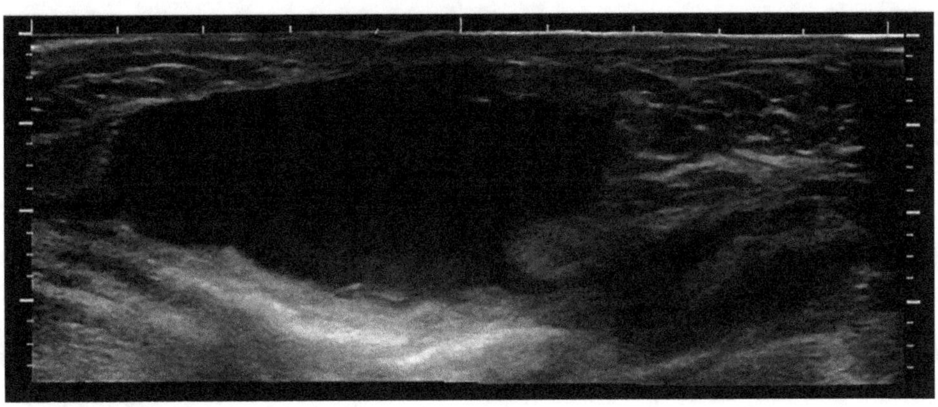

Figure 14. Seroma postinguinal hernia repair.

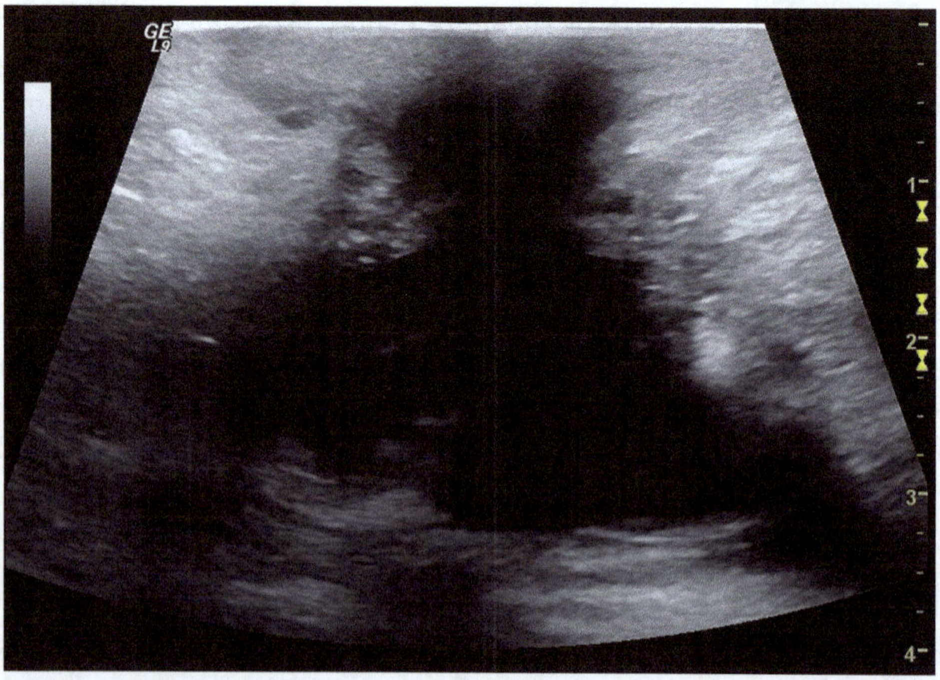

Figure 15. Seroma postumbilical hernia repair.

surrounding collections, and to exclude mesh failure, this is usually associated with dense posterior shadowing.

10. Magnetic resonance imaging.

The use of magnetic resonance imaging was recently suggested for occult inguinal hernias [12]. It may be considered as the alternative imaging of choice, only if ultrasound and computed tomography failed to answer the question about the suspected hernia site. Magnetic resonance imaging is an important multiplanar imaging, however, its use is only resorted to, only after other cheaper and more available imaging modalities, like ultrasound and CT [9].

Author details

Mohamed Abdelmohsen Bedewi[1]* and Mohamed El-sharkawy[2]

*Address all correspondence to: mohamedbedewi@yahoo.com

1 College of Medicine, Prince Sattam Bin Abdulaziz University, Alkharj, Kingdom of Saudi Arabia

2 King Khalid University Hospital, King Saud University, Riyadh, Kingdom of Saudi Arabia

References

[1] Bedewi MA, El-Sharkawy MS, Al Boukai AA, Al-Nakshabandi N. Prevalence of adult paraumbilical hernia. Assessment by high-resolution sonography: A hospital-based study. Hernia. 2012;**16**(1):59-62

[2] Aguirre DA, Santosa AC, Casola G, Sirlin CB. Abdominal wall hernias: Imaging features, complications, and diagnostic pitfalls at multi-detector row CT. Radiographics. 2005;**25**:1501-1520

[3] Harrison LA, Keesling CA, Martin NL, Lee KR, Wetzel LH. Abdominal wall hernias: Review of herniography and correlation with cross-sectional imaging. Radiographics. 1995;**15**:315-332

[4] Trainer V, Leung C, Owen RE, Venkatanarasimha N. External anterior abdominal wall and pelvic hernias with emphasis on the key diagnostic features on MDCT V. Clinical Radiology 2013; **38**:388-396

[5] Rettenbacher T, Hollerweger A, Macheiner P, Gritzmann N, Gotwald T, Frass R, Schneider B. Abdominal wall hernias: Cross-sectional imaging signs of incarceration determined with sonography. AJR American Journal of Roentgenology. 2001;**177**:1061-1066

[6] Herrington JK. Occult inguinal hernia in the female. Annals of Surgery. 1975;**181**(4):481-483

[7] Jaffe TA, O'Connell MJ, Harris JP, Paulson EK, DeLong DM. MDCT of abdominal wall hernias: Is there a role for Valsalva's maneuver? AJR American Journal of Roentgenology. 2005;**184**:847-851

[8] Smereczyński A1, Kołaczyk K1, Lubiński J1, Bojko S1, Gałdyńska M1, Bernatowicz E1. Sonographic imaging of Spigelian hernias. Journal of Ultrasonography. 2012;**12**(50):269-275

[9] Light D, Chattopadhyay D, Bawa S. Radiological and clinical examination in the diagnosis of Spigelian hernias. Annals of the Royal College of Surgens of England. 2013;**95**(2):98-100

[10] Suzuki S, Furui S, Okinaga K, et al. Differentiation of femoral versus inguinal hernia: CT findings. AJR Am J Roentgenol. 2007;**189**:W78-83

[11] Miller PA, Mezwa DG, Feczko PJ, et al. Imaging of abdominal hernias. Radiographics. 1995;15:333-347

[12] Light D, Ratnasingham K, Banerjee A, Cadwallader R, Uzzaman MM, Gopinath B. The role of ultrasound scan in the diagnosis of occult inguinal hernias. International Journal of Surgery. 2011;**9**(2):169-172

6

Robotic Ventral Hernia Repair

Kaylene Barrera, Paul Chung, Sarrina Shraga and Gainosuke Sugiyama

Abstract

Approximately 350,000 to 500,000 ventral hernias are repaired yearly in the United States. These hernias include congenital umbilical hernias, incisional hernias from previous surgeries, or epigastric hernias. The crux of hernia repair is honoring the principle of achieving a tension-free repair, often achieved with utilization of a synthetic mesh. Over the last quarter of this century, laparoscopic ventral hernia repair has established itself as a valuable tool in repair of ventral hernias, with the advantages of reduced postoperative complications. More recently, the adaptation of the robotic platform has given another tool to perform ventral hernia repairs. The aim of this chapter is to describe the evolution of ventral hernia repairs and highlight the robotic approaches to repair.

Keywords: robotic ventral hernia repair, incisional hernia, umbilical hernia, robotic surgery introduction

1. Introduction

Ventral hernias are a classification of hernias affecting the abdominal wall. Included in this definition are epigastric, umbilical, Spigelian, and incisional hernias [1]. Repair of these hernias remains one of the most commonly performed procedures with more than 350,000 performed per year in the United States (SAGES) [2]. In addition to the cosmetic detriment, these hernias also pose a risk for bowel ischemia and strangulation, which can result in grave consequences.

Early descriptions of ventral hernias were evident in tomb paintings from ancient Egypt. Servants and workmen were depicted with abdominal protrusions [3]. Historian George Moritz Ebers (1837–1898) obtained an ancient papyrus, now referred to as the "Ebers papyrus."

In that document, additional descriptions of hernias were given. In ancient Greece, Hippocrates (460–375 BC) also described inguinal hernias [4]. While attempts to operate on inguinal hernias have been well described through the Middle Ages to the nineteenth century, reports on ventral hernia repairs during this era were limited.

The first reports of surgical hernia repair were published in the late nineteenth and early twentieth centuries, mostly describing umbilical hernia repair. At the time, surgical repair of hernias was considered "radical," with most people preferring reduction with a pad or suspension of incarcerated hernias [5]. Dr. Lucas-Championniere was one of the first surgeons to describe the principle of excising the hernia sac and closure of the neck [6]. The next evolution in hernia repair came in circa 1901, when William Mayo described primary repair using overlapping layers of fascia, or "pants over vest" technique. He "advocated the overlapping of the aponeurotic structures which were already at hand, securing a wide area of adhesions in place of edge to edge union" [7]. Incisional hernias were also recognized in this era. Kenelm Winslow described the experience of surgeons at the time emphasizing prevention of these hernias by closing incisions in layers. He also noted that although the repair described by Mayo had become popular, recurrence was a persistent problem, especially with large hernias [8]. In the early 1960s, knitted polypropylene mesh was introduced, which revolutionized repair, allowing for decreased recurrence rates. This repair allowed for additional variations in repair based on the placement of the mesh including extraperitoneal versus intraperitoneal placement [9, 10].

The evolution of hernia repair continued with adaptation of minimally invasive surgery. The first laparoscopic ventral hernia repair was described in 1993 by LeBlanc and Booth [11]. Using 4 to 5 trocars, they repaired hernias in five patients using polytetrafluoroethylene (PTFE) mesh [8]. Laparascopic ventral hernia repair has become increasingly utilized in select cases, allowing for increased mesh overlap of defects and reduced postoperative complications compared to open repair. A limitation to laparoscopic ventral hernia repair, however, is that it remains a technically challenging procedure with a steep learning curve.

Robotic surgery allows for a way to alleviate the challenges presented by laparoscopic surgery. In 2000, the FDA approved the first robotic surgery system. The first robotic assisted ventral hernia repair was first described by Ballantyne et al. in 2003 [12] during which a PTFE mesh was placed and secured with a combination of sutures and tacks. Currently, the use of robotic ventral hernia repair is growing worldwide as a robotic platform allows for a more straightforward primary closure of the defect with the aid of wristed instruments. As the current body of literature is still evolving, the evaluation of its role as it relates to laparoscopic or open ventral hernia repairs is yet to be determined.

2. Indications

- Incisional hernia
- Umbilical hernia
- Spigelian hernia

- Epigastric hernia
- Incarcerated hernia

3. Contraindications

- Inability to tolerate general anesthesia
- Dense adhesions
- Bowel necrosis

4. Conversion to laparoscopic or open procedure

Conversion to conventional laparoscopy may be necessary if there is malfunction of the robotic components.

The surgeon should be prepared to convert to an open procedure in the event of significant hemorrhage, bowel injury, or limited accessibility due to diffuse adhesive disease.

5. Procedure

Materials

- da Vinci robotic platform
- Endo shears
- Blunt grasper
- Hook cautery
- Available energy source
- Mesh
- (optional) Sterile ruler; ruler provided with marking pen can be used
- (optional) Air seal

5.1. Patient setup

After administration of general anesthesia, the patient is placed in the supine position with arms tucked. The operating table can be rotated to accommodate positioning of the robotic tower (**Figures 1** and **2**). Three ports are placed on the contralateral (or any side if hernia is

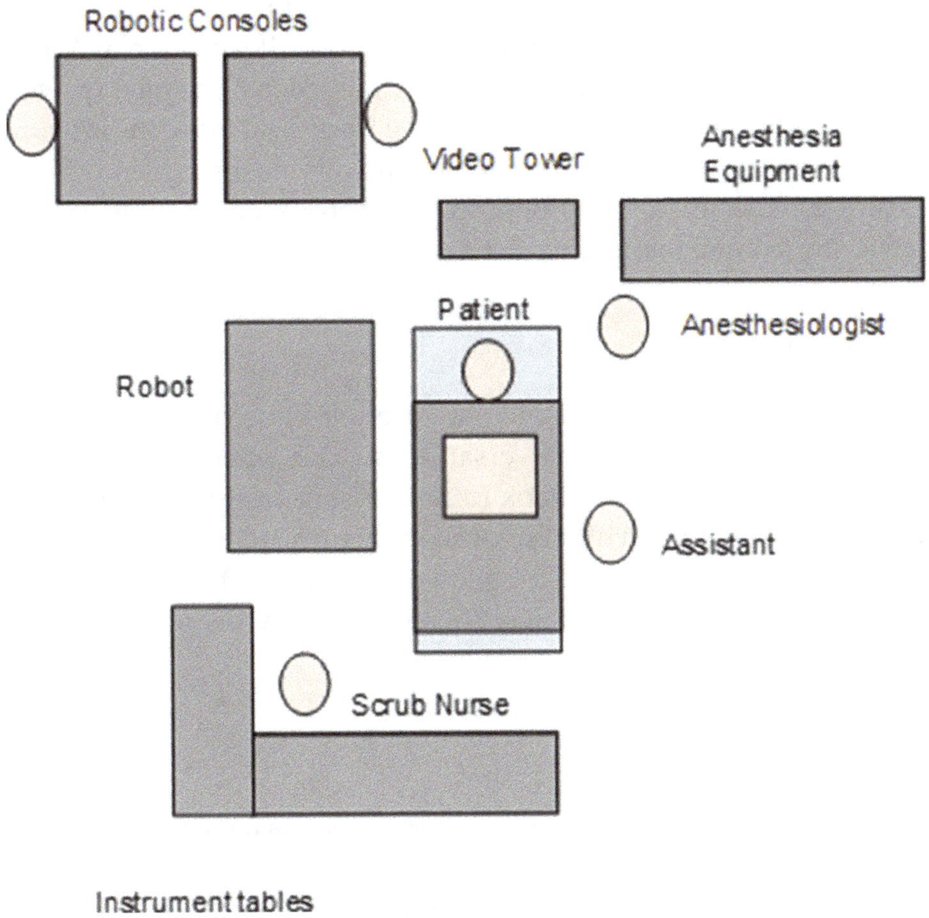

Figure 1. Operating room setup.

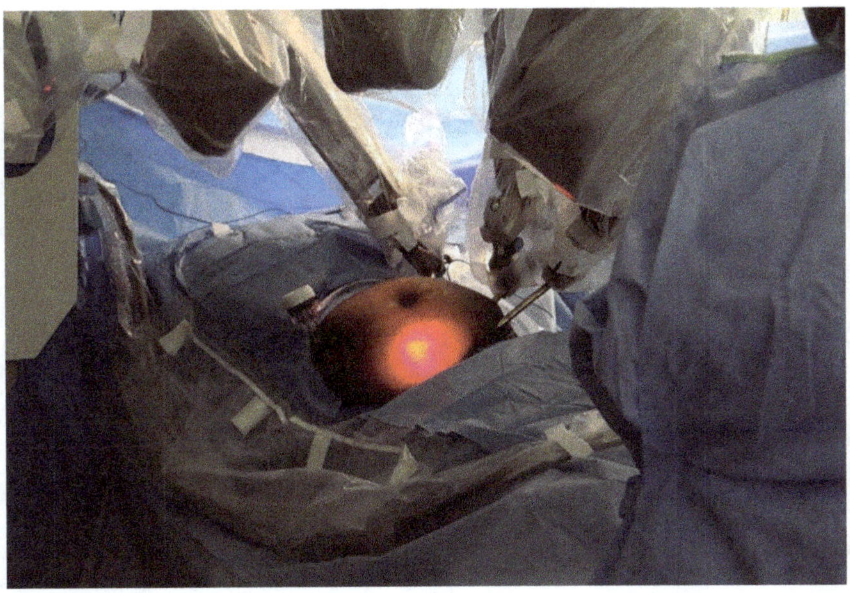

Figure 2. Docked robot with port placement.

midline) side to accommodate the instrument arms and camera. The ports are 5 or 8 mm wide and are placed 8 to 10 cm apart to avoid instrument collision. If using the da Vinci Si system, it may help to place bariatric trocar near the anterior superior iliac spine to avoid collision with the hip during dissection. Utilizing bariatric long trocar will move the instruments away from the hip, thus allowing for a free range of motion with the instruments. In our practice, we sometimes also include an accessory port on the opposite side to assist with instrument exchanges such as sutures and mesh introduction.

5.2. Dissection of the hernia sac

Adhesions are taken down using a combination of blunt dissection using a blunt grasper and Endoshears. The Endoshears have a versatile use, and when connected to an energy source, they can function in place of a hook cautery (using either with closed tips or with one jaw), control bleeding, or aid in blunt dissection (**Figure 3**). In our practice, we measure the defect by inserting a sterile ruler into the abdominal cavity. After insufflation is released to 5 to 8 mmHg, the dimensions of the defect are recorded to allow for adequate estimation of the defect.

5.3. Mesh selection

A 4- to 5-cm circumferential overlap is desirable for ventral hernia repairs and accommodates for related shrinkage. Products available include polypropylene and polyester mesh. At our institution, we most commonly use the polypropylene mesh. The mesh is rolled extracorporeally and secured with a single stay suture. It is then introduced into the cavity using an accessory

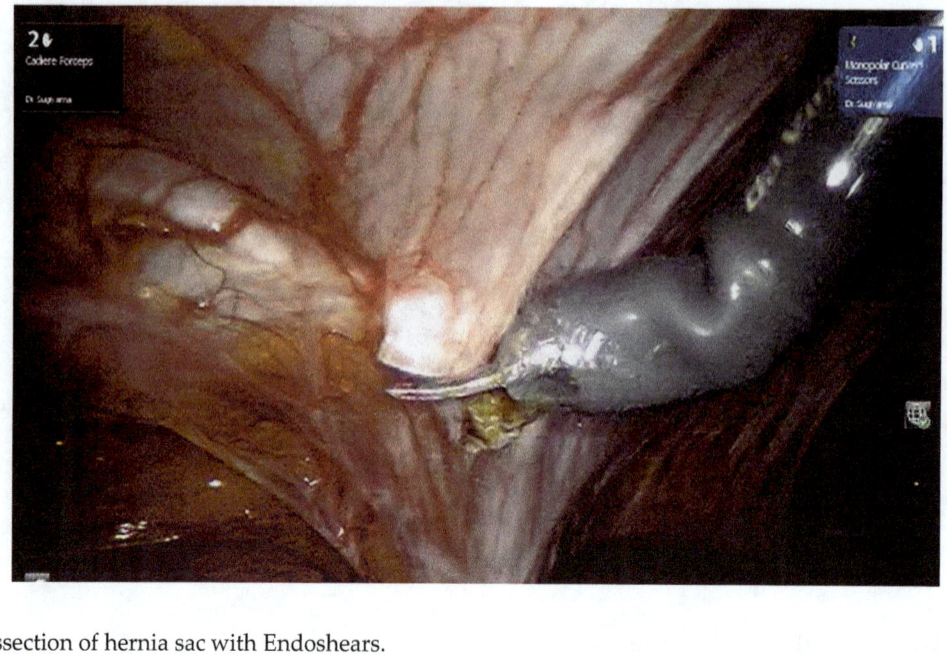

Figure 3. Dissection of hernia sac with Endoshears.

12-mm port. The mesh repair can then proceed using one of the following methods: intraperitoneal onlay mesh (IPOM), transabdominal preperitoneal (TAPP), transversus abdominis release (TAR), and retromuscular repair.

5.4. Intraperitoneal onlay mesh (IPOM)

Repairs using intraperitoneal onlay mesh originated with inguinal hernia repair and soon found a role in ventral hernia repair [13–15]. The repair is completed by positioning the mesh over the defect with 4 to 5 cm overlap. The mesh can be secured using permanent or absorbable tackers. This can be done using the standard laparoscopic technique. An advantage of the robotic platform is that with the degrees of freedom, the mesh can also be sewn in. In this method, two to four tacks can be used to position the mesh if needed. The mesh is secured with a running absorbable suture around the border.

Early hypotheses associated transfascial sutures and tacks with increased pain; however, there has been no significant difference in retrospective reviews. Transfascial sutures and tacking have demonstrated similar pain profiles in available series that analyzed postoperative pain, opiate use, and telephone interview follow-up (mean follow-up 30 months). Transfascial sutures were, however, associated with increased infection rate [16–18]. To date, there are no comparisons of prospective randomized controlled studies on running suture versus transfascial sutures or tacking.

5.5. Transabdominal preperitoneal (TAPP) repair

Given the concern for adhesions to mesh, potential for mesh migration, and other complications associated with intraperitoneal onlay mesh, there has been an increasing interest in more physiologic repairs. Preperitoneal repair for ventral hernia was first described in 2002, after it had already gained popularity in the repair of inguinal hernias [19]. In this technique, a peritoneal flap is created, and after the mesh is secured with tacks, the peritoneum is reconstructed with intracorporeal sutures. When compared to laparoscopic IPOM, there were no major differences in outcomes [20–22]. Despite the benefits of laparoscopic preperitoneal repair, the literature reflects a select few limited case series and case reports using this technique [23]. This may reflect the technical difficulty of laparoscopy in creating and closing the peritoneal flap. The articulating instruments and degree of freedom offered by robotic surgery can compensate for the difficult maneuvers required to perform a TAPP ventral hernia repair. The experience with robotic TAPP is evolving and has been demonstrated as a safe and feasible procedure in small retrospective case series [24]. The procedure starts with adhesiolysis and careful delineation of the hernia sac. Upon reduction of hernia sac, peritoneal flap creation starts. We typically start the dissection on the ipsilateral side of the port midway on the falciform ligament. By gently pulling down on the falciform ligament, a small area of peritoneum is opened and the dissection is initially carried out in superior to inferior dissection. Once the peritoneum is opened, the peritoneal flap creation is carried out laterally to accommodate the mesh with a 4- to 5-cm overlap. If enough peritoneum is dissected off of the posterior sheath, the peritoneum can be flexible enough to cover the mesh on the ipsilateral side to equally cover the mesh (**Figure 4A**). The flap can be created either through single docking with unilateral ports on one side or via double docking with ports on both sides of the abdomen. In our experience, TAPP repair for primary hernias such as epigastric

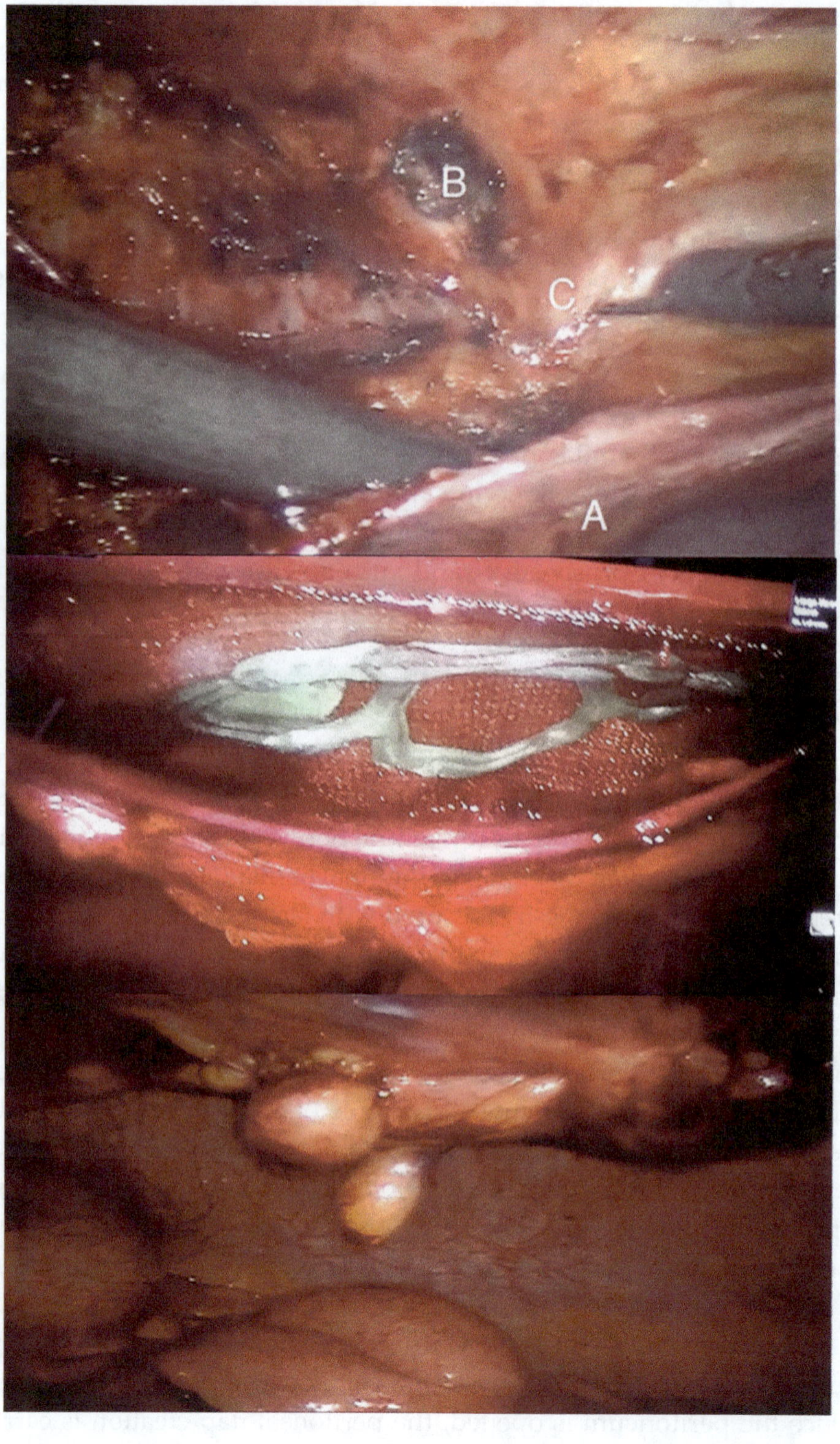

Figure 4. (Top) Creation of preperitoneal flap. (A) Lateral edge of peritoneal dissection. (B) Hernia defect and (C) lateral border of dissection. (Middle) Placement of mesh in preperitoneal space. (Bottom) Closure of peritoneum over the hernia defect.

and umbilical hernias can be accomplished using single docking; however, for the incisional hernias, it is preferable to employ double-docking technique by creating a flap starting in the midline. Upon completion of flap creation, the hernia defect can be primarily approximated using locking sutures. The mesh can then be placed in the preperitoneal space and secured to the posterior sheath with either sutures or absorbable tackers (**Figure 4B**). Upon completing mesh fixation, the peritoneal flap created can then be used to cover the mesh providing space for the mesh to integrate with posterior sheath and avoiding contact with intraperitoneal contents (**Figure 4C**) [30].

5.6. Transversus abdominis release (TAR)

Although tension-free repairs using mesh have been successful, the patient's posterior rectus provides a natural and less costly abdominal wall barrier. In this technique, after reduction of the hernia, the peritoneum and posterior rectus sheath are dissected from the rectus muscle. The dissection is then extended laterally and the transversus abdominis muscle aponeurosis is incised, producing component separation which allows for primary repair of the hernia defect. The primary repair can be completed using locking sutures, such as the STRATAFIX, which has been approved by the FDA for fascial closure [25].

5.7. Robotic retromuscular ventral hernia repair (RRVHR)

Component separation, a therapy for extensive abdominal wall defects, can also be achieved using minimally invasive techniques. Open component separation is still limited by recurrence and associated wound complications. Carbonell et al. reported release of the posterior rectus sheath in the retromuscular space and referred to it as posterior component separation technique (PCST) [26]. Posterior component separation was also adapted to minimally invasive techniques using the robot. When compared to laparoscopic ventral hernia repair in an analysis of Americas Hernia Society Quality Collaborative database, RRVHR was not significantly different in terms of direct hospital costs, narcotic requirements but was associated with increased incidence of seroma [27].

After the hernia is identified and reduced, edges of the hernia sac are delineated and edges are opened with electrocautery. Once the edges are opened, posterior sheath is separated from the rectus and the anterior sheath, and the dissection is carried out laterally until neurovascular bundles are found. Care must be taken to avoid disrupting the linea alba as the dissection is carried out. This should classically be done with ports on the bilateral flank. The initial dissection can start on one side, and once posterior sheath is separated on one edge of the hernia sac, additional ports are placed on the contralateral side. The above step is repeated to separate the posterior sheath from the rectus (**Figure 5**). Upon completely entering the retromuscular space, the hernia defect can be approximated using locking sutures and mesh reinforcement can be performed below the primary repair of the defect. The posterior sheath, which was separated, is then closed below the mesh using sutures to fully place the mesh in the retromuscular space. The peritoneum and posterior rectus fascia are both separated from

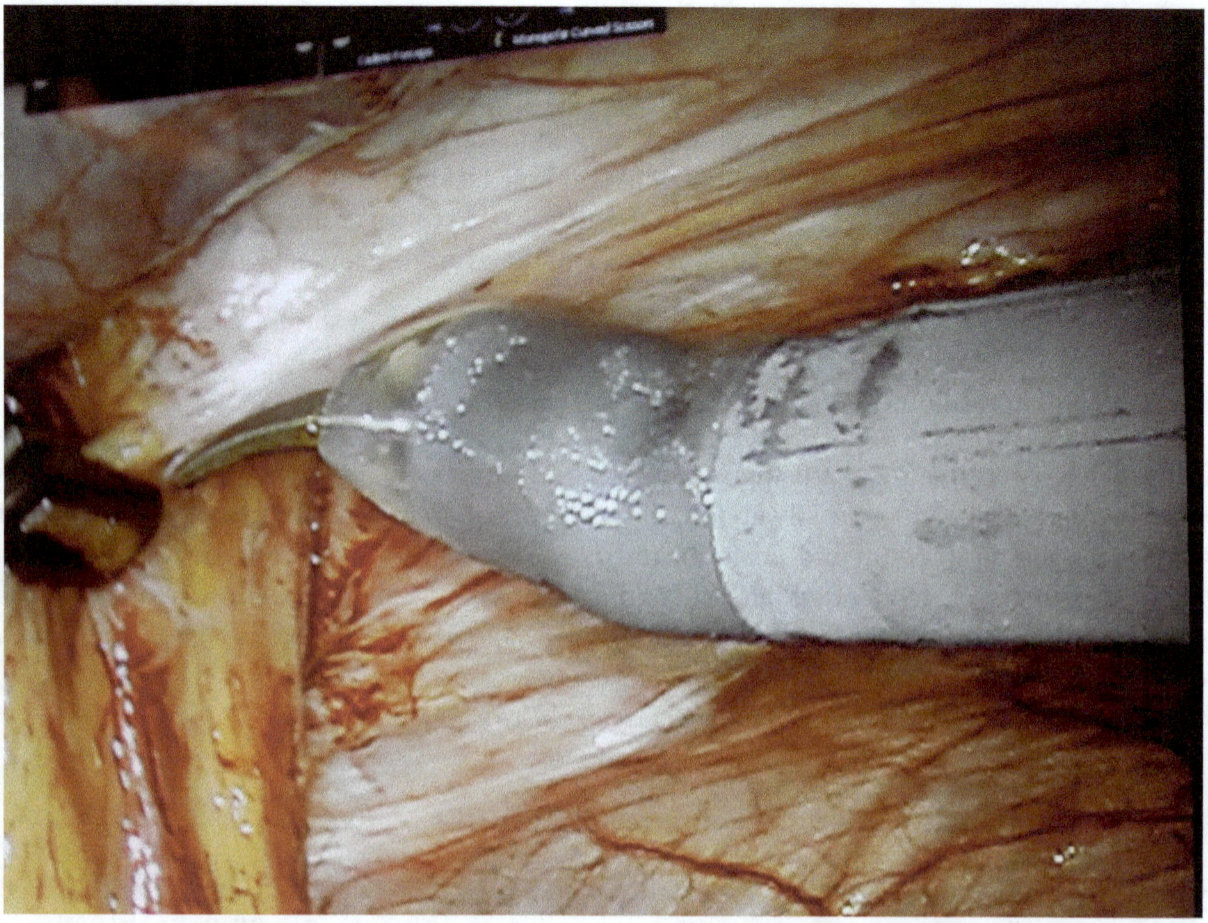

Figure 5. Dissection of the peritoneum and posterior rectus sheath to create a retromuscular space.

the posterior rectus muscle. A 4 to 5 cm perimeter is dissected. After repair of the primary defect, the polypropylene mesh is then placed inside the cavity and secured using a circumferential locking suture. The peritoneum and posterior fascia are then reapproximated using running locking suture.

6. Tips

- When securing the mesh during IPOM, avoid large gaps, which can allow bowel to become caught in the mesh
- To obtain an accurate measurement, we can use a sterile ruler with reduction in pneumoperitoneum (**Figure 6**)
- If complete closure of the peritoneum cannot be achieved, we can suture borders of peritoneum to preperitoneal mesh (**Figure 7**).

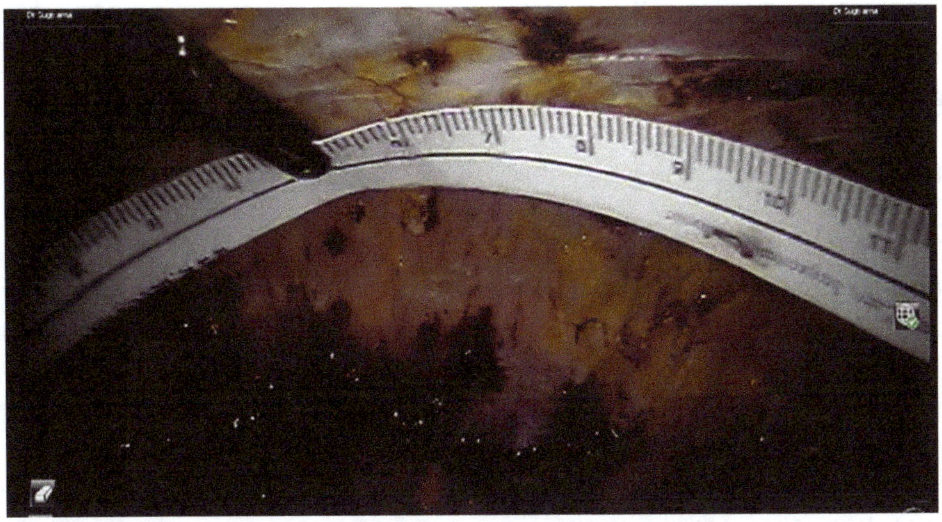

Figure 6. Intracorporeal measurement of the defect.

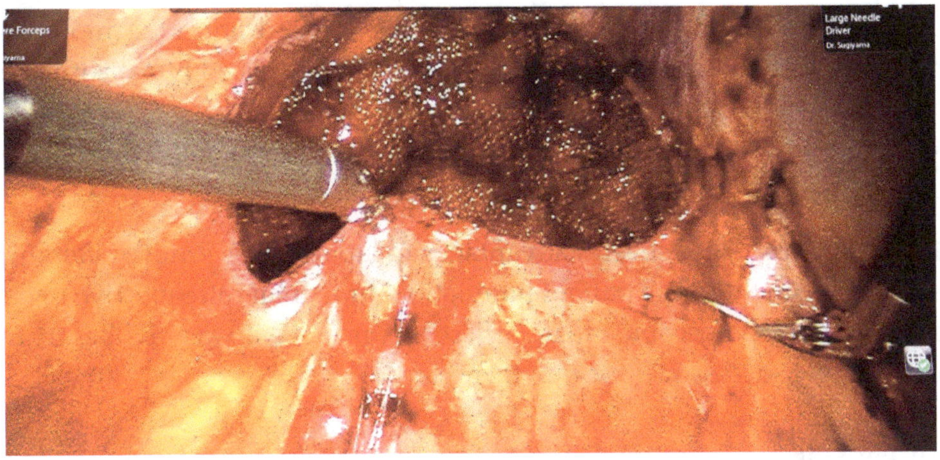

Figure 7. Partial peritoneal coverage of preperitoneal mesh.

7. Considerations

7.1. Cost

The cost benefit to laparoscopic ventral hernia repairs mirrors the clinical benefits of this approach. With decreased operative times and complications, accounting for readmissions and recurrences, laparoscopic ventral hernia repair was shown to be cost effective, including 1-year follow-up in analysis of both a statewide database and the National Inpatient Sample [28]. A concern of the use of robotic surgery is the cost of the technology. Consensus on the impact of cost has been a topic of controversy. As previously noted, laparoscopic and robotic retromuscular repairs do not significantly differ in terms of direct hospital costs in an analysis of a large multicenter database [27]. Differences in costs are multifactorial, and costs can be distributed in centers where multiple services are utilizing the robot. Kudsi et al., after finding improvement in operative times, suggested that this may also be an area of cost savings [29].

7.2. Obesity

Minimally invasive surgery in obese patients can be challenging. Body habitus and extensive subcutaneous tissue can hinder efforts to achieve pneumoperitoneum and maneuver laparoscopic instruments. Moreover, this population is at higher risk of developing recurrent incisional hernias and higher risks of complications following repair. Patients with a body mass index (BMI) ≥ 30 kg/m^2 have demonstrated poorer outcomes following ventral hernia repair, have higher rates of recurrence, more complications, and longer hospital stays [30]. The benefits of performing minimally invasive surgery in obese patients can compensate for the associated difficulties. Minimally invasive ventral hernia repair is associated with lower complication and recurrence rates. In a retrospective review of 163 obese patients (BMI ≥ 30 kg/m^2), Novitsky et al. found significantly lower rates of both complications and recurrences with laparoscopic PTFE mesh repair compared to open repair. The improved outcomes were associated with safe entry into abdomen via left upper quadrant, meticulous adhesiolysis, adequate mesh overlap (4 to 5 cm) and use of 4 to 6 equally spaced nonabsorbable sutures to secure the mesh [31]. Several other studies have reached similar conclusions, including more recent retrospective review in 2016 by Froylich et al., who found similar outcomes when comparing open to minimally invasive ventral hernia repair [32].

Robotic hernia repair provides several advantages to laparoscopy, but the literature is sparse for its use specifically in the obese patient population. In a small retrospective review comparing robotic-assisted to laparoscopic repair, where the mean BMI was 31.5 kg/m^2, the outcome showed a comparable success rate for robotic repair [33].

7.3. Pediatric patients

In our practice, we do not include pediatric patients; however, minimally invasive ventral hernia repair has been practiced in this population. The first series of minimally invasive ventral hernia repair in children was reported in 2006 using 3-mm ports and standard laparoscopic equipment with a mean age of 2 years in those with epigastric hernias and 4.2 years in patients with umbilical hernias, demonstrating that the procedure was safe and feasible [34]. Robotic ventral hernia repair is yet to be reported in this population; however, the scope of robotic surgery has expanded to include repair of congenital diaphragmatic hernias, cholecystectomy, and inguinal hernias.

8. Role of robotics in surgical education

As robotic surgery becomes increasingly integrated into various practices, including cardiothoracic surgery, oncologic surgery as well as urology and gynecology, it is also becoming important for trainees to become familiar with this technology. Simulation software included with the system allows trainees to develop skills. During live surgery, the ability to alternate between consoles provides a similar learning environment to standard open and laparoscopic surgery without affecting patient safety. A consensus on general surgery training and robotic training has not been described; however, in the field of urology, the importance of robotic training has been well recognized as a vital tool for trainees to grasp projecting that it will become basic skill in the future [35, 36]. In a recent survey addressing attitudes of general surgery attendings and residents, 73% of residents completed robotic simulator training, with 20% having experience as the primary console operator. One hundred percent of attending surgeons surveyed believed that robotic surgery training should be included in general surgery training programs [37].

9. Conclusions

The evolution of surgery for ventral hernias has followed developments in inguinal hernia repair. From trusses and external devices came open repair followed by minimally invasive techniques. The difficulties encountered with the limits of laparoscopic repair have been alleviated by the versatility offered by robotic surgery which includes enhanced dexterity, visualization, and ergonomics. Options for minimally invasive techniques include a wide variety of techniques reflecting the complexity of abdominal wall components and include intraperitoneal onlay mesh, transabdominal preperitoneal repair, transverse abdominis release, and retromuscular repairs. While the safety and efficacy of all of these modalities has been well validated, the type of repair should be patient centered.

While cost remains a concern in robotic ventral hernia repair, this is a topic of controversy. Assessing cost is a complex moving target and is sensitive to metrics such as operative times, utilization, and maintenance. Analysis of total robotic utilization across all specialties in an institution may be warranted to capture the true effect on healthcare costs.

As the use of robotic surgery has spread to include ventral hernia repair, it is likely that this can prove to be true for a broad range of procedures, making the techniques used in ventral hernia repair useful for building a basic skillset. For our current surgical trainees, this is especially true, and it is yet to be determined how this will shape general surgery curricula.

Author details

Kaylene Barrera, Paul Chung, Sarrina Shraga and Gainosuke Sugiyama*

*Address all correspondence to: gainosuke.sugiyama@downstate.edu

Downstate Medical Center, State University of New York, Brooklyn, New York, United States of America

References

[1] Jacob BP, Ramshaw B. The SAGES Manual of Hernia Repair. Los Angeles, CA: Society of American Gastrointestinal Endoscopic Surgeons; 2013

[2] Laparoscopic Ventral Hernia Repair Information from SAGES. n.d. Available from: https://www.sages.org/publications/patient-information/patient-information-for-laparoscopic-ventral-hernia-repair-from-sages/. January 22, 2017

[3] Nunn JF. Ancient Egyptian Medicine. Norman: University of Oklahoma Press; 1996

[4] Holzheimer RG. Surgical treatment: Evidence-based and problem-oriented. In: Holzheimer RG, Mannick JA, editors. Surgical Treatment: Evidence-Based and Problem-Oriented. W Zuckschwerdt Verlag: Munich; 2001

[5] Bullitt JB. III. Retrenchment of lipomatous abdominal wall combined with operation for radical cure of umbilical hernia. Annals of Surgery. 1900;**32**(5):663-667

[6] Keetley CB. The radical cure of hernia. Annals of Surgery. 1888;**8**(1):5-23

[7] Mayo WJ. VI. An operation for the radical cure of umbilical hernia. Annals of Surgery. 1901;**34**(2):276-280

[8] Winslow K VI. The aponeuroses the supporting structures of the abdominal wall; their approximation for the prevention and cure of hernia. Annals of Surgery. 1904;**39**(2): 245-255

[9] Cassar K, Munro A. Surgical treatment of incisional hernia. The British Journal of Surgery. 2002;**89**(5):534-545

[10] Usher FC. Hernia repair with knitted polypropylene mesh. Surgery, Gynecology & Obstetrics. 1963;**117**:239-240

[11] LeBlanc KA, Booth WV. Laparoscopic repair of incisional abdominal hernias using expanded polytetrafluoroethylene: Preliminary findings. Surgical Laparoscopy & Endoscopy. 1993 Feb;**3**(1):39-41

[12] Ballantyne GH, Hourmont K, Wasielewski A. Telerobotic laparoscopic repair of incisional ventral hernias using intraperitoneal prosthetic mesh. Journal of the Society of Laparoendoscopic Surgeons. 2003;**7**(1):7-14

[13] Fitzgibbons RJ, Jr, Salerno GM, Filipi CJ, Hunter WJ, Watson P. A laparoscopic intraperitoneal onlay mesh technique for the repair of an indirect inguinal hernia. Annals of Surgery. 1994;**219**(2):144-156

[14] Chan AC, Lee TW, Ng KW, Chung SC, Li AK. Early results of laparoscopic intraperitoneal onlay mesh repair for inguinal hernia. The British Journal of Surgery. 1994;**81**(12):1761-1762

[15] Tsimoyiannis EC, Tassis A, Glantzounis G, Jabarin M, Siakas P, Tzourou H. Laparoscopic intraperitoneal onlay mesh repair of incisional hernia. Surgical Laparoscopy & Endoscopy. 1998;**8**(5):360-362

[16] Nguyen SQ, Divino CM, Buch KE, Schnur J, Weber KJ, Katz LB, Reiner MA, Aldoroty RA, Herron DM. Postoperative pain after laparoscopic ventral hernia repair: A prospective comparison of sutures versus tacks. Journal of the Society of Laparoendoscopic Surgeons. 2008;**12**(2):113-116

[17] Kitamura RK, Choi J, Lynn E, Divino CM. Suture versus tack fixation of mesh in laparoscopic umbilical hernia repair. Journal of the Society of Laparoendoscopic Surgeons. 2013;**17**(4):560-564

[18] Brill JB, Turner PL. Long-term outcomes with transfascial sutures versus tacks in laparoscopic ventral hernia repair: A review. The American Surgeon. 2011;**77**(4):458-465

[19] Sarli L, Pietra N, Choua O, Costi R, Cattaneo G. Laparoscopic hernia repair: A prospective comparison of TAPP and IPOM techniques. Surgical Laparoscopy & Endoscopy. 1997;**7**(6):472-476

[20] Miserez M, Penninckx F. Endoscopic totally preperitoneal ventral hernia repair. Surgical Endoscopy. 2002;**16**(8):1207-1213

[21] Prasad P, Tantia O, Patle NM, Khanna S, Sen B. Laparoscopic transabdominal preperitoneal repair of ventral hernia: A step towards physiological repair. Indian Journal of Surgery. 2011;**73**(6):403-408

[22] Prasad P, Tantia O, Patle NM, Khanna S, Sen B. Laparoscopic ventral hernia repair: A comparative study of transabdominal preperitoneal versus intraperitoneal onlay mesh repair. Journal of Laparoendoscopic and Advanced Surgical Techniques A. 2011;**21**(6):477-483

[23] Luque JA, Luque AB, Menchero JG, Grau JM, Moreno JG, Gomez AT, Jurado JG. Safety and effectiveness of self-adhesive mesh in laparoscopic ventral hernia repair using transabdominal preperitoneal route. Surgical Endoscopy. 2017;**31**(3):1213-1218

[24] Sugiyama G, Chivukula S, Chung PJ, Alfonso A. Robot-assisted transabdominal preperitoneal ventral hernia repair. Journal of the Society of Laparoendoscopic Surgeons. 2015;**19**(4):e2015.00092

[25] Krause D. Letter to Donna Marshall. Ethicon Incorporated a Johnson and Johnson Company Inc.; 2015. Available from: https://www.accessdata.fda.gov/cdrh_docs/pdf15/K151200.pdf

[26] Carbonell AM, Cobb WS, Chen SM. Posterior components separation during retromuscular hernia repair. Hernia: The Journal of Hernias and Abdominal Wall Surgery. 2008;**12**(4):359-362

[27] Warren JA, Cobb WS, Ewing JA, Carbonell AM. Standard laparoscopic versus robotic retromuscular ventral hernia repair. Surgical Endoscopy. 2017;**31**(1):324-332

[28] Funk LM, Perry KA, Narula VK, Mikami DJ, Melvin WS. Current national practice patterns for inpatient management of ventral abdominal wall hernia in the United States. Surgical Endoscopy. 2013;**27**(11):4104-4112

[29] Kudsi OY, Paluvoi N, Bhurtel P, McCabe Z, El-Jabri R. Robotic repair of ventral hernias: Preliminary findings of a case series of 106 consecutive cases. American Journal of Robotic Surgery. 2015;**2**(1):22-26

[30] Kaoutzanis C, Leichtle SW, Mouawad NJ, Welch KB, Lampman RM, Wahl WL, Cleary RK. Risk factors for postoperative wound infections and prolonged hospitalization after ventral/incisional hernia repair. Hernia: The Journal of Hernias and Abdominal Wall Surgery. 2015;**19**(1):113-123

[31] Novitsky YW, Cobb WS, Kercher KW, Matthews BD, Sing RF, Heniford BT. Laparoscopic ventral hernia repair in obese patients: A new standard of care. Archives of Surgery 2006;**141**(1):57-61

[32] Froylich D, Segal M, Weinstein A, Hatib K, Shiloni E, Hazzan D. Laparoscopic versus open ventral hernia repair in obese patients: A long-term follow-up. Surgical Endoscopy. 2016;**30**(2):670-675

[33] Allison N, Tieu K, Snyder B, Pigazzi A, Wilson E. Technical feasibility of robot-assisted ventral hernia repair. World Journal of Surgery. 2012;**36**(2):447-452

[34] Albanese CT, Rengal S, Bermudez D. A novel laparoscopic technique for the repair of pediatric umbilical and epigastric hernias. Journal of Pediatric Surgery. 2006;**41**(4):859-862

[35] Grover S, Tan GY, Srivastava A, Leung RA, Tewari AK. Residency training program paradigms for teaching robotic surgical skills to urology residents. Current Urology Reports. 2010;**11**(2):87-92

[36] Patel HR, Linares A, Joseph JV. Robotic and laparoscopic surgery: Cost and training. Annals of Surgical Oncology. 2009;**18**(3):242-246

[37] Nolan HR, Christie DB III, Ashley DW. Comparison of attending and resident surgeons' opinions of robotic surgery training in general surgery residency. The American Surgeon. 2015;**81**(8):303-305

7

Parastomal Hernia

Suleyman Utku Celik, Akin Firat Kocaay and
Cihangir Akyol

Abstract

Parastomal hernia (PSH) is a type of incisional hernia defined as a protrusion of abdominal contents through a weakness in the abdominal wall. PSH is the most common and significant complication following enterostomy construction, with an incidence of 30–50%. The risk is higher in colostomies than in ileostomies. Diagnosis of PSH is based on clinical examination or imaging. Most patients with PSH are usually asymptomatic. On the other hand, PSHs may affect an individual's physical function and decrease their quality of life. Surgical repair is indicated in 10–30% of patients with PSH. For repair, no single technique is superior to another. Therefore, several surgical methods have been developed and attempted, including primary repair, stoma relocation, and repair with different types of mesh either via the open or laparoscopic approach. However, high recurrence rates have been reported after repair. Because this is a difficult and problematic entity, the prevention of PSH occurrence is clearly the most appropriate management approach.

Keywords: parastomal hernia, repair, Sugarbaker, laparoscopy, prevention, mesh

1. Introduction

Ostomy creation is usually associated with potential weakness of the abdominal wall, and parastomal hernia (PSH) is a common complication of permanent stoma formation [1, 2]. PSH is a type of incisional hernia located near an intestinal stoma (**Figure 1**). Although PSH is rare (ranges from 0 to 3%) in the early postoperative period, it occurs most commonly within the first 2 years after surgery, with a prevalence of 30–50%, and the risk persists for more than 20 years [2–4]. Ostomy creation and one of its major complications, PSH may negatively affect an individual's physical function and quality of life (QoL) [5]. There is no current consensus on the surgical procedure or optimal technique for stoma formation [1, 6]. On the other hand, high recurrence rates have been reported after repair [1, 3, 7]. Presently, the prevention of PSH development is clearly considered the best management approach for this difficult and problematic entity [1–4, 8]. In this chapter, an overview of parastomal hernia will be presented, and its clinical features, incidence and risk factors, preventive strategies, and surgical management techniques will be discussed.

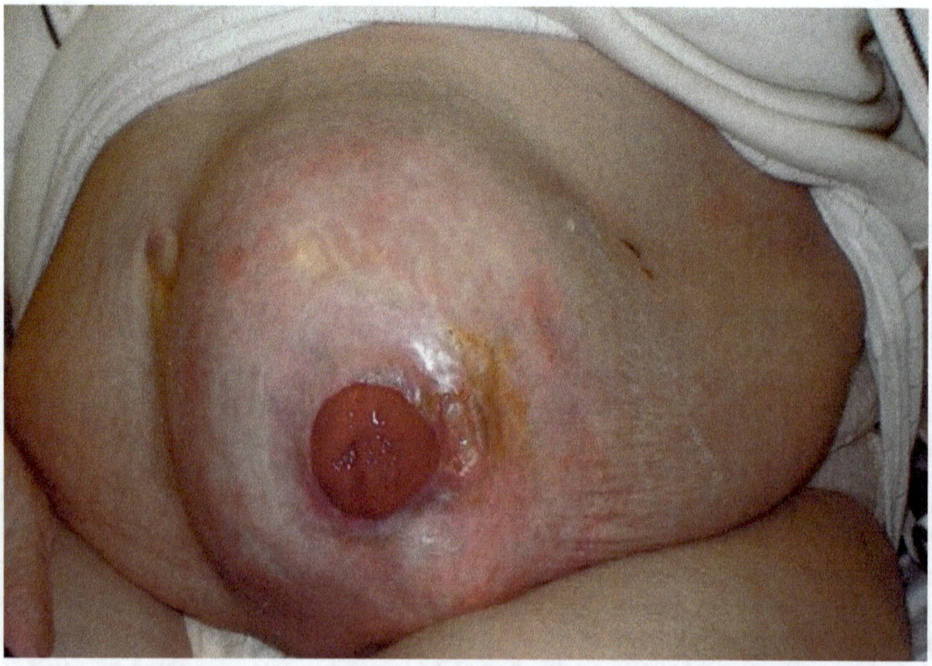

Figure 1. A patient with parastomal hernia on the left side of the abdominal wall.

2. Incidence and risk factors

It is difficult to establish the exact incidence of PSH; however, it has been estimated at 4–48% for colostomies and 2–28% for ileostomies in surgical practice [1, 6] (**Table 1**). This discrepancy is presumably because of the lack of a consistent definition of PSH, variations in clinical or radiological diagnostic methods (which have yet to be standardized), variations in follow-up time, and small or heterogeneous patient groups [4, 6, 9–11]. The use of imaging methods, such as ultrasonography (US) or computed tomography (CT), may have contributed to the high PSH rates reported during the last years because they can detect smaller hernias that are not apparent at clinical examination [2, 4, 6]. Cingi et al. [12] reported a PSH incidence of 52% at physical examination, while it was up to 78% with the addition of CT scan. Although majority of parastomal hernias most commonly occur within the first 2 years, the risk of herniation persists for up to 20 years following stoma creation [3, 6]. The lower rate for loop stoma, especially loop ileostomy, is most probably associated with the temporary nature of loop ostomies and the short follow-up period [1]. Rates of PSH after laparoscopic stoma formation are low and have been reported in the range of 0–6.7% [1, 8]. However, there is some evidence that PSHs are more common after laparoscopic surgery than after open surgery

(18 vs. 2%, respectively; $p = 0.04$), especially when the specimen is removed from the future ostomy site [13].

Development of parastomal herniation has been associated with patient- and technical-related risk factors (**Table 2**). Patient-related risk factors for parastomal hernia include female sex; age >60 years; obesity (waist circumference of >100 cm or body mass index of >25 kg/m^2); smoking; comorbidities such as hypertension, chronic respiratory disease, and ascites; poor nutritional status; inflammatory bowel disease; immunosuppression; corticosteroid use; postoperative sepsis; concomitant incisional hernia; and increases in intra-abdominal pressure [8, 10, 11, 14, 15]. Surgery or technique-specific factors that should be taken into consideration include emergency stoma placement, the type of stoma (**Table 1**), surgical technique for ostomy construction, the diameter of the trephine, or size of the aperture in the abdominal wall, bringing the stoma out through the resection site, placement of prophylactic mesh, and position of the stoma [2, 6, 7, 10, 16]. However, the exact pathogenesis of PSH formation remains unclear. A reduction ratio of mature type I collagen to immature type III collagen during healing is thought to be a contributing factor to PSH formation [8, 17].

Type of enterostomy	**Incidence of PSHs (%)**
Loop ileostomy	0–6.2
Loop colostomy	0–30.8
End ileostomy	1.8–28.3
End colostomy	4–48.1
Laparoscopic stoma formation	0–6.7
Trephine stoma formation	6.7–12
Placement of prophylactic mesh	0–8.3

Table 1. Incidence of parastomal hernias for different types of enterostomies.

Patient-related risk factors		**Technique-specific factors**
Age	Hypertension	Emergency surgery
Female gender	Steroids	Colostomy > ileostomy
Obesity	Immunosuppression	End stoma > loop stoma
Malnutrition	Postoperative sepsis	Stoma aperture size
Smoking	Ascites	Trephine size
Inflammatory bowel disease	Concomitant incisional hernia	Preventing mesh placement
Chronic obstructive pulmonary disease	Increased intra-abdominal pressure	Stoma placement - Transrectal > lateral pararectal

Table 2. Risk factors for the development of a parastomal hernia.

3. Clinical features, diagnosis, and classification

PSHs are mostly asymptomatic; as with other types of hernias, patients generally present with a bulge or a protrusion near the stoma. However, some patients may complain of mild abdominal discomfort or pain, intermittent cramping, distention, difficulty with device application, and life-threatening complications such as strangulation, perforation, and obstruction [1, 5, 7, 9, 10]. Furthermore, in almost all patients with PSH, a significant decline in QoL is observed [5].

As a rule, PSHs are typically diagnosed clinically by history and physical examination [2, 4, 15, 18]. However, in case of doubt, imaging studies such as CT scan and US should be performed as an adjunct to clinical evaluation [2, 4, 10, 12, 18, 19] (**Figure 2**). Assessment of the patient in the upright and supine positions is important for an adequate physical examination. The Valsalva maneuver in the standing position, straight leg raising in the supine position, or coughing can increase the detection of PSHs and should be performed in this evaluation [2, 15, 17]. In addition, Jänes et al. [20] claimed that CT scan in the prone position and placement of the stoma in the center of an inflatable plastic ring produced a stronger correlation with clinical findings than that of conventional tomography.

There are several classification systems for PSH that are based on clinical, radiological, or intraoperative criteria; however, none of the classification proposals have been universally adopted because each has its own limitations (**Table 3**). Although these classification systems may be useful in academic research, there is little requirement for them in clinical practice because assessment, management, and diagnosis are usually based on symptoms and clinical

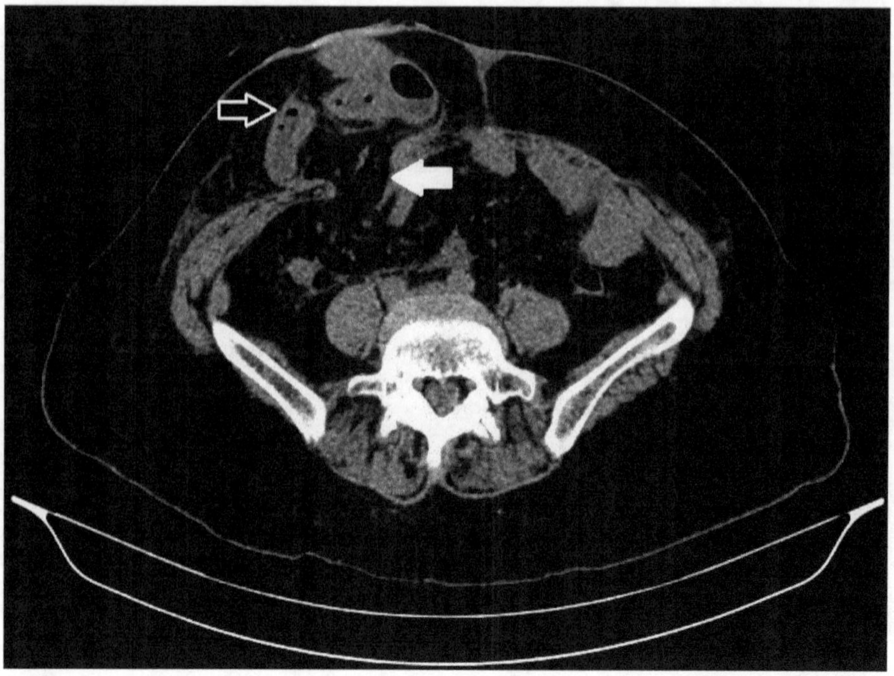

Figure 2. An axial CT scan showing a fascial defect (white arrow) and a parastomal hernia (black/white arrow).

examination. More recently, the European Hernia Society assembled to review the existing classification systems and expanded upon the definitions proposed by Gil and Szczepkowski to include a size cutoff of 5 cm; however, this new system has not yet been validated as a clinical tool [8, 18, 19, 21–24].

Author and year	Classification proposals
Devlin (1983) [22] • Intraoperative findings • Clinical validation: Yes	Type I: interstitial hernia Type II: subcutaneous hernia Type III: intrastomal hernia Type IV: peristomal hernia (stoma prolapse)
Rubin (1993) [23] • Intraoperative findings • Clinical validation: No	Type I: true PSH Type Ia: interstitial Type Ib: subcutaneous Type II: intrastomal hernia Type III: subcutaneous
Moreno-Matias (2007) [19] • Tomography findings • Clinical validation: Yes	Type 0: peritoneum follows the wall of the bowel forming the stoma, with no formation of a sac Type Ia: bowel forming the colostomy with a sac of <5 cm Type Ib: bowel forming the colostomy with a sac of >5 cm Type II: sac containing omentum Type III: intestinal loop other than bowel forming the stoma
Gil and Szczepkowski (2011) [24] • Physical examination • Clinical validation: Yes	Type I: isolated small PSH Type II: small PSH with cIH (without any wall deformity) Type III: isolated large PSH (with abdominal wall deformity) Type IV: large PSH with cIH (with abdominal wall deformity)
Śmietański (2013) [21] • Intraoperative findings • Clinical validation: No	Type I: PSH <5 cm without cIH Type II: PSH 5 cm with cIH Type III: PSH >5 cm without cIH Type IV: PSH >5 cm with cIH P → primary PSH R → recurrent PSH

Abbreviations: PSH, parastomal hernia; cIH, concomitant incisional hernia.

Table 3. Hernia types in different classifications with basis of classification and clinical validation.

4. Treatment strategies

4.1. Conservative management

Most patients with PSH are usually asymptomatic; therefore, they can be managed conservatively [1, 2, 6, 13, 16, 25]. Conservative management is preferred because surgical treatment can be challenging, with no guarantee of success. Patients who agreed to be followed up with nonoperative approaches should be educated about life-threatening signs and symptoms and should be prompted to seek medical assistance to avoid a delay in diagnosis. The uses of stomal-supporting devices, such as abdominal support belts especially while undertaking heavy work during the first year after the surgery, patient education regarding the avoidance of lifting heavy objects, weight loss, diet changes, and abdominal exercises to strengthen the abdominal muscle, are successful strategies for conservative management of PSHs [2, 15, 18, 26]. Unfortunately, despite all attempts, one-third of all patients with PSH require surgical repair [15, 17, 27–29].

4.2. Surgical treatment

Urgent or emergent surgical repair is indicated for patients who develop acute PSH-related complications, such as bowel obstruction, incarceration or strangulation of hernia content, stomal ischemia, fistulization, and prolapse, and for those with chronic symptoms that impair the QoL [1–4, 8, 30, 31]. Other indications are relative and include failure of conservative measures, chronic abdominal pain related to the PSH, ulceration of the surrounding skin, and dissatisfaction with the aesthetic appearance [18]. For repair, there is no single technique that is superior to another [1, 6, 31]. These surgical techniques include local repair of enlarged fascial defects, relocation of stoma to a new site, and prosthetic mesh repair via laparotomy or laparoscopic approach [2, 8, 10, 16, 17, 31, 32]; all are associated with high rates of hernia recurrence (57.6–69.4% vs. 24–86% vs. 6.9–17.8%, respectively) and high rates of overall complication ranging from 24–88% [7, 8, 30, 31, 33].

4.2.1. *Primary fascial repair without mesh*

Primary local fascial repair is technically simple, does not require a laparotomy or dissection, and has low morbidity [8]. However, the results are disappointing, with recurrence rates up to 50%, thus limiting its clinical applicability [3, 4, 7, 8, 30–33]. A systematic review by Al Shakarchi and Williams [7] reported an overall complication rate of 14.1%, wound infection rate of 9.4%, and PSH recurrence rate of 57.6% at a mean follow-up of 30 months (range, 7–65 months). Therefore, primary fascial repair of PSHs has been largely abandoned and should be performed only in exceptional circumstances because of the significantly higher recurrence rate than that of mesh repairs; it should also be performed in patients with small defects for whom there is a strong desire to avoid prosthetic mesh or more extensive surgery [2, 3, 18, 30].

4.2.2. *Repair by stoma relocation*

Stoma relocation is another choice for repair of PSH, and it is associated with a high recurrence rate (range, 24–86%), morbidity rate (23%), and an additional risk of incisional hernia development in the midline or at the old ostomy site of 20% [4, 8, 34]. This technique usually requires a formal laparotomy or peristomal incision, dissection of the PSH along with other parts of the bowel, and mobilization of the intestine to enable stoma repositioning [18]. Although short-term outcomes seem to be favorable, the recurrence rates appear to be significantly high with longer follow-up periods [3]. Hernia recurrence rate for stoma relocation is lower than that for primary fascial repair; however, the complication rate is higher with longer hospitalization [3, 4, 18]. Moreover, stomas relocated to the contralateral side of the abdomen appear to have a decreased risk of subsequent herniation compared with the risk for those relocated to the same side [4, 15]. Patients treated with relocation of the stoma should be carefully selected because this approach may be difficult, especially in patients with intra-abdominal adhesions [18].

4.2.3. *Repair with mesh*

Mesh repair is well established as the method of choice for repairing PSHs [1, 25, 28]. Recurrence rates for PSH with mesh repair are in the range of 6.9–17.8%, which compares favorably to those for both direct repair and relocation [30]. Meshes can be implanted in several different layers of the abdominal wall: onlay, inlay, sublay (retromuscular), or underlay (intraperitoneal onlay). Onlay mesh is placed subcutaneously and fixed onto the anterior rectus aponeurosis. Inlay mesh is placed in the abdominal wall defect and sutured to fascial edges. Sublay mesh is placed between the rectus abdominis muscle and posterior rectus sheath. With an underlay technique (both keyhole and Sugarbaker techniques), the mesh is placed intra-abdominally onto the peritoneum [4].

The advantage of the onlay technique is that a laparotomy is not required. The disadvantages are the high risk of mesh infection and impaired wound healing or superficial skin ischemia [2, 4, 25]. This technique has been associated with an overall morbidity rate of 12.7%, a wound infection rate of 1.9%, a mesh infection rate of approximately 2%, and a PSH recurrence rate of 14.8–17.2%. The sublay and intraperitoneal onlay mesh (IPOM) techniques may be theoretically more effective in preventing recurrent PSH formation because the mesh is located on the high-pressure side of the abdominal wall, and this pressure supports the mesh fixed to the fascia [7, 35, 36]. Perhaps because of this, the sublay and IPOM techniques appear to have lower recurrence rates (6.9–7.9 and 7.2–9.2%, respectively) than that of the onlay technique; however, this difference is not statistically significant (**Table 4**). Although laparotomy is necessary for both techniques, the IPOM technique may have the added risk of adhesions between the mesh and bowel, mesh infection, and fistula formation. Despite the advantages and disadvantages of each technique, there are no differences in recurrence, wound infection, and other complication rates between the methods [7]. The inlay mesh technique has already been abandoned in PSH repair because of the high failure and recurrence rates [30].

4.2.4. *Laparoscopic repair*

Laparoscopic PSH repair techniques have been gaining popularity over the past several decades. According to the American College of Surgeons National Surgical Quality Improvement Program data records, only approximately 10% of the PSH cases are repaired laparoscopically [27]. The main advantages of laparoscopic surgery over open repair are less postoperative pain, reduced rate of wound infection, shorter hospital stay, fast recovery, and the possibility of diagnosis and treatment of other abdominal wall hernias [2, 4, 7, 8, 27]. Additionally, it has been shown that laparoscopic repair of a PSH is both safe and feasible and enables better visualization of the abdomen [15]. Presently, three methods have been described for laparoscopic PSH repair that apply the synthetic mesh intraperitoneally: the modified Sugarbaker technique, keyhole technique, and "sandwich" technique (which combines the first two techniques). In the modified Sugarbaker approach, a mesh is placed to cover the stoma site, fascial defect, and the lateralized bowel segment going to the stoma of ≥5 cm beyond the edge of the defect. When the keyhole technique is used, the bowel is inserted through a 2–3 cm funnel in the center of the mesh. The sandwich repair uses two pieces of mesh; the first mesh is placed in a keyhole configuration, and the larger second mesh covers the first mesh, stoma site,

Author	Technique	Number of study/ patient	Follow-up duration	Recurrence	Complications
Hansson et al. [30]	Primary repair	5/106	27 months[a]	69.4%*	WI: 11.8%*
	Onlay mesh	7/157	36 months[a]	17.2%	WI: 1.9% MI: 2.6%
	Sublay mesh	3/42	12 months[a]	6.9%	WI: 4.8% MI: 0%
	Underlay mesh	4/45	28 months[a]	7.2%	WI: 2.2% MI: 2.2%
Al Shakarchi et al. [7]	Primary repair	7/141	30 months[b]	57.6%*	WI: 9.4%*
	Onlay mesh	13/216	40 months[b]	14.8%	WI: 1.9% MI: 1.9%
	Sublay mesh	4/76	24 months[b]	7.9%	WI: 3.9% MI: 0%
	Underlay mesh	5/65	38 months[b]	9.2%	WI: 3.1% MI: 1.5%

Abbreviations: WI, wound infection; MI, mesh infection.
*Statistically significant.
[a]Median.
[b]Mean.

Table 4. The results of recently published meta-analyses on open parastomal hernia repair techniques.

and lateralized bowel and reinforces the weak point of the lateral abdominal wall using the Sugarbaker technique [2, 4, 37].

For parastomal hernias, recurrence rates are significantly lower for laparoscopic Sugarbaker technique (10.2–11.6%) than for the keyhole technique (27.9–34.6%), as shown in recent studies [30, 37]. Additionally, the laparoscopic sandwich technique has been reported to have the lowest rate of recurrence (2.1%) [38]. In laparoscopic procedures, DeAsis et al. [37] reported rates for wound infection, mesh infection, and other complications (such as ileus, pneumonia, or urinary tract infection) of 3.8, 1.7, and 16.6%, respectively and a conversion to open repair rate of 3.1%. According to the recent studies, there was no difference in postoperative morbidity between any of the laparoscopic procedures, except for recurrence rates [8, 15]. Therefore, it appears that global trends are shifting toward the use of the modified Sugarbaker technique rather than the keyhole technique. Open and laparoscopic repairs also have been found to be comparable in terms of short- and long-term results [15, 17].

Currently, several mesh types are being used for PSH repair; however, available data are insufficient to determine the optimal mesh type and remain controversial [4, 8, 38]. Expandable polytetrafluoroethylene (ePTFE) mesh is the most widely preferred prosthetic material in laparoscopic PSH repair [39]. It is softer and more flexible, has lower shrinkage, and causes fewer tissue adhesions and less fistula formation than does the polypropylene mesh, which has been predominantly used in the past. The only drawback of using ePTFE meshes is the high infection risk when it is used in a contaminated field [2, 6, 39, 40]. Therefore, biological prostheses have gained popularity in PSH repair because of their resistance to mesh infection in potentially contaminated areas [3, 14, 36]. However, it cannot be concluded that biologic meshes are preferred over synthetic prostheses for reducing the rates of short- or long-term complications [36]. Biological grafts are also very expensive and associated with higher rates of seroma formation than those of synthetic meshes [40]. In addition, a recent systematic review showed that biological grafts have recurrence rates comparable to those of synthetic meshes [2, 36].

5. Prevention

The recurrence rate after PSH repair is reported up to 50% even after successful repair [6]. Thus, the prevention of PSH occurrence from the very beginning, at the time of stoma creation, appears to be more rational and ideal approach than repairing the defect [1, 4, 8, 10, 33–35, 38]. This method was first implemented by Bayer et al. in the late 1980s and favorable short- and long-term outcomes have been reported [2, 3]. In view of these encouraging preliminary results, an increasing number of clinical studies have documented the safety and effectiveness of prophylactic placement of mesh. Very recently, four meta-analyses (**Table 5**) have shown that prophylactic mesh application at the time of stoma creation is a promising method and may reduce the incidence of PSH, without an increased risk of mesh-related peristomal complications [33, 41–43]. These results have been evident when obtained using either clinical (6.5–10.8 vs. 28.8–32.4%) or radiological (34 vs. 55%) outcome measures [33, 43]. Mesh reinforcement as prophylaxis at initial stoma creation has also been shown to have a lower incidence of PSH requiring surgical repair (2.3 vs. 8.4%; $p = 0.005$) than that of a control group [33]. However, these four recent meta-analyses demonstrated no significant increases in stoma-related complications such as parastomal infection [33, 42, 43], wound infection [43], stomal prolapse [33], stricture [33], necrosis [42, 43], and stenosis [43].

In one of these studies, Cornille et al. [41] reported that the use of synthetic meshes as prophylaxis resulted in a significantly lower PSH occurrence (23.4 vs. 54.7%, $p = 0.008$) than that for biological meshes (10.2 vs. 15.9%, $p = 0.510$), when the different types of mesh were separately compared with controls (no mesh). In another study, Lee et al. [44] demonstrated a cost-effectiveness analysis and reported that prophylactic mesh insertion might be cost-effective unless the incidence of mesh infection and the cost of the mesh were high.

Another point of interest is the worldwide increase in the use of laparoscopic approach for the prevention of PSHs. As in open intraperitoneal repairs, the modified Sugarbaker and keyhole techniques can be utilized laparoscopically in addition to the sandwich technique [25, 45]. Placement of a mesh using the modified Sugarbaker technique has been shown to be effective and safe in the prevention of PSH [45]. Furthermore, promising new devices and techniques such as the stomaplasty ring (Koring™), three-dimensional funnel mesh, and stapled mesh stoma reinforcement technique (SMART) have been developed to prevent PSH occurrence [46–48]. Despite these significant advancements, the determination of the optimal mesh type, the best position of implantation, and cost-effectiveness are yet to be established.

Author	No. of cases (m - c)	Follow-up duration	Definition of PSH	Incidence of PSH (m - c)	Complications (m - c)
Cornille et al. [41]	430 (217 - 213)	30 days to 83 months	I: 1 study C: 1 study C+R: 6 studies	19.4–43.2%*	6.9–7.0%
Chapman et al. [33]	432 (218 - 214)	Min. 12 months	C: 2 studies R: 2 studies C+R: 3 studies	C: 10.8–32.4%* R: 34.6–55.3%*	PSI: 2.0–1.5% Prolapse: 0.6–2.9% Stricture: 4.5–1.8% PSH repair: 2.3–8.4%*
Cross et al. [42]	649 (324 - 325)	12 months to 5 years	C: 2 studies R: 2 studies C+R: 6 studies	16.4–36.6%*	PSI: 2.2–3.4% Stenosis: 4.9–1.4% Necrosis: 4.7–5.7% PSH repair: 2.5–8.9%*
Zhu et al. [43]	522 (259 - 263)	3–60 months	C: 3 studies R: 2 studies C+R: 3 studies	C: 6.5–28.8%* R: 34.1–54.9%*	PSI: 1.5–3.1% WI: 6.1–8.4% Stenosis: 2.4–1.2% Necrosis: 4.4–8.6% PSH repair: 2.2–8.8%*

Abbreviations: No., number; PSH, parastomal hernia; m - c, mesh - control; I, intraoperative findings; C, clinical examination; R, radiological imaging; min., minimum; PSI, parastomal infection; WI, wound infection.
*Statistically significant.

Table 5. The characteristics and outcomes of four recently published meta-analyses on prophylactic mesh placement.

6. Conclusion and summary

- A parastomal hernia is a type of incisional hernia occurring at the site of stoma formation, with an incidence of 30–50%.
- Risk factors are comparable to those recognized for incisional hernia and include female sex, advancing age (>60 years), obesity, chronic respiratory disease, inflammatory bowel disease, chronic or recurrent increases in intra-abdominal pressure, poor nutritional status, type of stoma, size of the aperture in the abdominal wall, and placement of the prophylactic mesh.
- Most patients with PSHs are asymptomatic. As a rule, PSHs are typically diagnosed clinically by history and physical examination. In case of doubt, imaging studies should be performed as an adjunct to clinical evaluation.
- For open repairs, the use of mesh in a sublay or an intraperitoneal position is favored; in laparoscopic repairs, the recurrence rate for the Sugarbaker technique is lower than that for the keyhole technique.
- Although biological grafts are associated with lower rates of infection, their costs are much higher than those of synthetic meshes.

- Prevention of PSH occurrence from the very beginning appears to be more rational and better approach than defect repair. Therefore, prophylactic meshes can be effectively used in various anatomical locations to dramatically decrease subsequent parastomal herniation without increasing perioperative morbidity, especially in patients with high-risk factors for PSH.

Author details

Suleyman Utku Celik, Akin Firat Kocaay and Cihangir Akyol*

*Address all correspondence to: cihangirakyol@gmail.com

Department of General Surgery, Ankara University School of Medicine, Ankara, Turkey

References

[1] Carne PWG, Robertson GM, Frizelle FA. Parastomal hernia. British Journal of Surgery. 2003;**90**(7):784-793. DOI: 10.1002/bjs.4220

[2] Aquina CT, Iannuzzi JC, Probst CP, Kelly KN, Noyes K, Fleming FJ, Monson JR. Parastomal hernia: A growing problem with new solutions. Digestive Surgery. 2014; **31**(4-5):366-376. DOI: 10.1159/000369279

[3] Kwiatt M, Kawata M. Avoidance and management of stomal complications. Clinics in Colon and Rectal Surgery. 2013;**26**(2):112-121. DOI: 10.1055/s-0033-1348050

[4] Israelsson LA. Parastomal hernias. Surgical Clinics of North America. 2008;**88**(1):113-125. DOI: 10.1016/j.suc.2007.10.003

[5] van Dijk SM, Timmermans L, Deerenberg EB, Lamme B, Kleinrensink GJ, Jeekel J, Lange JF. Parastomal hernia: Impact on quality of life? World Journal of Surgery. 2015;**39**(10):2595-2601. DOI: 10.1007/s00268-015-3107-4

[6] Hotouras A, Murphy J, Thaha M, Chan CL. The persistent challenge of parastomal herniation: A review of the literature and future developments. Colorectal Disease. 2013;**15**(5):e202-e214. DOI: 10.1111/codi.12156

[7] Al Shakarchi J, Williams JG. Systematic review of open techniques for parastomal hernia repair. Techniques in Coloproctology. 2014;**18**(5):427-432. DOI: 10.1007/s10151-013-1110-z

[8] Shah NR, Craft RO, Harold KL. Parastomal hernia repair. Surgical Clinics of North America. 2013;**93**(5):1185-1198. DOI: 10.1016/j.suc.2013.06.011

[9] Helgstrand F, Rosenberg J, Kehlet H, Jorgensen LN, Wara P, Bisgaard T. Risk of morbidity, mortality, and recurrence after parastomal hernia repair: A nationwide study. Diseases of the Colon & Rectum. 2013;**56**(11):1265-1272. DOI: 10.1097/DCR.0b013e3182a0e6e2

[10] Sohn YJ, Moon SM, Shin US, Jee SH. Incidence and risk factors of parastomal hernia. Journal of Korean Society of Coloproctology. 2012;**28**(5):241-246. DOI: 10.3393/jksc.2012.28.5.241

[11] Pilgrim CH, McIntyre R, Bailey M. Prospective audit of parastomal hernia: Prevalence and associated comorbidities. Diseases of the Colon & Rectum. 2010;**53**(1):71-76. DOI: 10.1007/DCR.0b013e3181bdee8c

[12] Cingi A, Cakir T, Sever A, Aktan AO. Enterostomy site hernias: A clinical and computerized tomographic evaluation. Diseases of the Colon & Rectum. 2006;**49**(10):1559-1563. DOI: 10.1007/s10350-006-0681-4

[13] Randall J, Lord B, Fulham J, Soin B. Parastomal hernias as the predominant stoma complication after laparoscopic colorectal surgery. Surgical Laparoscopy Endoscopy & Percutaneous Techniques. 2012;**22**(5):420-423. DOI: 10.1097/SLE.0b013e31825d36d7

[14] Ripoche J, Basurko C, Fabbro-Perray P, Prudhomme M. Parastomal hernia. A study of the French federation of ostomy patients. Journal of Visceral Surgery. 2011;**148**(6):e435-e441. DOI: 10.1016/j.jviscsurg.2011.10.006

[15] Bafford AC, Irani JL. Management and complications of stomas. Surgical Clinics of North America. 2013;**93**(1):145-166. DOI: 10.1016/j.suc.2012.09.015

[16] Hardt J, Seyfried S, Weiß C, Post S, Kienle P, Herrle F. A pilot single-centre randomized trial assessing the safety and efficacy of lateral pararectus abdominis compared with transrectus abdominis muscle stoma placement in patients with temporary loop ileostomies: The PATRASTOM trial. Colorectal Diseases. 2016;**18**(2):O81-O90. DOI: 10.1111/codi.13251

[17] Skibiński R, Pasternak A, Szura M, Solecki R, Matyja M, Matyja A. Parastomal hernia—Contemporary methods of treatment. Polski Przeglad Chirurgiczny. 2015;**87**(10):531-537. DOI: 10.1515/pjs-2015-0100

[18] Mizrahi H, Geron N, Parker MC. Parastomal hernia is a problem yet to be solved. Journal of Current Surgery. 2015;**5**(2-3):151-156. DOI: 10.14740/jcs268w

[19] Moreno-Matias J, Serra-Aracil X, Darnell-Martin A, Bombardo-Junca J, Mora-Lopez L, Alcantara-Moral M, Rebasa P, Ayguavives-Garnica I, Navarro-Soto S. The prevalence of parastomal hernia after formation of an end colostomy. A new clinico-radiological classification. Colorectal Diseases. 2009;**11**(2):173-177. DOI: 10.1111/j.1463-1318 2008.01564.x

[20] Jänes A, Weisby L, Israelsson LA. Parastomal hernia: Clinical and radiological definitions. Hernia. 2011;**15**(2):189-192. DOI: 10.1007/s10029-010-0769-6

[21] Śmietański M, Szczepkowski M, Alexandre JA, Berger D, Bury K, Conze J, Hansson B, Janes A, Miserez M, Mandala V, Montgomery A, Morales Conde S, Muysoms F. European Hernia Society classification of parastomal hernias. Hernia. 2014;**18**(1):1-6. DOI: 10.1007/s10029-013-1162-z

[22] Devlin HB. Peristomal hernia. In: Dudley H, editor. Rob & Smith's Operative Surgery: Alimentary Tract and Abdominal Wall. 4th ed. London: Butterworths; 1983. pp. 441-443

[23] Rubin MS, Bailey HR. Parastomal hernias. In: MacKeigan JM, Cataldo PA, editors. Intestinal Stomas: Principles, Techniques and Management. 1st ed. St. Louis: Quality Medical Publishing; 1993. pp. 245-267

[24] Gil G, Szczepkowski M. A new classification of parastomal hernias—From the experience at Bielański Hospital in Warsaw. Polski Przeglad Chirurgiczny. 2011;**83**(8):430-437. DOI: 10.2478/v10035-011-0067-8

[25] Garvey EM, Harold KL. Parastomal hernia. In: Pawlik TM, Maithel SK, Merchant NB, editors. Gastrointestinal Surgery – Management of Complex Perioperative Complications. 1st ed. New York: Springer-Verlag New York; 2015. pp. 427-441. DOI: 10.1007/978-1-4939-2223-9_41

[26] Thompson MJ. Parastomal hernia: Incidence, prevention and treatment strategies. British Journal of Nursing. 2008;**17**(2):16, 18-20. DOI: 10.12968/bjon.2008.17.Sup1.28145

[27] Halabi WJ, Jafari MD, Carmichael JC, Nguyen VQ, Mills S, Phelan M, Stamos MJ, Pigazzi A. Laparoscopic versus open repair of parastomal hernias: An ACS-NSQIP analysis of short-term outcomes. Surgical Endoscopy. 2013;**27**(11):4067-4072. DOI: 10.1007/s00464-013-3062-9

[28] Brandsma HT, Hansson BM, Aufenacker TJ, van Geldere D, van Lammeren FM, Mahabier C, Steenvoorde P, de Vries Reilingh TS, Wiezer RJ, de Wilt JH, Bleichrodt RP, Rosman C. Prophylactic mesh placement to prevent parastomal hernia, early results of a prospective multicentre randomized trial. Hernia. 2016;**20**(4):535-541. DOI: 10.1007/s10029-015-1427-9

[29] Lambrecht JR, Larsen SG, Reiertsen O, Vaktskjold A, Julsrud L, Flatmark K. Prophylactic mesh at end-colostomy construction reduces parastomal hernia rate: A randomized trial. Colorectal Diseases. 2015;**17**(10):O191-O197. DOI: 10.1111/codi.13065

[30] Hansson BM, Slater NJ, van der Velden AS, Groenewoud HM, Buyne OR, de Hingh IH, Bleichrodt RP. Surgical techniques for parastomal hernia repair: A systematic review of the literature. Annals in Surgery. 2012;**255**(4):685-695. DOI: 10.1097/SLA.0b013e31824b44b1

[31] Târcoveanu E, Vasilescu A, Cotea E, Vlad N, Palaghia M, Dănilă N, Variu M. Parastomal hernias—Clinical study of therapeutic strategies. Chirurgia (Bucuresti). 2014;**109**(2):179-184

[32] Shabbir J, Chaudhary BN, Dawson R. A systematic review on the use of prophylactic mesh during primary stoma formation to prevent parastomal hernia formation. Colorectal Diseases. 2012;**14**(8):931-936. DOI: 10.1111/j.1463-1318.2011.02835.x

[33] Chapman SJ, Wood B, Drake TM, Young N, Jayne DG. Systematic review and meta-analysis of prophylactic mesh during primary stoma formation to prevent parastomal hernia. Diseases of the Colon & Rectum. 2017;**60**(1):107-115. DOI: 10.1097/DCR.0000000000000670

[34] Brandsma HT, Hansson BM, V-Haaren-de Haan H, Aufenacker TJ, Rosman C, Bleichrodt RP. PREVENTion of a parastomal hernia with a prosthetic mesh in patients undergoing

permanent end-colostomy; the PREVENT-trial: Study protocol for a multicenter randomized controlled trial. Trials. 2012;**13**:226. DOI: 10.1186/1745-6215-13-226

[35] O'Neill CH, Borrazzo EC, Hyman NH. Parastomal hernia repair. Journal of Gastrointestinal Surgery. 2015;**19**(4):766-769. DOI: 10.1007/s11605-014-2717-8

[36] Slater NJ, Hansson BM, Buyne OR, Hendriks T, Bleichrodt RP. Repair of parastomal hernias with biologic grafts: A systematic review. Journal of Gastrointestinal Surgery. 2011;**15**(7):1252-1258. DOI: 10.1007/s11605-011-1435-8

[37] DeAsis FJ, Lapin B, Gitelis ME, Ujiki MB. Current state of laparoscopic parastomal hernia repair: A meta-analysis. World Journal of Gastroenterology. 2015;**21**(28):8670-8677. DOI: 10.3748/wjg.v21.i28.8670

[38] Berger D, Bientzle M. Polyvinylidene fluoride: A suitable mesh material for laparoscopic incisional and parastomal hernia repair! A prospective, observational study with 344 patients. Hernia. 2009;**13**(2):167-172. DOI: 10.1007/s10029-008-0435-4

[39] Hansson BM, Morales-Conde S, Mussack T, Valdes J, Muysoms FE, Bleichrodt RP. The laparoscopic modified Sugarbaker technique is safe and has a low recurrence rate: A multicenter cohort study. Surgical Endoscopy. 2013;**27**(2):494-500. DOI: 10.1007/s00464-012-2464-4. Erratum in: Surgical Endoscopy. 2016;**30**(9):4160

[40] St. Germaine N, McCormick J. Parastomal hernias: Laparoscopic management. Seminars in Colon & Rectal Surgery. 2012;**23**(1):31-36. DOI: 10.1053/j.scrs.2011.10.008

[41] Cornille JB, Pathak S, Daniels IR, Smart NJ. Prophylactic mesh use during primary stoma formation to prevent parastomal hernia. Annals of the Royal College of Surgeons of England. 2017;**99**(1):2-11. DOI: 10.1308/rcsann.2016.0186

[42] Cross AJ, Buchwald PL, Frizelle FA, Eglinton TW. Meta-analysis of prophylactic mesh to prevent parastomal hernia. British Journal of Surgery. 2017;**104**(3):179-186. DOI: 10.1002/bjs.10402

[43] Zhu J, Pu Y, Yang X, Zhang D, Zhao K, Peng W, Xing C. Prophylactic mesh application during colostomy to prevent parastomal hernia: A meta-analysis. Gastroenterology Research Practice. 2016;**2016**:1694265. DOI: 10.1155/2016/1694265

[44] Lee L, Saleem A, Landry T, Latimer E, Chaudhury P, Feldman LS. Cost effectiveness of mesh prophylaxis to prevent parastomal hernia in patients undergoing permanent colostomy for rectal cancer. Journal of the American College of Surgery. 2014;**218**(1):82-91. DOI: 10.1016/j.jamcollsurg.2013.09.015

[45] López-Cano M, Serra-Aracil X, Mora L, Sánchez-García JL, Jiménez-Gómez LM, Martí M, Vallribera F, Fraccalvieri D, Serracant A, Kreisler E, Biondo S, Espín E, Navarro-Soto S, Armengol-Carrasco M. Preventing parastomal hernia using a modified Sugarbaker technique with composite mesh during laparoscopic abdominoperineal resection: A randomized controlled trial. Annals in Surgery. 2016;**264**(6):923-928. DOI: 10.1097/SLA.0000000000001684

[46] Guarnero V, Hoffmann H, Hetzer F, Oertli D, Turina M, Zingg U, Demartines N, Ris F, Hahnloser D. A new stomaplasty ring (Koring™) to prevent parastomal hernia: An observational multicenter Swiss study. Techniques in Coloproctology. 2016;**20**(5):293-297. DOI: 10.1007/s10151-016-1452-4

[47] Köhler G, Hofmann A, Lechner M, Mayer F, Wundsam H, Emmanuel K, Fortelny RH. Prevention of parastomal hernias with 3D funnel meshes in intraperitoneal onlay position by placement during initial stoma formation. Hernia. 2016;**20**(1):151-159. DOI: 10.1007/s10029-015-1380-7

[48] Williams NS, Hotouras A, Bhan C, Murphy J, Chan CL. A case-controlled pilot study assessing the safety and efficacy of the Stapled Mesh stomA Reinforcement Technique (SMART) in reducing the incidence of parastomal herniation. Hernia. 2015;**19**(6):949-954. DOI: 10.1007/s10029-015-1346-9

8

Hernia in Ambulatory Surgery Centre

Ivan Šeparović and Goran Augustin

Abstract

Surgical treatment of hernia is one of the most common procedures in general population. Since it was traditionally treated as "non-complex" operation, it is an ideal procedure for ambulatory surgery settings. Ambulatory surgery is superior to in-hospital treatment due to faster patient flow, reduced patient stress, early mobilization, and lower overall costs. Unforeseen hospitalization can be avoided with meticulous patient selection, education and preparation, use of local anesthesia whenever possible, and avoidance of opioids in early postoperative period.

Keywords: inguinal hernia, ambulatory surgery, day surgery, hernia repair, antibiotic prophylaxis, thromboprophylaxis, mesh, hernia sac, laparoscopy, local anesthesia, PONV

1. Introduction

Hernia surgery is one of the most frequently performed surgeries and one of the most fre-quently performed operations in the ambulatory surgery settings. However, setting up and performing hernia procedures in ambulatory surgery often present a challenge both to the sur-geon and to the patient. Only by challenging the unproven dogma, which still exists regard-ing the routine management of outpatients undergoing ambulatory surgery procedures, one will advance current practices in the future. Maximizing the use of minimally invasive technology and new prosthetic devices, more complex surgical procedures can be performed in the ambulatory setting. By reducing postoperative complications related to surgery (and anesthesia), patient care can be improved with reduced costs for the healthcare system.

1.1. Definition

Ambulatory surgery, also known as outpatient surgery, same-day surgery, day case, or day surgery is surgery that does not require an overnight hospital stay, meaning surgery patients may go home and do not need an overnight hospital bed. The purpose of the outpatient surgery is to keep hospital costs down, as well as saving the patient's time that would otherwise be wasted in the hospital. There are numerous benefits of such approach, which are as follows:

- **Convenience:** Usually, recovery at home is easier and more convenient than in-hospital recovery.
- **Lower cost**: With no in-hospital stay, standard hospital expenses (nursing, medications, food, hospital room expenses, etc.) per patient are much lower for outpatient surgery.
- **Reduced stress:** Given its predictable nature and distance from seriously ill patients, outpatient surgery is less stressful than inpatient surgery. Of course, that is especially true for children who are afraid of being away from their parents and home (hospitalism syndrome). Recovery at home also reduces stress in most people.
- **Scheduling:** No emergency surgeries and long and complicated procedures as in in-hospital setting make ambulatory surgery very predictable. With less complex and routine procedures, day surgery unit can generally maintain it schedule.

Ambulatory surgery centers also known as **ASCs** are modern healthcare facilities focused on providing same-day surgical care, including diagnostic and preventive procedures. Hernia procedures, as procedures of "low intensity and high frequency" are ideal for day surgery.

1.2. Historical perspective

Some of the first procedures in general anesthesia fall under what is now called a one-day surgery. Even in 1899, James H. Nicoll in Glasgow Royal Hospital for Sick Children in general anesthesia operated on children, of which 460 were cleft palate and lip, and these children were discharged same day.

In 1912, Ralph Waters based his Downtown Anesthesia Clinic in Iowa, which deal mainly with one-day surgery under general anesthesia. After these early pioneers, interest in one-day surgery was reduced to the 1950s of the twentieth century when centers for outpatient and day surgery started to open in South Africa, Canada, and the United States.

In 1994, about 60% of all surgical procedures in the United States were performed as one-day surgery. In 2001, depending on the hospital, in England and Wales, around 45% of procedures were performed as one-day surgery. The Ministry of Health of the United Kingdom estimates that up to 75% of surgical procedures could be performed in one-day surgery setting [1].

1.3. Patient selection criteria

Probably the most important difference of ambulatory from in-hospital surgery is home recovery with no nursing or medical assistance. Since that means the patient needs to manage himself in postoperative period, his cooperation is essential and his selection and education are very important for outpatient surgery success.

Patient assessment for day surgery falls into three main categories as follows.

1.3.1. Surgical criteria

The major factors that determine whether or not a given operation can be performed on a day case basis are as follows:

1. The degree of tissue damage, and hence pain
2. The extent of blood and fluid loss
3. The extent of postoperative care and complications.

Although arbitrary time limits have been suggested in the past, modern anesthesia allows acceptably rapid recovery after procedures lasting several hours. Therefore, operating time should not be a limit for one-day surgery.

After the operation is completed, there should be no continuing blood loss or requirements for fluid therapy and no need for complex postoperative care, which is difficult to provide in the community.

1.3.2. Social criteria

Although patients will not be discharged from the day unit until they are stable (see Section 5.5), one cannot say that they have completely recovered, especially because it may take several hours to completely regain precise motor control and fine judgment. Therefore, patient needs to have in company responsible and physically able adult person who can help them during first postoperative day, have phone line nearby and react and call for help in the case of complication.

Social factors are an increasingly common reason for excluding patients from day surgery. For example, single, elderly patients without caregivers, patients with little children, etc., but with adequate planning, lots of these limitations can be overcome.

Although surgery increases risk for thromboembolic events, there is no firm evidence to preclude long journeys or air travel, except in patients with risk factors for venous thromboembolism (VTE) who should consider graduated compression stockings and/or LMWH for flights longer than 6 h after day surgery [2].

Moreover, if rapid return to the hospital in case of emergency is not possible, facilities for emergency care must be available at the final destination.

1.3.3. Medical criteria

Selection of patients should be based on their overall physiological status and not governed by arbitrary limits such as age, weight, or American Society of Anesthesiologists (ASA) status.

For any pre-existing condition, the patient may have its nature, stability, and functional limitation should all be evaluated. The conditions should be under control and any medical treatment must be optimized. It is also important to ask whether the patient's management or outcome of the procedure would be improved by hospitalization. Unless this would be the case, surgery should take place in day surgery setting [3].

Regarding age of the patients, both medical and social problems tend to increase with age, but these should be considered independently, without any arbitrary upper age limit [4].

The American Society of Anesthesiologists (ASA) classification is a simple index of chronic health but it is far too nonspecific for use in day surgery settings. For example, patient with ASA III status experiences no more complications than patients with ASA grade I or II. While specific conditions should always be assessed on an individual basis, in general, patients of ASA grade I–III should be suitable for day surgery unless there are other contraindications. Even some ASA IV patients will be acceptable, provided their surgery produces minimal postoperative disturbance, as will often be the case when performed under local anesthesia [3].

Obesity is a challenge, but is not a contraindication in ambulatory surgery. In expert hands, even morbidly obese patients can be safely managed, of course, appropriate resources provided. It is well known that increasing BMI increases the incidence of complications during the operation or in the early recovery phase, but these problems would still occur in the case of in-hospital procedures and would have usually been successfully resolved by the time a day case patient would be discharged. Moreover, short-duration anesthetic techniques and early mobilization associated with day surgery benefit obese patients [5].

Patients with stable chronic disease such as diabetes, asthma, or epilepsy are often better managed as day cases because of minimal disruption to their daily routine.

2. Anesthesia

There are three categories of anesthesia available:

1. General anesthesia
2. Spinal or epidural anesthesia
3. Local anesthesia

For hernia repair, all three types of anesthesia are used. Choice of anesthesia primarily depends on expertise, traditions, and whether the institution has specific interest in hernia surgery. Because of that local anesthesia use varies in different countries, from almost 100% in specialized institutions, dedicated to hernia surgery to 18% in Denmark and a few percent in Sweden [6].

2.1. General anesthesia

Theoretically, general anesthesia is ideal for the operator, providing patient immobility and muscular relaxation if required. Large, complex, or incarcerated hernias can be repaired in the confident knowledge that any unforeseen intraoperative difficulty can be dealt with. In addition, general anesthesia can be combined with regional anesthetics infiltration for better postoperative pain control [7, 8].

General anesthesia has, however, a number of disadvantages. Systemic and sedative effects of the anesthetic can delay recovery so an unplanned overnight stay needs to be provided. This type of anesthesia can result with postoperative nausea and vomiting (PONV) and urinary retention in elderly patients or in children who also prolong recovery. Of course, not negligible is the factor that the use of general anesthesia is significantly more expensive than local anesthesia [9].

The use of endotracheal tube (ET tube or ETT) has been a standard method of providing secure airway during general anesthesia. ET reliably provides a pathway from an outside source of air to the lungs, when placed correctly. ET makes easier to use and adjust ventilator and breathing parameters, deeper levels of anesthesia possible and offers good protection from aspiration and aspiration pneumonia. However, the use of ET is not without risks, such as failed intubation resulting in broken teeth, sore throat, injuries of lips, mouth or pharynx, and damage to vocal cords, can result in hoarse voice, exacerbation of asthma in susceptible people, increased or decreased heart rate, and changes in blood pressure due to nervous system effects, injuries of spinal cord, and even brain damage or death.

Introduction of the laryngeal mask airway (LMA) has been a revolutionary development in airway management over the last decades. It was used clinically in 1981 by A. Brain for the first time and has been widely used in Germany since 1990. Originally intended as a substitute for conventional mask respiration for short periods of general anesthesia, the laryngeal mask is in the meantime used in many areas as an alternative to elective endotracheal intubation as well as an option for controlling difficult airways. Advantages over endotracheal intubation that these devices offer make them excellent choice for outpatient anesthesia. Placement and management of LMA requires lower dose of anesthetic than an endotracheal tube. In addition, the use of neuromuscular blocking agents is rarely necessary; the incidence of airway morbidity is lower; and the use of LMA may facilitate faster recovery and earlier discharge of patients. Two limitations of LMAs are incomplete protection against aspiration of gastric contents and inadequate delivery of positive pressure ventilation. Newer variants of the original laryngeal mask airway as well as an array of other recently developed supraglottic airway devices (SGAs), which aim to address these limitations. Their utility and safety in specific patient populations (e.g., the morbidly obese) and during certain procedures (e.g., laparoscopic surgery) remain to be determined [10]. It is suggested that general anesthesia should be combined with ilioinguinal nerve block for better postoperative pain control and faster mobilization of patients [8].

2.2. Spinal or epidural anesthesia

Great intraoperative analgesia and relaxation can be achieved with spinal anesthesia. Local vasoconstriction in the inguinal and pelvic regions (compensation from lower limb vasodilation as a result from sympathetic block) provides excellent operating conditions with dry operative field. However, spinal anesthesia may produce a prolonged duration of sensory and motor block, and arterial hypotension so discharge from hospital may be delayed. This has stimulated the development of alternative agents, including combinations of local anesthetics and opioids. Intrathecal opioids added to low-dose local anesthetics produce a synergistic effect without increasing the sympathetic block or delaying discharge. Attention to technique, reduction of dose, and addition of fentanyl to lidocaine result in effective spinal anesthesia with rapid recovery and a low incidence of significant side effects or complications [11, 12]. If the limb is protected and adequate support is available at home, patients may safely be discharged with some residual sensory or motor blockade. Of course, patients must receive written instructions about their behavior until normal power and sensation returns and explanations about nature and expected duration of the blockade.

2.3. Local anesthesia

Local infiltration of anesthetics with or without local nerve blocks and system sedation gives excellent intraoperative analgesia, and it is undoubtedly the method of choice for repairing uncomplicated primary inguinal hernias in most patients [13]. Because there is no motor block and no systemic effect (provided sedation has not been given in excess), mobilization is rapid, and the technique is thus ideally suited to ambulatory surgery. Furthermore, local anesthesia administered before the incision produces longer postoperative analgesia because local infiltration, theoretically, inhibits build-up of local nociceptive molecules and, therefore, there is better pain control in the postoperative period.

Today, lidocaine (that provides fast onset of anesthesia) in combination with bupivacaine (provides longer duration of anesthesia—up to 6 h) is anesthetics of choice in hernia surgery. Reduction in onset time has been reported with the addition of sodium bicarbonate 1 mEq per 10 mL of lidocaine [13, 14].

Recent efforts in decreasing concentrations of local anesthetics, reducing local and systemic toxicity, and prolonging their effect have resulted in encapsulation in liposomes, complexation in cyclodextrins, and to a little extent in gold nanoparticles. However, with the promising future of lipid nanoparticles application in biomedical fields, more multicenter clinical trials are needed to be carried out [15].

In spite of everything, local anesthesia is admittedly more demanding of the surgeon, requiring accurate sharp dissection and gentle handling of tissues. Moreover, teaching hernia repair to the trainee with an awake patient presents its own challenges, especially when application of most local anesthetics results in different degrees of local vasodilation, and, after administration of large doses, this contributes to the hypotension Local anesthetics must be respected alsoas central nervous system depressants, and they can enhance respiratory depression usually connected with opioids and sedatives. In addition, seizures provoking concentrations of local anestetics are lower if patient has elevated carbon dioxide in blood (hypercarbia) [14].

However, some patients are unsuitable for local anesthesia. It is certainly not suitable for patients with large inguinoscrotal, incarcerated, or complex recurrent hernias, for excessively obese patients, children, or for mentally impaired patients [7]. Although elderly or medically unfit patients may be ideal candidates for local anesthesia, they may be far from ideal for ambulatory surgery.

3. Preoperative preparation

Preoperative preparation (also known as preoperative assessment) consists of major components:

1. Education of patients and their caregiver about ambulatory surgery settings.
2. Information about planned procedures and postoperative care (important information should be given in written form)—which is helping patients to make informed decisions.
3. Identification of risk factors, optimization of patient's health condition.

Member of the multidisciplinary team, trained in preoperative assessment for ambulatory surgery, needs to prepare patients for day surgery.

Patients ASA grade I or II, younger than 70 years, with unilateral inguinal hernias are amendable for examination, assessment, and treatment in the same day. This is called one-stop (single-stop surgery) protocol. Such protocols are developed for reduction of patient visits to the hospital. Many more hernia repairs and other day case procedures could be carried out using similar protocols [16, 17].

3.1. Fasting

The European Society of Anesthesiologists (ESA) in its guidelines says that it is safe to consume:

- Clear liquids (water, clear tea, black coffee, mineral drinks, and clear fruit juice) up to 2 h before surgery. Milk in large quantities curdles in the stomach and acts like a solid, but smaller quantities are handled like other liquids and are safe.
- Solid food, up to 6 h before surgery.

An operation should not be cancelled or delayed just because the patient is chewing gum, sucking a boiled sweet, or smoking immediately before anesthesia administration, but above is based solely on effects on gastric emptying and nicotine intake (including smoking, nicotine gum, and patches) should be discouraged before elective surgery [18].

Regarding chronic medications, American Society of Anesthesiologists Committee prepared extensive list of medications that are allowed prior surgery [19]. Prophylactic antibiotics are not recommended in laparoscopic or open surgery, except in the presence of risk factors for wound infection based on patient (recurrence, advanced age, immunosuppressive conditions) or surgical (expected long operating times, use of drains) factors [7].

3.2. Thromboprophylaxis

According to the thromboembolism risk stratification of the latest edition of the American College of Chest Physicians (ACCP) guideline, deep venous thrombosis (DVT) risk is low, less than 10% without thromboprophylaxis. For day surgery patients who undergo open or laparoscopic procedure, early mobilization and ambulation are preferred over routinely administered pharmacological thromboprophylaxis.

Of course, a detailed venous thromboembolism (VTE) risk assessment must be a routine practice. Using pharmacological prophylaxis (if bleeding risk is not increased) is justified in patients with VTE risk factor at the time of surgical procedure (for example, a previous episode of VTE) [20].

4. Surgical techniques

The choice of technique used in inguinal hernia repair depends on the following factors.

- **Patient condition:** Open approach under local anesthesia is maybe better choice in elderly patients or in patients in poor health who are too weak to safely have a general anesthesia.
- **Surgical experience:** Not all surgeons are experienced enough in laparoscopic surgery so they are prone to open hernia repair.

According to European Hernia Society, laparoscopic surgery is recommended in patients with bilateral or recurrent hernias after open surgery. Unilateral or recurrent hernias after laparoscopic surgery are eligible for open approach in local anesthesia, if possible [7].

Management of hernia sac during procedure depends of intraoperative findings.

In most cases, it recommended that the hernia sac should be left intact to avoid increase in postoperative pain [21]. In patient with ascites, resection of hernia sac leads to complications such as persistent leakage of ascitic fluid [22].

In addition, injury of the spermatic cord structures should be avoided. In prevention of ischemic orchitis, resection of the hernia sac is recommended with distal hernia sac left *in situ* in the case of large inguinoscrotal hernias. All patients should have long-acting local anesthetic wound infiltration for postoperative pain control [7].

According to traditional teaching, ilioinguinal nerve should be preserved at all times in fear of the supposed morbidity associated with cutaneous sensory loss or chronic groin pain that can follow injury of the nerve. However, most patients reported minimal morbidities following excision of ilioinguinal nerve. Moreover, ilioinguinal nerve excision is an effective and very well-documented treatment of chronic inguinal pain following hernia surgery. Neurectomy of ilioinguinal nerve during operation is associated with a lower incidence of chronic inguinal pain after the procedure according to newer retrospective studies [23].

Surgical experience needed for surgical procedures in ambulatory surgery is not properly specified. However, according to European Hernia Society guidelines, the learning curve for open Lichtenstein repair is shorter than for endoscopic inguinal hernia repair (especially totally extraperitoneal technique) which is between 50 and 100 procedures (the first 30–50 are the most critical). Careful patient selection and adequate surgical training might minimize the risks for possible serious complications in the learning curve of endoscopic surgery.

Interestingly, there does not seem to be a negative effect on outcome when resident instead of surgeon performs an operation [7].

5. Postoperative management

5.1. Recovery

Recovery from surgery and anesthesia is divided into three parts:

1. **First stage:** Duration of the first stage ends when the patient is awake, pain is under control and with protective reflexes recovered. First stage of recovery should be spent in a recovery room with educated nurses—postanesthesia care unit (PACU). Most patients who undergo surgery with a local anesthetic block can bypass the first stage recovery area.
2. **Second stage:** Lasts until the patient is meeting postoperative discharge criteria. Second stage should be in premises near to the ambulatory surgery theatre. Of course, these premises need to be equipped and personnel need to be educated to deal not only with usual postoperative problems (pain, PONV) but also with emergencies (for example, cardiovascular events or hemorrhages). In addition, the anesthesiologist must be in contact to help with problems if they arise.
3. **Third stage:** Ends when the patient has made a full physiological and psychological recovery from the procedure. This may take several weeks or months from procedure.

Since the PACU is high dependency area and may contribute for a significant portion of the perioperative costs, efforts have been invested to develop strategies to skip first stage recovery area. These strategies are variously called fast track surgery.

Fast track surgery uses different techniques in the care of patients undergoing ambulatory procedures. That means the use of regional or spinal anesthesia, minimally invasive surgery, excellent control of pain, and fast rehabilitation (early oral nutrition and mobilization). This type of surgery shortens recovery time by reducing patient stress response and accompanying organ dysfunction.

Effectiveness of fast track surgery generally depends on three groups of factors as follows:

- **Preoperative factors:** Careful patient assessment and selection, careful explanation about the procedure, and what will happen at every stage of the perioperative pathway, including early mobilization and resumption of food and drink.
- **Intraoperative factors:** The use of regional anesthesia where possible, combined with minimal invasive surgery, avoidance of long-acting opioids, nasogastric tubes, and surgical drains. Intraoperative fluid therapy should be goal directed to avoid sodium or fluid overload, and attention should be paid to maintaining normothermia.
- **Postoperative factors:** Effective analgesia that minimizes the risk of PONV and allows early mobilization. Systemic opioids should be avoided where possible and regular oral

(or intravenous) analgesia with simple analgesics (paracetamol and NSAIDs) should be used. Hydration should be maintained with intravenous fluids but discontinued as soon as the patient returns to oral fluids, and PONV should be treated aggressively using a multimodal approach to therapy [5].

5.2. PONV avoidance and treatment

Postoperative nausea and vomiting (PONV) is frequent but distressing consequence of anesthesia. Incidence of PONV can be as high as 80% in high-risk patients with incidence of vomiting about 30% and nausea about 50% [24]. PONV can result in extended postanesthesia care unit (PACU) stay with unforeseen hospital admission so we see that PONV results in a significant increase in overall care costs.

Research in PONV risk factors started in the 1990s. The identification of PONV high-risk patients can reduce the number of potential candidates for prophylactic antiemetic pharmacotherapy, so reducing costs and antiemetic side effects for patients unlikely to benefit.

Several risk factors have systematically proved to be PONV-independent factors [25].

1. *Patient-related independent factors*

- **Female gender**

  It is unclear why female gender is more prone to PONV, especially during menstruation and preovulatory phase of the menstrual cycle. Maybe because of sensitization of the chemoreceptor trigger zone (CTZ) and vomiting center to estrogen and follicle-stimulating hormone (FSH). This gender difference in PONV does not exist in children or patients older than 60 years.

- **Nonsmoking**

  Nonsmokers are almost twice as likely as smokers to have PONV. Chronic exposure to smoke produces changes in liver enzymes that may affect the metabolism of drugs used in the perioperative period and the ability of these drugs to produce PONV.

- **History of PONV, motion sickness, or migraine**

  Patients with previous history of PONV, motion sickness, or migraine are more likely to suffer from PONV.

- **Age**

  In pediatric age, the PONV rate is highest in the 6- to 10-year age group and then decreases with the start of puberty and further decreases with progressing age.

- **Obesity**

  A body mass index (BMI) of more than 30 in patients had been traditionally associated with PONV. Recent findings suggest that PONV risk is not in relation with increased BMI, but in patients with other risk factors, increased BMI may increase chance of PONV [26].

2. *Anesthesia-related independent predictors*

- **Use of opioids**

  Risk of PONV is almost doubled with the postoperative use of opioids. It appears to be more significant total dose than exact type of drug. If the patient already feels pain, the use of opioids does not significantly increase the chance of PONV.

- **Inhalational anesthetics and use of nitrous oxide (N_2O)**

  Volatile induction maintenance anesthesia (VIMA) is associated with lesser PONV than balanced anesthesia using opioids but with no differences in incidence of PONV among the individual volatile anesthetics. Avoiding N_2O, which has emetogenic effect, can lead to reduction in risk of PONV.

- **Duration of anesthesia**

  Increasing the operative duration by 30 min may increase the risk of PONV by 60%.

Although the type of surgery has been identified as a risk factor in numerous reports, its status is still somewhat controversial; the specific procedures implicated as particularly emetogenic sometimes vary among studies [25].

The risk of PONV should be estimated for each patient. No prophylaxis is recommended for patients at low risk for PONV. For patients at moderate to high risk for PONV, regional anesthesia should be considered. If this is not possible or contraindicated and a general anesthesia is used, a multimodal approach that combines pharmacologic and nonpharmacological prophylaxis to minimize risk of PONV should be adopted [25, 27].

Postdischarge nausea and vomiting (PDNV) defined from 24 h postdischarge up to 72 h has an incidence of up to 55% and it appears that it has different risk factors than those for PONV [27].

5.3. Postoperative urinary retention

Postoperative urinary retention (POUR), inability to void in the presence of a full bladder immediately after surgery, is relatively common and can occur in 0.2–25% of patients after inguinal hernia repair [28]. The widely varying reported incidence of POUR reflects its multifactorial etiology and the lack of uniform defining criteria. This complication leads to increased length of stay, increased discomfort, need for invasive catheterizations, and increased costs.

To minimize POUR risk, physician must be aware of preoperative risk factors such as age greater than 50 years, postoperative narcotic medications, concurrent neurologic diseases such as stroke, poliomyelitis, cerebral palsy, multiple sclerosis, spinal lesions, and diabetic and alcoholic neuropathy and over 2 h anesthesia duration [28–30].

History of benign prostate hyperplasia, unilateral versus bilateral hernia repair, body mass index, and laparoscopic hernia repair are also found significant in some studies [28, 31].

Bladder catheterization is the standard treatment of POUR and is recommended in high-risk patients for 24 h under adequate antibiotic prophylaxis. Low-risk patients can be discharged without voiding (see Section 5.5) [30, 32].

5.4. Postoperative management of pain

Postoperative pain experience is affected by multiple factors, such as the type of surgery, age, pain threshold, and expectations. Patients can experience postoperative pain for more than 3 days and have reduced quality of life for more than 7 days after operation [33].

Although many patients continue to experience pain and discomfort after discharge, 30–50% patients do not take adequate analgesia because of misunderstandings and insufficient information. For example, pain in elderly patients is often underrecognized and underassessed. It is important to understand that pain perception and threshold do not decrease with aging and that elderly patients influenced by their attitude and beliefs may refrain from reporting pain. To increase compliance, especially among elderly patients, patients with poor education and those without a strong social network, information on postoperative analgesia should be conveyed both verbally and in written form thus helping patients assimilate information.

The use of analgesics that provide effect with different mechanisms results in synergistic or additive analgesia. That allows lower doses for each of analgesics, so diminishing side effects. Multimodal remains the recommended approach for pain management [34]. Of course, obvious measures to minimize postoperative pain include minimally invasive surgical techniques and the use of regional and spinal anesthesia. Reliance on long-acting opioids may exacerbate PONV and delay recovery and discharge.

Choice of analgesics

- **Paracetamol:** Paracetamol (also available in combination with opioids) is an analgesic with few side effects but with a desired opioid-sparing effect (when a nonopioid is combined with an opioid, the opioid dose can be lowered without compromising pain relief). Oral paracetamol is 80–90% absorbed from the gastrointestinal tract and displays peak plasma concentration within 30–60 min with onset of pain relief after 5–10 min. However, there is a possibility of higher risk of toxicity from intravenous paracetamol in patients with renal or hepatic insufficiency.

- **NSAIDs:** Nonsteroidal anti-inflammatory drugs (NSAIDs) have an established role as effective analgesics for day-case surgery and can, provided there are no contraindications, be prescribed to all patients. To allow time for strongest analgesic effect, NSAIDs need to be use either preoperatively or early during surgery because of slower start of analgesia in comparison with opioids. Use of nonselective NSAIDs or the more selective COX-2 inhibitors in the first 3 postoperative days has been shown to produce adequate analgesia, reduce the need for opioids, and facilitate a faster recovery compared with opioid-based analgesia. Additionally, studies indicate synergistic effects on opioid reduction when paracetamol and NSAIDs are prescribed together [34].

- **Opioids:** Opioids such as fentanyl or morphine can be used for moderate-to-severe pain in the PACU setting. However, incidence of PONV is significantly higher in patients who received opioids and higher in patients who received morphine instead of fentanyl. Other side effects of opioids are sedation, constipation, pruritus, respiratory depression, and urinary retention. A reliance on opioids for perioperative pain management may even cause acute opioid-induced hyperalgesia in some patients. Therefore, multi-modal analgesia is preferable and use of long-acting opioid is discouraged [34].

- **Ketamine:** This N-methyl D-aspartate (NMDA) receptor antagonist provides significant opioid-sparing effects that can be long lasting. Low doses (0.1–0.15 mg/kg) make it possible to achieve this desirable analgesic outcome without the significant adverse effects, such as dissociation and hallucinations [35]. However, one must be careful because the known side effects, such as hypotension, bradycardia, postoperative dizziness, and sedation, can occur thus delaying mobilization and discharge [34].

5.5. Discharge

As mentioned in Section 5.1, there are three stages of recovery. With patient discharge from hospital, second stage of recovery is completed. Patient is fit for discharge when meets discharge criteria that can be medical and nonmedical.

Medical criteria are as follows:

- Stable vital signs
- Orientated to preoperative stage
- Minimal nausea and vomiting
- Controllable pain
- No significant bleeding having regard to the procedure.

Nonmedical criteria are as follows:

- An adult to accompany the patient home and to be with them at home for the first 24 h following surgery.
- Access to a functioning telephone at home.

Physicians experienced in outpatient surgery can use their knowledge and experience to decide when a patient has recovered sufficiently for discharge. Common anesthetic reasons for hospital transfer were inadequate recovery, nausea and vomiting, hypotension, and syncope. Surgical reasons for hospital transfer included bleeding, extensive surgery, perforated viscus, and further treatment. The decision to discharge a patient after day surgery is a major decision because postoperative care and assistance needs to be provided as if the patient is in a long-term hospital stay. Because of that, the use of an objective evaluation system for safe discharge is essential. Post Anaesthetic Discharge Scoring System (PADSS) was developed by Chung et al. at the Toronto hospital, where it has been used extensively to determine when patients can be discharged home safely and it has proved to be a reliable guide [36]. PADSS considers five criteria: vital signs, ambulation, nausea/vomiting, pain, and bleeding. Requirements to drink and void have been removed from newer version of PADSS [32].

5.6. Follow-up

Most surgeons ask that their patients to return in about a week for a follow-up visit. At this time, all stitches will be removed and patient will receive further instructions regarding behavior, workload, etc. To further reduce patient time and expense for travel and free clinic time for new patients, some institutions tend to substitute the standard postoperative clinic visit with telehealth where patients are contacted via telephone, and stitches are removed at their GP office [37, 38].

6. Conclusion

Hernia repair in ambulatory surgery center is a trend that is rapidly evolving and it is logical to expect a further increase in the number of operations, as well as the variety of surgical procedures in these settings. Despite the enormous progress in the field of one-day surgery, there is still room for further reduction in postoperative pain, potential to speed-up recovery of patients with further lowering the costs of treatment(s).

Author details

Ivan Šeparović[1] and Goran Augustin[2*]

*Address all correspondence to: augustin.goran@gmail.com

1 University Hospital Centre Zagreb, Zagreb, Croatia

2 University Hospital Centre Zagreb and School of Medicine, University of Zagreb, Zagreb, Croatia

References

[1] Thomas WEG, Senninger N, editors. Short Stay Surgery. Springer-Verlag Berlin Heidelberg. 2008. ISBN 9783540411017

[2] Philbrick JT, Shumate R, Siadaty MS, Becker DM. Air travel and venous thromboembolism: A systematic review. Journal of General Internal Medicine. 2007;**22**:107-114. DOI:10.1007/s11606-006-0016-0

[3] Smith I. Day surgery for all: Updated selection criteria. Current Anaesthesia & Critical Care. 2007;**18**:181-187. DOI: 10.1016/j.cacc.2007.07.003

[4] Chung F, Mezei G, Tong D. Adverse events in ambulatory surgery. A comparison between elderly and younger patients. Canadian Journal of Anesthesia. 1999;**46**:309-321. DOI: 10.1007/BF03013221

[5] Verma R, Alladi R, Jackson I, et al. Day case and short stay surgery: 2. Anaesthesia. 2011;**66**:417-434. DOI: 10.1111/j.1365-2044.2011.06651.x

[6] Callesen T. Inguinal hernia repair: Anaesthesia, pain and convalescence. Danish Medical Journal. 2003;**50**:203-218. DOI: 10.1007/s10029-011-0888-8

[7] Simons MP, Aufenacker T, Bay-Nielsen M, Bouillot JL, Campanelli G, Conze J. European Hernia Society guidelines on the treatment of inguinal hernia in adult patients. Hernia. 2009;13:343-403. DOI: 10.1007/s10029-009-0529-7

[8] Vizcaíno-Martínez L, Gómez-Ríos MÁ, López-Calviño B. General anesthesia plus ilio-inguinal nerve block versus spinal anesthesia for ambulatory inguinal herniorrhaphy. Saudi Journal of Anaesthesia. 2014;**8**:523-528. DOI: 10.4103/1658-354X.140883

[9] Nordin P, Zetterström H, Carlsson P, Nilsson E. Cost-effectiveness analysis of local, regional and general anaesthesia for inguinal hernia repair using data from a randomized clinical trial. British Journal of Surgery. 2007;**94**:500-505. DOI: 10.1002/bjs.5543

[10] Luba K, Cutter TW. Supraglottic airway devices in the ambulatory setting. Anesthesiology Clinics. 2010;**28**:295-314. DOI: 10.1016/j.anclin.2010.02.004

[11] Urmey WF. Spinal anaesthesia for outpatient surgery. Best Practice & Research: Clinical Anaesthesiology. 2003;**17**:335-346. DOI: 10.1016/S1521-6896(03)00015-6

[12] Goel S, Bhardwaj N, Grover VK. Intrathecal fentanyl added to intrathecal bupivacaine for day case surgery: A randomized study. European Journal of Anaesthesiology. 2003;**20**:294-297. DOI: 10.1097/00003643-200304000-00004

[13] Amid PK, Shulman AG, Lichtenstein IL. Local anesthesia for inguinal hernia repair: Step-by-step procedure. Annals of Surgery. 1994;**220**:735-737. DOI: 10.1097/00000658-199412000-00004

[14] Becker DE, Reed KL. Essentials of local anesthetic pharmacology. Anesthesia Progress. 2006;**53**:98-109. DOI:10.2344/0003-3006(2006)53[98:EOLAP]2.0.CO;2

[15] Beiranvand S, Eatemadi A, Karimi A. New updates pertaining to drug delivery of local anesthetics in particular bupivacaine using lipid nanoparticles. Nanoscale Research Letters. 2016;**11**:307. DOI:10.1186/s11671-016-1520-8

[16] Carty N, Curtis NJ, Ranaboldo CJ. Single hospital visit day case laparoscopic hernia repair without prior outpatient consultation is safe and acceptable to patients. Surgical Endoscopy. 2016;**30**:5565. DOI:10.1007/s00464-016-4929-3

[17] Putnis S, Merville-Tugg R, Atkinson S. "One-stop" inguinal hernia surgery-day-case referral, diagnosis and treatment. Annals of the Royal College of Surgeons of England. 2004;**86**:425-427. DOI:10.1308/147870804506

[18] Smith I, Kranke P, Murat I, Smith A, O'Sullivan G, Søreide E, Spies C, in't Veld B. Perioperative fasting in adults and children: Guidelines from the European Society of Anaesthesiology. European Journal of Anaesthesiology. 2011;**28**:556-569. DOI: 10.1097/EJA.0b013e3283495ba1

[19] Apfelbaum JL, Caplan RA, Connis RT, Epstein BS, Nickinovich DG, Warner MA. Practice guidelines for preoperative fasting and the use of pharmacologic agents to reduce the risk of pulmonary aspiration: Application to healthy patients undergoing

elective procedures: An Updated Report by the American Society of Anesthesiologists Committee on Standards and Practice Parameters. Anesthesiology. 2011;**114**:495-511. DOI: 10.1097/ALN.0b013e3181fcbfd9

[20] Alessandro S, Achille V. Thromboprophylaxis in day surgery. International Journal ofSurgery. 2008;6(Suppl 1):S29–S30. DOI: 10.1016/j.ijsu.2008.12.020

[21] Shulman AG, Amid PK, Lichtenstein IL. Ligation of hernial sac. A needless step in adult hernioplasty. International Journal of Surgery. 1993;**78**:152-153

[22] Overview of treatment for inguinal and femoral hernia in adults [Internet]. Available from: https://www.uptodate.com/contents/overview-of-treatment-for-inguinal-and-femoral-hernia-in-adults [Accessed: April1,2017]

[23] Lik-Man Mui W, Ng CSH, Ming-Kit Fung T, et al. Prophylactic ilioinguinal neurectomy in open inguinal hernia repair: A double-blind randomized controlled trial. Annals of Surgery. 2006;**244**:27-33. DOI:10.1097/01.sla.0000217691.81562.7e

[24] Gan TJ, et al. Consensus guidelines for the management of postoperative nausea and vomiting. Anesthesia & Analgesia. 2014;**118**:85-113. DOI: 10.1213/ANE.0000000000000002

[25] Chatterjee S, Rudra A, Sengupta S. Current concepts in the management of postoperative nausea and vomiting. Anesthesiology Research and Practice. 2011;**2011**:748031. DOI:10.1155/2011/748031

[26] Kranke P, Apefel CC, Papenfuss T, Rauch S, Löbmann U, Rübsam B, Greim CA, Roewer N. An increased body mass index is no risk factor for postoperative nausea and vomiting. A systematic review and results of original data. Acta Anaesthesiologica Scandinavica. 2001;**45**:160-166. DOI: 10.1034/j.1399-6576.2001.450205.x

[27] Chandrakantan A, Glass PSA. Multimodal therapies for postoperative nausea and vomiting, and pain. British Journal of Anaesthesia. 2011;**107**:i27-i40. DOI: 10.1093/bja/aer358

[28] Hudak KE, Frelich MJ, Rettenmaier CR, et al. Surgery duration predicts urinary retention after inguinal herniorrhaphy: A single institution review. Surgical Endoscopy. 2015;**29**:3246-3250. DOI:10.1007/s00464-015-4068-2

[29] Patel JA, Kaufman AS, Howard RS, Rodriguez CJ, Jessie EM. Risk factors for urinary retention after laparoscopic inguinal hernia repairs. Surgical Endoscopy. 2015;**29**:3140-3145. DOI: 10.1007/s00464-014-4039-z.

[30] Baldini G, Bagry H, Aprikian A, Carli F, Phil M. Postoperative urinary retention: Anesthetic and perioperative considerations. Anesthesiology. 2009;**110**:1139-1157. DOI: 10.1097/ALN.0b013e31819f7aea

[31] Sivasankaran MV, Pham T, Divino CM. Incidence and risk factors for urinary retention following laparoscopic inguinal hernia repair. American Journal of Surgical. 2014;**207**:288-292. DOI: 10.1016/j.amjsurg.2013.06.005

[32] Marshall SI, Chung F. Discharge criteria and complications after ambulatory surgery. Anesthesia & Analgesia. 1999;**88**:508-517. DOI: 10.1097/00000539-199903000-00008

[33] Beauregard L, Pomp A, Chinire M. Severity and impact of pain after day surgery. Canadian Journal of Anesthesia. 1998;**45**:304-311. DOI: 10.1007/BF03012019

[34] Tharakan L, Faber P. Pain management in day-case surgery. Continuing Education in Anaesthesia, Critical Care & Pain. 2014;**15**:180-183. DOI: 10.1093/bjaceaccp/mku034

[35] Kamming D, Chung F, Williams D, McGrath BM, Curti B. Pain management in ambulatory surgery. Journal of PeriAnesthesia Nursing. 2004;**19**:174-182. DOI:10.1016/j.jopan.2004.03.001

[36] Chung F, Chan VW, Ong D. A post-anesthetic discharge scoring system for home readiness after ambulatory surgery. Journal of Clinical Anesthesia. 1995;**7**:500-506. DOI: 10.1016/0952-8180(95)90087-X

[37] Hwa K, Wren SM. Telehealth Follow-up in lieu of postoperative clinic visit for ambulatory surgery. Results of a pilot program. JAMA Surgery. 2013;**148**:823-827. DOI:10.1001/jamasurg.2013.2672

[38] Eisenberg D, Hwa K, Wren SM. Telephone Follow-Up by a midlevel provider after laparoscopic inguinal hernia repair instead of Face-to-Face clinic visit. JSLS: Journal of the Society of Laparoendoscopic Surgeons. 2015;**19**:e2014.00205. DOI:10.4293/JSLS.2014.00205

9

All-in-One Mesh Hernioplasty: A New Procedure for Inguinal Hernia Repair

Angelo Guttadauro, Matteo Maternini,
Nicoletta Pecora, Marco Chiarelli,
Valentina Riggio and Francesco Gabrielli

Abstract

Since the 1970s, when biocompatible meshes were introduced with the consequent decrease of recurrence, one of the priorities in inguinal hernia surgery was that of minimizing postoperative chronic pain. All technical variations, proposed during the past years in order to improve patient's comfort, reported a variable incidence of chronic neuralgia. The procedure we describe, applicable to all cases of primary inguinal hernia, employs a smaller pre-cut single mesh that covers all weak areas of the inguinal canal and is enveloped in a fibro-cremasteric sheath, avoiding contact of the prosthesis with neural structures. The new procedure, already performed on 250 patients, aims to improve patients' comfort and to reduce the incidence of chronic neuralgia.

Keywords: inguinal hernioplasty, tension-free hernia repair, hernioplasty technique, mesh for groin hernia, neuralgia posthernioplasty

1. Introduction

A major goal of modern surgery is to achieve better outcomes with less invasive techniques while sparing functional tissue and reducing pain and long-term complications. Pain and restriction of daily activity rank high among patient concerns. The variety of surgical procedures for inguinal hernia repair might arouse suspicion that, because none to date has proven effective, old techniques need to be refined and new ones developed.

In 1974, Lichtenstein revolutionized hernia surgery with the use of tension-free mesh repair that would eventually supplant sutured procedures (Bassini, Shouldice) in which the area of weakness is strengthened by overlapping and suturing the musculoaponeurotic structures of the inguinal canal. Placement of an easy-to-use, biocompatible mesh prosthesis allowed for inguinal hernia repair was tension-free and so could potentially reduce its recurrence [1]. In the Lichtenstein procedure, a prosthetic mesh is placed under the external oblique muscle fascia (**Figure 1**) and fixed without tension to the surrounding musculoaponeurotic structures, thus reducing the rate of hernia recurrence. Later, Trabucco developed a pre-shaped monofilament polypropylene mesh that is inserted under the aponeurosis of the external oblique muscle where it is held in place by intra-abdominal pressure. This sutureless, tension-free technique also entails the placement of a "plug" prosthesis to reinforce the area of weakness of the floor of the inguinal canal after the hernia sac has been reduced in the abdominal cavity (**Figure 1**) [2]. Fibroblastic proliferation through the mesh and formation of fibrin already hours after prosthesis implantation, together with precipitation of collagen, provide for a natural seal of the mesh and tension-free hernioplasty.

Several problems remain, however:

- Persistent postoperative pain that may progress to chronic neuropathic or somatic pain

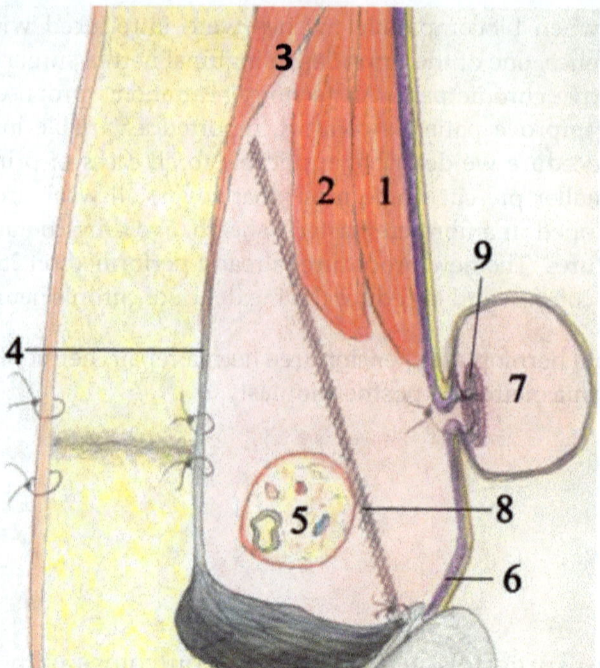

Figure 1. (1) Transverse muscle, (2) internal oblique muscle, (3) external oblique muscle, (4) aponeurosis of external oblique muscle, (5) spermatic cord, (6) transversalis fascia, (7) reduced direct inguinal hernia and sutured transversalis fascia, (8) prosthetic mesh placed according to Lichtenstein procedure, (9) prosthetic plug inserted into point of weakness according to Trabucco repair, (10) pubic tubercle.

- Severe complications, albeit rare, due to plug migration
- Long-term risk of recurrence

Postoperative pain is usually transient and subjective and varies from one patient to another. Somatic pain arises from the presence of a foreign body (prosthetic mesh) which, owing to its size and implantation site, may affect muscles. Chronic neuropathic pain is often debilitating and generally caused by nerve entrapment in the subaponeurotic layer [3, 4], which is why some authors have underlined the need to isolate or transect nerves to prevent the development of chronic pain [5, 6]. Nerve resection is known to alter sensation of the skin area where the nerve has been resected and may induce a neuralgic effect, with the formation of a neuroma that causes chronic pain. Over the years, a variety of "plugs and patches," as well as surgical techniques (e.g., laparoscopy), have been developed without substantially changing the situation [7–10].

In 2012 a newly designed surgical technique began to be standardized for the placement of a pre-cut mesh prosthesis that would reinforce the areas of weakness of the inguinal canal without affecting the nerve structures of the inguinal canal. To better illustrate this system, a brief anatomic review is given below.

2. Anatomy of the inguinal region

The inguinal canal is located at the midpoint of the inguinal ligament that runs between the anterior superior iliac spine (ASIS) and the pubic tubercle. It is about 5 cm long and passes obliquely downward and inward. It is bounded by four walls: anteriorly, the aponeurosis of the external oblique muscle; posteriorly, the transversalis fascia; superiorly (roof), the fascia of the internal oblique and transverse abdominal muscles (joined by the conjoint tendon in 5% of cases); and inferiorly (floor), the rolled up portion (lacunar ligament) of the inguinal ligament. The deep inguinal ring is an opening in the transversalis fascia; it is located between the epigastric vessels and the fascia of the internal oblique and the transverse muscles and reinforced by Hesselbach's ligament. The superficial inguinal ring is a triangular opening formed by the external oblique where it inserts on the pubic crest and the pubic tubercle. It is bounded on either side by the margins of the opening in the aponeurosis, the crura of the ring. Lying superficial to the inguinal aponeurosis and deep to the superficial abdominal ring is Colles' ligament (reflected inguinal ligament), a triangular fibrous connective tissue band running from the pubic bone and lacunar ligament medially and upward to the linea alba [11–13].

The posterior wall of the inguinal canal is reinforced laterally by Hesselbach's (interfoveolar) ligament, medially by the conjoint tendon, and the reflected part of Colles' ligament at the distal end of Henle's ligament (formed by the union of the inferior terminal fibers of the aponeurosis of the transverse muscle and the iliopubic band) and is present only in the central part of the transversalis fascia. This oval area is particularly weak between the lower edge of the aponeurosis of the transverse muscle superiorly, the iliopubic band (thickening of the transversalis fascia near the inguinal ligament) inferiorly, Henle's ligament at the medial end, the junction of the inferior edge of the transverse muscle, and the iliopubic band at the lateral end (**Figure 2**) [11–13].

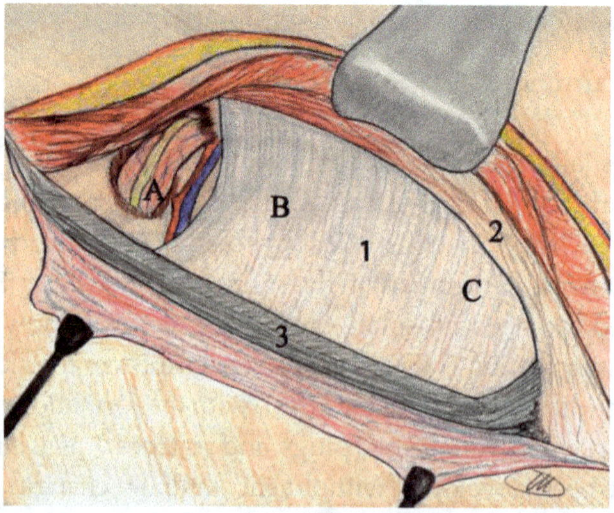

Figure 2. (1) Transversalis fascia (inguinal hiatus), (2) falx inguinalis, (3) inguinal ligament (iliopubic band), (A) lateral fossa (origin of external oblique inguinal hernia), (B) middle fossa (origin of direct inguinal hernia), (C) medial fossa (origin of internal oblique inguinal hernia.

This area of weakness comprises the deep inguinal ring, the site of indirect hernias, the area underlying it, and the site of direct hernias. Topographically, beneath the transversalis fascia, the inferior epigastric vessels run vertically and medially to the deep inguinal ring. Medial to the epigastric vessels and passing outward and downward is the remnant of the umbilical artery. Based on their relationship with the epigastric vessels and the remnant of the umbilical artery (**Figure 3**), three types of hernia can be distinguished:

1. External oblique hernia originates from the deep inguinal ring in an area of weakness termed the lateral fossa.

2. Direct hernia originates from an aperture in the posterior wall of the inguinal canal between the epigastric vessels and the remnant umbilical artery in an area of weakness termed the middle fossa.

3. Internal oblique hernia protrudes medially to the site of direct hernia in an area of weakness between the remnant of the umbilical artery and the urachus, termed the medial fossa. This type of hernia occurs rarely owing to the protective effect of the conjoint tendon, Colles' ligament, and Henle's ligament.

This universally recognized classification of inguinal hernia was recently simplified by the European Hernia Society into two areas of weakness of the inguinal canal floor: the medial area (direct hernias) and the lateral area (indirect hernias) [14].

Detailed anatomic study of the inguinal region shows how the transversalis fascia, together with the aponeurosis of the oblique internal and transverse abdominal muscles, by virtue of their anatomic structure and function, works to retain the content of the abdominal cavity. The aponeurosis of the external oblique muscle appears to have two roles: to cover and to oppose intra-abdominal pressure. In 1884 Edoardo Bassini conceived of a method to reinforce

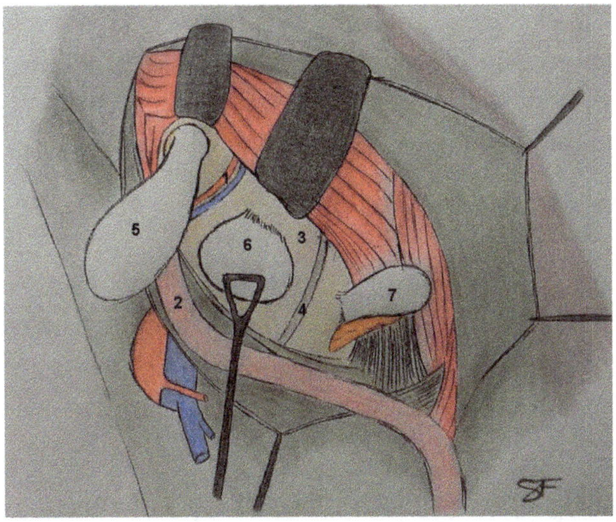

Figure 3. (1) Epigastric vessels, (2) spermatic cord, (3) transversalis fascia, (4) remnant of umbilical artery, (5) external oblique inguinal hernia, (6) direct inguinal hernia, (7) internal oblique inguinal hernia.

the wall using a triple layer in which the transversalis fascia, along with the internal oblique and the transverse muscles, was sutured to the posterior border of the inguinal (Poupart's) ligament. The drawback to this technique was that tension on the sutures led to high rates of hernia recurrence. To demonstrate the retainment capability of the transversalis fascia, Bassini showed that incidence of recurrence was higher when a double layer comprising only the internal oblique and the transverse muscles was employed to repair the defect. Later, Lichtenstein and Trabucco independently understood the need to reinforce the wall weakness using instead of sutures a mesh prosthesis with or without placing a "plug" in the weak point of the transversalis fascia. The drastic reduction in recurrence rates with the use of these techniques has made prosthesis hernioplasty the gold standard in inguinal hernia repair [1, 2].

Observing the anatomy of the transversalis fascia, we can imagine it as a thin layer lining the abdominal cavity, contracting relationships with the muscles and aponeurotic and bony structures. Cephalad fuses with the diaphragmatic fascia, in contact with the lower ribs, the first lumbar vertebrae, and the lumbodorsal fascia. Inferolaterally, it is continuous with the psoas fascia and the quadratus lumborum muscles and anteriorly with the rectus abdominis muscles and the aponeurosis of the transverse muscle. The image is that of a sac hung on the musculoaponeurotic and bony structures of the upper abdomen, with posterior and lateral connections in which the only area of passage is the semicircular arch of Douglas. The transversalis fascia then thickens medially (Henle's ligament) at the lateral concave edge (he called it the falx inguinalis) which inserts at its base in Cooper's ligament and anteriorly attaches to the conjoint tendon [11–13].

More lateral to the arch of Douglas is a thickening that continues to Hesselbach's (interfoveolar) ligament and inserts between the two fossas, the superficial inguinal ring and the medial fossa. It then inserts in the inguinal ligament after having circled the deep inguinal ring inferiorly. More laterally, the transversalis fascia forms a U-shaped sling around the ring and is continuous with the internal spermatic fascia. The so-called transversalis fascial sling, on contraction of the transverse muscle due to increased intra-abdominal pressure, is flattened at its base, producing partial closure of the ring. The transversalis fascia performs a containing function by virtue of its bony and musculoaponeurotic attachments, particularly in the upper abdomen, attachment of Henle's ligament to Cooper's ligament and Hesselbach's ligament, and its attachment to the transverse muscle (transversalis fascial sling) and valve mechanism.

Other structures that assist in this function include:

- The internal oblique muscle surrounding the deep inguinal ring superiorly and then forming the medial wall of the inguinal canal. Contraction of the transversus abdominis causes this structure to move down toward the inguinal (Keith) ligament in a kind of protective shutter mechanism, which reinforces the weakest area of the groin on elevation of intra-abdominal pressure.
- The transverse muscle, which forms the medial wall of the inguinal canal and, together with the internal oblique muscle, unites in the conjoint tendon. The conjoint tendon then forms a lateral concavity and inserts on the pubic symphysis, the pubic tubercle, and Cooper's ligament. Posteriorly, it fuses with Henle's ligament (falx inguinalis). When the transverse muscle contracts, the deep inguinal ring narrows via the action of Hesselbach's ligament (Lytle's sling), another protective mechanism.
- Colles' ligament is made of fibers of the aponeurosis of the contralateral external oblique muscle that crosses at the midline.

The falx inguinalis, together with the inguinal ligament, forms the curved upper edge of the inguinal hiatus; its base is formed by the inguinal ligament (**Figure 2**). In healthy conditions, the falx inguinalis and the transversalis fascia contribute synergistically to retainment of the walls of the inguinal canal [11–13].

Three principal nerve structures pass through the inguinal canal:

1. The iliohypogastric nerve (anterior branch) runs along the internal oblique muscle, parallel and cranial to the spermatic cord; it exits the inguinal canal through a small aperture above the superficial inguinal ring.
2. The ilioinguinal nerve runs along the anterosuperior border of the spermatic cord between the cremasteric fibers.
3. The genital branch of the genitofemoral nerve enters the inguinal canal medial to the deep inguinal ring and runs along the posterolateral cremasteric fascia together with the external spermatic vessels [11–13].

2.1. Pathophysiological aspects

Changes in strength and resistance of anatomical structures, often associated with congenital or acquired degenerative disorders, and remodeling of collagen and elastic fibers can lead to widening of the deep inguinal ring and weakening of the posterior wall of the inguinal canal by increased intra-abdominal pressure. The abdominal cavity can be compared to a container holding a dense, viscous content. Since its walls are subject to the laws of plasticity, the content of the abdominal cavity exerts a force per unit area perpendicularly to a surface, commonly defined as pressure. An imbalance between the force of intra-abdominal pressure and resistance of the inguinal wall at an area of weakness of the inguinal canal can result in plastic deformation that will increase even when the pressure remains unchanged [15]. It is this deformation at the points of weakness of the transversalis fascia that leads to its weakening.

The work by Wegh and Read showed that the fascia of hernia patients had low hydroxyproline content [16]. Histology demonstrated in many cases degeneration of collagen and elastic fibers in the musculoaponeurosis of the transverse muscle, like that seen in patients with Marfan syndrome [17, 18], apparently due to collagen catabolism because of a metabolic defect [18]. The use of prosthetic material that can promote rapid fibroblast proliferation is therefore required for reinforcing the inguinal wall and renders its resistance enough to ensure mesh stability after the patient has left the operating table, assumes the upright position, and begins to go about his daily activities.

Lichtenstein procedures are performed in part directly on the transversalis fascia since the mesh is placed in the subaponeurotic space (anterior wall of the inguinal canal) [1], and Trabucco procedures involve the floor of the inguinal canal through the application of plugs. The use of isolated plugs does not reduce the risk of recurrence at the site of insertion nor recurrence at other sites due to differences in the distribution of pressure. Hence, there is a need to apply also a prosthetic mesh to reinforce the aponeurosis of the external oblique muscle [2]. The support mechanism is similar to that provided by hernia support garments that apply targeted compression to prevent failure of the inguinal canal floor due to elevation of intra-abdominal pressure.

The absence of tension on the musculoaponeurotic layer after application of a prosthetic mesh under the anterior wall of the inguinal canal has reduced hernia recurrence rates; however, this type of mesh can cause pain due to contact with the musculoaponeurotic and nerve structures or induce a foreign body sensation due to wrinkling of the mesh. Analysis of hernia recurrence causes shows that they always occur in an area beneath a subaponeurotic mesh that has become well integrated with the anterior wall of the inguinal canal. In a review of 1276 patients operated on for hernia recurrence, Lichtenstein found a hernia defect near the pubic tubercle in 47% of cases, at the deep inguinal ring in 40%, and involving the entire suture in 13% [1].

This gave rise to the idea of a tension-free mesh prosthesis designed to provide direct reinforcement of the entire area of weakness of the inguinal canal floor, thus restoring its normal function. In addition, a technique was developed to apply a mesh that would not interfere with nerves and muscles in the area. Mesh shape and size were derived from repeated measurement of the inguinal canal floor for targeted application. No isolated plugs or subaponeurotic patches are needed. The mesh conforms to anatomy, with the less use of foreign body material, thus reducing the risk of pain and increasing patient comfort.

Furthermore, the presence of a missed hernia sac, which may be the cause of early hernia recurrence after a Lichtenstein or Trabucco procedure, is no longer possible. The areas of weakness of the transversalis fascia at the floor of the inguinal canal are contemporaneously reinforced by apposition of a single prosthetic mesh designed to conform to the anatomy and function of the inguinal canal. The resulting rapid integration of fibroblasts into the mesh and the transversalis fascia strengthens the new wall, rendering the entire area of weakness of the inguinal canal floor more resistant to weakening under elevated intra-abdominal pressure.

3. Surgical technique

A skin incision is made, the aponeurosis of the external oblique muscle is opened, and the spermatic cord is identified. The subaponeurotic nerves (iliohypogastric and ilioinguinal nerves) need not be identified. Using a diathermy coagulator, a longitudinal medial incision is made along the cremasteric muscle and external spermatic cord fascia (fibrous cremasteric sheath); these are then separated from the spermatic cord to the inguinal ligament. The cremaster muscle, a continuation of the internal oblique abdominal muscle, arises at the pubic tubercle and the inguinal ligament. It forms the middle covering layer of the spermatic cord between the external and internal spermatic fascias, as it passes through the inguinal canal and distally to the common tunica vaginalis, an extroflexion of the transverse fascia.

The medial borders of the cremasteric sheath are grasped with Klemmer clamps (**Figure 4**), and the hernia sac is identified and separated from the spermatic cord. In direct or internal oblique inguinal hernia, the sac should be isolated from the surrounding anatomical structures and the transversalis fascia up to its neck when present. The area of weakness is then flattened by plicating the transversalis fascia. The deep internal inguinal ring is then prepared for applying section A of the mesh (**Figure 5**). In external oblique inguinal hernia, the hernia sac should be freed from the deep inguinal ring so that it can be completely reduced in the abdominal cavity. If present, a

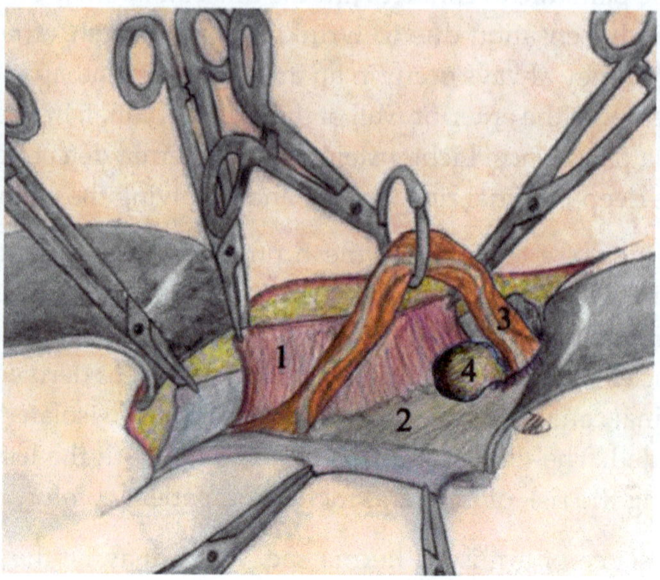

Figure 4. (1) Cremasteric sheath, (2) transversalis fascia, (3) spermatic cord, (4) external oblique inguinal hernia.

voluminous prehernia lipoma can be resected or reduced in the abdominal cavity together with the hernia sac. If necessary, the deep inguinal ring is then narrowed with resorbable interrupted sutures. In all cases, the posterior wall is reinforced with the prosthetic mesh, as shown in **Figure 5**.

This innovative, semiresorbable pre-cut mesh (70% polyglycolic acid and 30% polypropylene) is designed to reinforce the entire floor of the inguinal canal. It is shaped to conform to anatomy without the risk of wrinkling or need to trim it. Polypropylene is noted for its ability to induce an inflammatory fibrous reaction that promotes rapid, firm adhesion of the mesh onto tissues [19]. The mesh is available as a large-pore woven mesh that promotes infiltration and integration of connective tissue [16, 20, 21]. Less susceptible to bacterial colonization, the mesh can be left in place in case of infection [20, 22, 23].

Section A of the mesh is applied to surround the spermatic cord contents and form a cone around them by overlapping the two tails (A1 and A2). The length of the tails can be shortened to adjust the opening of the cone apex to the diameter of the spermatic cord. If present, diffuse lipomatosis

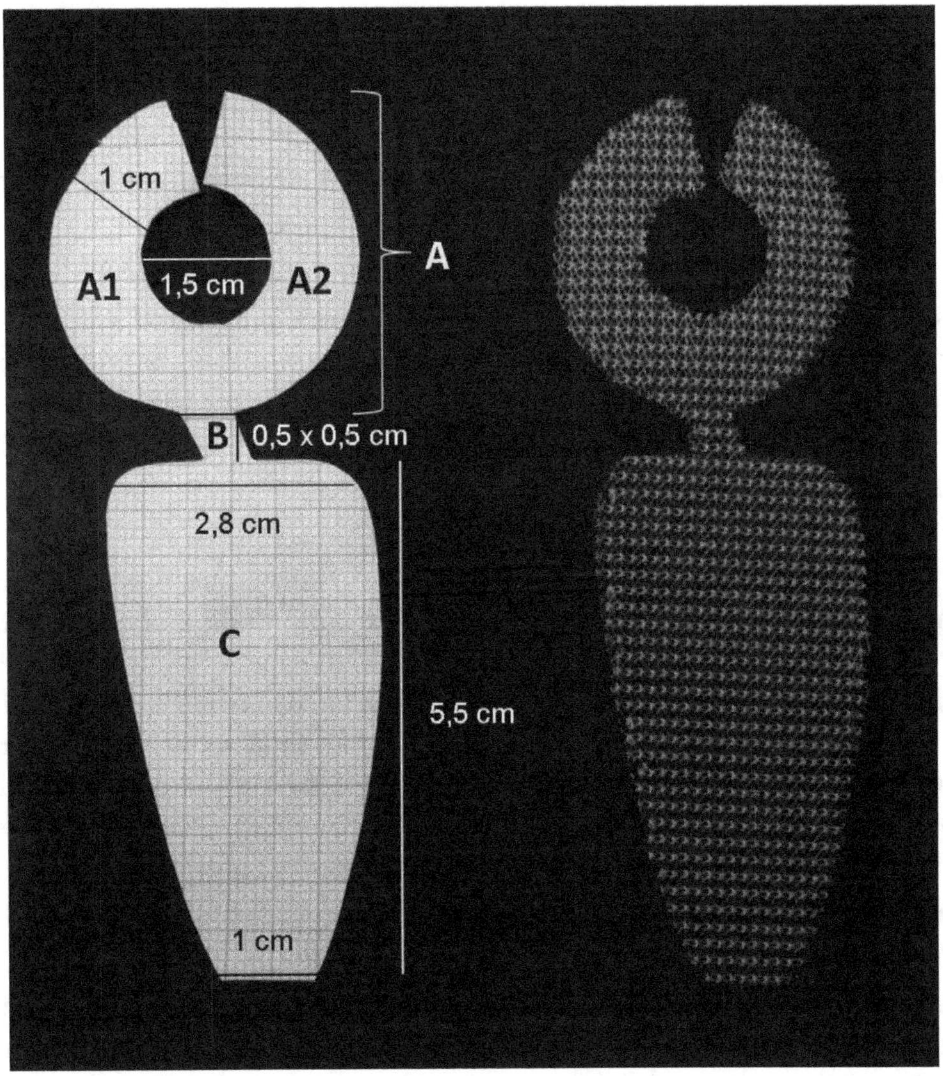

Figure 5. "All-in-one mesh" device.

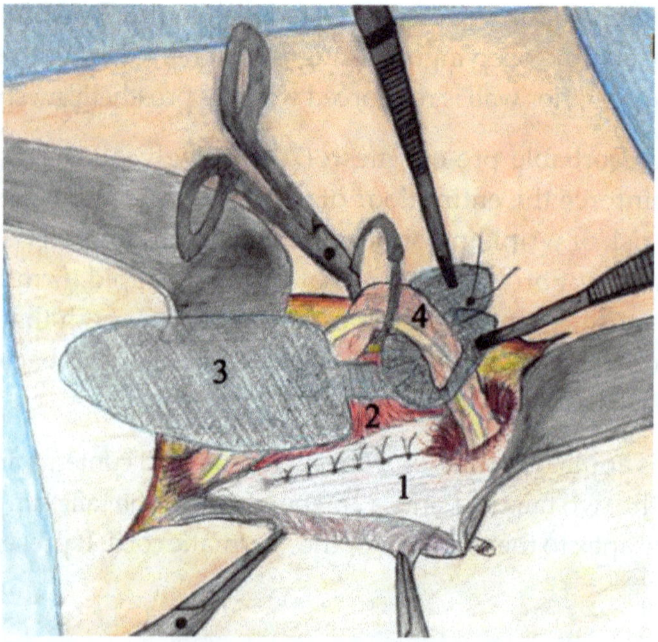

Figure 6. (1) Transversalis fascia after flattening the direct inguinal hernia, (2) isolation of the cremasteric sheath, (3) prosthetic mesh reinforcing the inguinal hiatus, (4) spermatic cord.

of the spermatic cord can be resected. The cone is closed with a suture tying the overlapping tails. While the assistant elevates the spermatic cord with Bottini forceps, the surgeon inserts the prosthetic ring into the deep inguinal ring using two anatomic forceps (**Figure 6**).

The cone serves to strengthen the area of weakness at the deep inguinal ring. When inserted into the ring, the cone depth is such that the implant does not interfere with or compromise the many underlying vessels, including the iliac vein medial to the artery and collateral vessels. Bendavid reported that the distance between the iliac vein and the transversalis fascia at the deep inguinal ring is between 0.8 and 1.2 cm [24]. A plug inserted any deeper would certainly comprise vessel function.

Sections B and C of the mesh are placed on the transversalis fascia. Section B connects section A in a medial angle to section C, which covers the entire floor of the inguinal canal and reinforces the middle and the medial fossa. So applied, the mesh sits laterally with its lesser convexity abutting the concavity of the inguinal ligament and extends medially to the conjoint tendon or above it, depending on the length of the canal, so as to avoid mesh wrinkling. A smooth mesh surface prevents the formation of dead spaces that delay fibroblast infiltration to the site and increase the risk of mesh-related infection and hernia recurrence. The distal end of section C (about 1 cm) is fixed to the pubic tubercle (not the periosteum) using resorbable suture (**Figure 7**). The shape of the mesh is configured so that it can be used for left- and right-sided inguinal hernia repair.

The medial edge of the previously identified cremasteric muscle is retrieved and sutured to the musculoaponeurotic structures using a running resorbable suture to cover the mesh (**Figure 8**). The cremaster serves only as a cover to prevent contact between the spermatic cord and the underlying mesh. If the muscle is injured during dissection, it can be repaired with

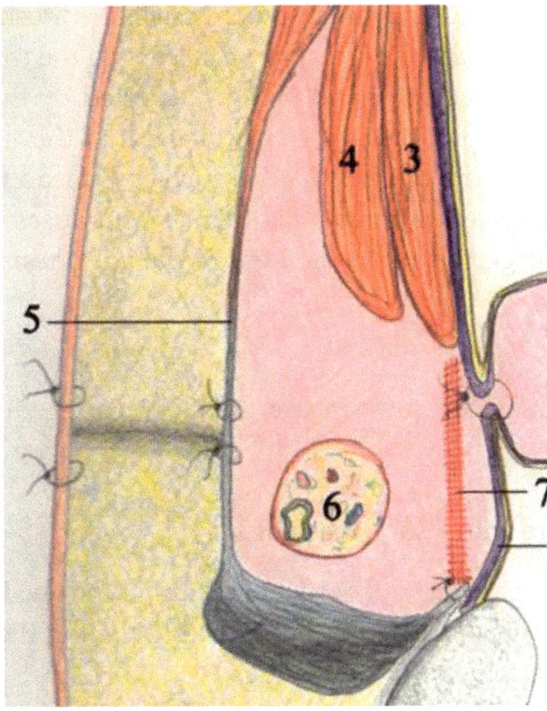

Figure 7. (1) Transversalis fascia, (2) reduced direct inguinal hernia flattened by suturing the transversalis fascia, (3) transverse muscle, (4) internal oblique muscle, (5) aponeurosis of the external oblique muscle, (6) spermatic cord, (7) all-in-one mesh placed as described in the text. The special mesh configuration allows for deployment in left and right hernioplasty.

a resorbable suture. The spermatic cord is returned to its natural position, and the external oblique aponeurosis is closed over the cord with interrupted resorbable sutures, as are the superficial layers.

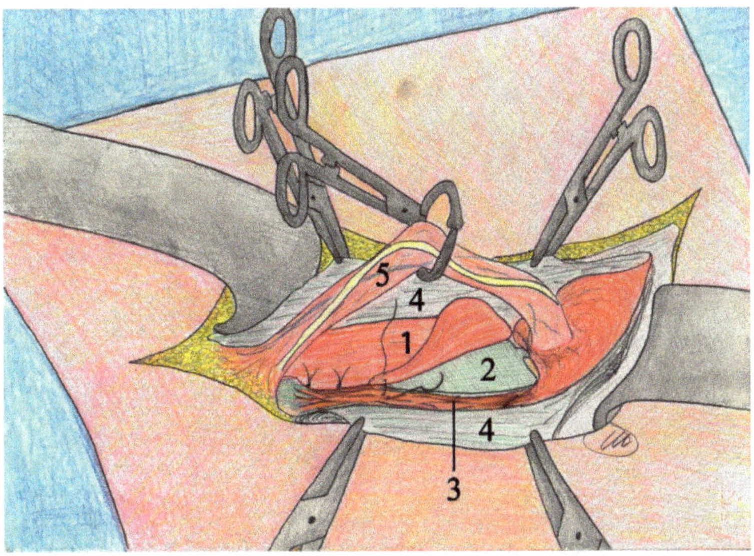

Figure 8. (1) Cremaster, (2) prosthetic mesh, (3) musculoaponeurotic layer, (4) external oblique muscle fascia, (5) spermatic cord.

Fixed between the deep inguinal ring and the pubic tubercle, the mesh reinforces the posterior inguinal wall as it extends between the cremaster muscle and the transversalis fascia. The spermatic cord, subaponeurotic structures, and pressure exerted by the tissues compress it. Rapid fibroblast infiltration of the prosthesis incorporates it into the tissues to form a triple retaining layer, without the formation of dead space which could lead to the development of hematoma and/or seroma or nerve entrapment, all of which are causes of chronic pain that is notoriously difficult to treat. Surgery is performed with local anesthesia [25].

3.1. Advantages

Compared with other techniques currently in use, this novel procedure has the following advantages:

1. A relatively simple procedure with a short learning curve.
2. Shorter operating time and greater ease of execution, without the need to isolate nerves, prepare the site for subaponeurotic placement, trim the mesh, fix it to the surrounding musculoaponeurotic structures, or apply one or more plugs.

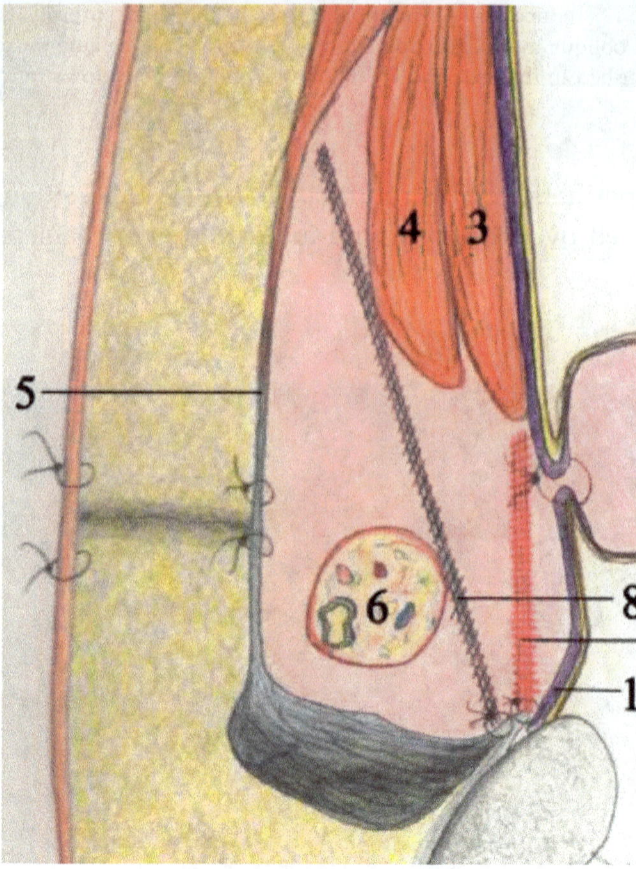

Figure 9. (1) Transversalis fascia, (2) reduced direct inguinal hernia flattened by suturing the transversalis fascia, (3) transverse muscle, (4) internal oblique muscle, (5) aponeurosis of the external oblique muscle, (6) spermatic cord, (7) all-in-one mesh placed as described in the text, (8) mesh prosthesis placed according to Lichtenstein procedure or modifications thereof.

3. Reduced surgical trauma, with no or minimal postoperative pain and rapid return to activities of daily living.
4. Minimal use of mesh material and elimination of problems related to mesh wrinkling.
5. Early hospital discharge.
6. Reduced risk of chronic neuropathic or somatic pain caused by contact of mesh prosthesis with nerves and surrounding musculoaponeurotic structures.
7. No plugs used; no risk of plug migration.
8. Potential reduction of hernia recurrence since the mesh covers the entire area of weakness of the floor of the inguinal canal and does not come into contact with the overlying layer, as occurs with the Lichtenstein and Trabucco procedures (**Figure 9**).

4. Personal case

4.1. Population

We considered a cohort of patients suffering from primary unilateral inguinal hernia that underwent the "all-in-one" mesh hernioplasty technique consecutively, at our institution. Hernias were divided according to the European Hernia Society criteria (**Table 1**). The work described has been carried out in accordance with the code of ethics of the World Medical Association. Written informed consent was obtained from each patient included in the study. All data of the cohort were registered in a specific database. Spinal anesthesia was adopted, and 2.0 g cefazolin was administrated intravenously over 30 minutes before the incision for all patients, and the procedure was performed on a 1-day surgery basis. From September 2012 to August 2015, we treated 250 adult patients for primary inguinal hernia, 241 males and 9 females with an average age of 61.7 years (range, 22–90).

4.2. Follow-up

Postoperative pain was gauged on the ward by a surgeon of the team. At discharge, all patients received a data sheet designed for the evaluation of postoperative pain using visual analogue scale (VAS) score, quantity of pain medication, and any postoperative discomfort. The patient's discomfort was assessed in terms of limitation of daily activities during the postoperative period, and return to work, and sports. Patients were asked for an overall opinion on the operation, on the postoperative period, and on the final result. These data were recorded by patients themselves on data sheet after 1, 2, and 3 weeks from discharge. The first clinical evaluation was made 7 days after surgery by a member of the surgical team. The second and third week interviews were made on the phone. The postoperative data registered by patients were collected. Follow-up, made to evaluate local signs, any kind of chronic pain, any sensation of foreign body, and recurrence, took place at 3, 6, 12, 18, and 24 months after surgery in the outpatient clinic by a surgeon of the team. All patient data were collected in a database of our institution.

Type	No. of patients
P L1M0F0	53
P L2M0F0	53
P L3M0F0	33
P L2M2F0	24
P L1M1F0	20
P L0M2F0	16
P L0M1F0	12
P L3M3F0	12
P L1M2F0	12
P L0M3F0	8
P L1M3F0	3
P L2M1F0	2
P L2M3F0	1
P L3M2F0	1

Table 1. Hernias were divided according to the European hernia society classification.

4.3. Results

Three (1.2%) patients complained of urinary retention, 2 (0.8%) of orchitis, and 14 (5.6%) showed bruising of the external genitalia. No other early complications were reported. Pain reported by patients in the immediate postoperative period was slight (mean VAS score = 2.1). A total of 79 (31.6%) patients required no pain medication, while the remaining 171 (68.4%) were given nonnarcotic analgesics. Average VAS score during the first postoperative week 171 was 1.2, and 119 (47.6) patients took no medication (**Table 2**). During the second postoperative week, 8 (3.2%) subjects still complained of slight pain referred to the wound

VAS 0	46.8% (117 pts)
VAS 1	17.6% (44 pts)
VAS 2	17.6% (44 pts)
VAS 3	10.8% (27 pts)
VAS 4	3.2% (8 pts)
VAS 5	3.2% (8 pts)
VAS 6	0.8% (2 pts)
Average pain VAS 1.2; SD 1.5.	

Table 2. Postoperative pain in the first week.

VAS 0	96.8% (242 pts)
VAS 1	0.8% (2 pts)
VAS 2	1.2% (3 pts)
VAS 3	1.2% (3 pts)
Average pain VAS 0.06; SD 0.4.	

Table 3. Postoperative pain in the second week.

(average VAS score = 0.06). None of the patients took medication (**Table 3**). During the third postoperative week, only 0.4% (1) of patients complained of slight pain (average VAS score 0.01) which needed no medication (**Table 4**). Only 23 (9.2%) subjects experienced slight limitations of normal activities during the first week (**Table 5**). Thirty (20.1%) patients were able to engage in sports as early as 1 week from surgery, while 46 (30.9%) started between 7 and 21 days after surgery. Patients underwent to planned follow-up at 3 months (50 patients), 6 months (35 patients), 12 months (25 patients), 18 months (35 patients +1 patient lost), and 24 months (104 patients). Average follow-up is 15 months. None of our patients suffered from postoperative neuralgia, sensation of foreign bodies, or even simply discomfort. One recurrence was seen. All patients seemed satisfied with the operation, the recovery, and the final result [25].

4.4. Discussion

Tension-free techniques dramatically reduced recurrence rates making them the standard in hernia surgery. A not negligible incidence of postoperative chronic neuralgia [8, 26, 27] brought the attention of surgeons to new precautions even with the use of meshes [28].

Postoperative pain is temporary, usually controlled by medication. When persistent after 3–6 months from surgery, pain becomes disabling and may compromise the patient's quality of life. Pain may be related to the presence of the mesh that, because of size and location, takes contact with muscular structures or caused by fibrotic entrapment of nerves by a subfascial prosthesis [4, 13]. Studies conducted on animals also showed perineural alterations with myelinic degeneration due to contact between nervous structures and mesh [29]. Therefore, there is a necessity of identifying and dissecting subfascial nerves [30] and even of dividing them to avoid chronic pain [5, 6]. New surgical techniques and numerous kinds of meshes were proposed in the past years in the attempt to reduce postoperative neuralgia; nevertheless, the results of these new procedures were not completely satisfactory [7–10].

VAS 0	99.6% (249 pts)
VAS 1	0.4% (1 pt)
Average pain VAS 1.2; SD 1.5.	

Table 4. Postoperative pain in the third week.

	First week n. pt	Second week n. pt	Third week n. pt
No restriction	227	246	250
Slight restriction	23	4	0
Severe restriction	0	0	0

Table 5. Restriction in daily activities.

This led to the setting of guidelines for prevention and treatment of this situation [31].

If we consider the areas of weakness within the inguinal canal from which the three types of hernia arise, we see an oval-shaped surface surrounded by known muscular and fascial structures on the canal's floor and a further weak zone in proximity to the deep inguinal ring (**Figure 2**).

The transversalis fascia is an important restraining element for both structure and functionality in a region lacking overlying muscular structures. Then, the idea of a prosthesis specifically shaped to obtain containment by acting directly on the weak areas of the transversalis fascia without involving muscular or nervous structures avoiding to place a subaponeurotic mesh. This allows the procedure more anatomical with minimal foreign body implantation.

The prosthesis size, defined after numerous measurements of the inguinal canal made at the operating table, is notably smaller than the ones used as of now, allowing a precise and smooth positioning in a different plane to where the nerves lie.

The weak areas along the transversalis fascia are strengthened, all at once, by the prosthesis (all-in-one mesh), so that losing a hernia sac can no longer happen [2].

Polypropylene was chosen because of its capacity of inducing a lively inflammatory and fibrotic response with quick and strong adhesion to adjacent tissues. A prompt fibroblastic reaction between transversalis fascia and mesh immediately takes place because of the absence of any dead space and quickly forms a new wall.

This new technique is simple to perform and guarantees quick discharge and return to normal activities without any long-term discomfort. The average operative time was 25 min. The surgeon needs not dissect the cremaster, which may cause damage to the nerves, nor create a subfascial "nest," because no mesh is inserted at that level.

Furthermore, no plugs nor mesh trimming are necessary, and the prosthesis does not have to be sutured to adjacent structures. The use of a smaller quantity of prosthetic material allows the envelopment of the mesh by the fibro-cremasteric sheath, avoiding contact with surrounding nerves. Because of its shape, the mesh is placed in a deeper site directly over the weak areas of the floor of the inguinal, canal and, although smaller, it seems not to increase rate of recurrence.

The most common technique of Lichtenstein provides a prosthesis which, to remain on the transversalis fascia, must be fixed to the sides and becomes necessarily under aponeurotic in the upper third.

In our technique, the prosthesis is positioned and remains on the transversalis fascia because it is coated with the fibro-cremasteric sheath and it remains anchored on the inguinal floor with a single fixing point at the pubic level and with the prosthetic conical ring on the deep inguinal ring. It is not directly under-aponeurotic at any point, and it stays in place and therefore does not require lateral fixation.

In addition, the prosthesis is not in contact with the ilioinguinal and iliohypogastric nerves. Our paper is an observational cohort study with only midterm (2 years) follow-up. Clinical trials comparing the "all-in-one mesh" hernioplasty to the most common surgical techniques are required to obtain a validation of our procedure. Indeed, a much longer follow-up could highlight the actual recurrence rate of the new procedure.

5. Conclusion

This new procedure claims many technical advantages and helps the less experienced surgeon to avoid pitfalls in dealing with nerves. According to our series, "all-in-one mesh" hernioplasty presents a low rate of long-term complications. Employing a smaller amount of prosthetic material, placed where no contact with nerves occurs, avoids neuralgia and sensation of foreign body.

A multicenter study is underway to compare this new procedure with the most common techniques.

Author details

Angelo Guttadauro[1*], Matteo Maternini[1], Nicoletta Pecora[1], Marco Chiarelli[2], Valentina Riggio[3] and Francesco Gabrielli[1]

*Address all correspondence to: angelo.guttadauro@unimib.it

1 Department of Medicine and Surgery, General Surgery Unit, Istituti Clinici Zucchi, University of Milano-Bicocca, Monza, Italy

2 General Surgery Unit, Ospedale di Lecco, Italy

3 Department of Medicine and Surgery, University of Milano-Bicocca, Italy

References

[1] Lichtenstein IL. Herniorrhaphy. A personal experience with 6321 cases. American Journal of Surgery. 1987;**153**(6):553-559

[2] Trabucco E, Trabucco A, Rollino R, et al. L'ernioplastica inguinale tension-free con rete presagomata senza suture secondo Trabucco. Chirurgia. 1998;**11**:142-148

[3] Canzani M, Frattini F, Cavalli, et al. Trattamento chirurgico nel dolore cronico posternio-plastica. Atti del 110 Congresso SIC; 2008

[4] Heise CP, Starling JR. Mesh inguinodynia: A new clinical syndrome after inguinal herni-orrhaphy? Journal of the American College of Surgeons. 1998;**187**:514-518

[5] Karakayali F, Oksuz E, Turk E, et al. Effectiveness of multiple neurectomies to prevent chronic groin pain after tension-free hernia repair. International Surgery. 2010;**95**:40-48

[6] Mui WL, Ng CS, Fung TM, et al. Prophylactic ilioinguinal neurectomy in open inguinal hernia repair: A double-blind randomized controlled trial. Annals of Surgery. 2006;**244**:27-33

[7] Amid PK. Groin hernia repair: Open techniques. World Journal of Surgery. 2005;**29**: 1046-1051

[8] Valenti G, Baldassarre E, Testa A, et al. Dynamic self-regulating prosthesis (protesi autoregolantesi dinamica): The long-term results in the treatment of primary inguinal hernias. The American Surgeon. 2006;**72**:244-248

[9] Koeninger J, Redecke J, Butters M. Chronic pain after hernia repair: A randomized trial comparing Shouldice, Lichtenstein and TAPP. Langenbeck's Archives of Surgery. 2004;**389**:361-365

[10] Birk D, Hess S, Garcia-Pardo C. Low recurrence rate and low chronic pain associated with inguinal hernia repair by laparoscopic placement of Parietex ProGrip™ mesh: Clinical outcomes of 220 hernias 340 with mean follow-up at 23 months. Hernia. 2013;**17**:313-320

[11] Testut L, Jacob O. Trattato di Anatomia Topografica. In: UTET, editor. Torino. 1967. Vol. II 405-431, Vol. III 568-576

[12] Terranova O, Battocchio F. La chirurgia delle ernie della regione inguinale e crurale. Anatomia. Padova: La Garangola; 1988

[13] Pellissier E. Tecniche Chirurgiche Addominali. Anatomia Chirurgica Dell'inguine. Elsevier; 40-105. DOI: 10.1016/S1283-0798(07)49266-X

[14] Miserez M, Alexandre JH, Campanelli G, et al. The European hernia society groin hernia classification: Simple and easy to remember. Hernia. 2007;**11**:113-116

[15] Hoffman CH, Vinton Traverso A. Preperitoneal prosthetic herniorrhaphy. One surgeon's successful technique. Archives of Surgery. 1993;**128**(9):964-969

[16] Campanelli G, Bottero L, Leopaldi E, et al. Cosa sta cambiando nella chirurgia dell'ernia inguinale. Chir Arch Trim. 1993;**17**:13-17

[17] Campanelli G, Bottero L, Campagnoli P, et al. L'approccio pre-peritoneale in anestesia locale nella chirurgia delle recidive di ernia inguinale. Atti SPIGC; 1992

[18] Nyhus LM, Pollak R, Bombeck CT, et al. The pre-peritoneal approach and prosthetic buttress repair for recurrent hernia. The evolution of a technique. Annals of Surgery. 1988;**208**(6):733-737

[19] Bendavid R. L'intervento di Shouldice. Una tecnica per la riparazione dell'ernia inguinale. In: Terranova O, Battocchio F, editors. La chirurgia delle ernie della regione inguinale e crurale. La Garangola; 1988. pp. 76-83

[20] Shulman AG, Amid PK, Lichtenstein IL. The "plug" repair of 1402 recurrent inguinal hernias. 20-year experience. Archives of Surgery. 1990;**125**(2):265-267

[21] Shulman AG, Amid PK, Lichtenstein IL. Prosthetic mesh plug repair of femoral and recurrent inguinal hernias: The American experience. Annals of the Royal College of Surgeons of England. 1992;**74**(2):97-99

[22] Gilbert A. Sutureless repair of inguinal hernia. American Journal of Surgery. 1992;**163** (3):331-335

[23] Barnes JP Jr. Inguinal hernia repair with routine use of Marlex mesh. Surgery, Gyne cology & Obstetrics. 1987;**165**(1):33-37

[24] Bendavid R. The space of Bogros and the deep inguinal iliac circulation. Surgery, Gynecology & Obstetrics. 1992;**174**(5):356-357

[25] Guttadauro A, Maternini M, Frassani S, et al. "All-in-one mesh" hernioplasty: A new procedure for primary inguinal hernia open repair. Asian Journal of Surgery. 2017; Aug 26. pii: S1015-9584(17)30162-8. DOI: 10.1016/j.PMID:28851612

[26] Campanelli G, Sfeclan C, Cavalli M, et al. Reducing postoperative pain: The use of Tisseel for mesh fixation in inguinal hernia repair. Surgical Technology International. 2012;**22**:134-139

[27] Bueno J, Serralta A, Planells M, et al. Inguinodynia after two inguinal herniorrhaphy methods. Surgical Laparoscopy, Endoscopy & Percutaneous Techniques. 2004;**14**:210-214

[28] Lionetti R, Neola B, Dilillo S, et al. Sutureless hernioplasty with light-weight mesh and fibrin glue versus Lichtenstein procedure: A comparison of outcomes focusing on chronic postoperative pain. Hernia. 2012;**16**:127-131

[29] Demirer S, Kepenekci I, Evirgen O, et al. The effect of polypropylene mesh on ilioinguinal nerve in open mesh repair of groin hernia. The Journal of Surgical Research. 2006;**131**:175-181

[30] Alfieri S, Rotondi F, Di Miceli D, et al. Chronic pain after inguinal hernia mesh repair: Possible role of surgical manipulation of the inguinal nerves. A prospective multicentre study of 973 cases. Chirurgia Italiana. 2006;**58**:23-31

[31] Alfieri S, Amid PK, Campanelli G, et al. International guidelines for prevention and management of post-operative chronic pain following inguinal hernia surgery. Hernia. 2011;**15**:239-249

10

Individualized Treatment of Inguinal Hernia in Children

Jie Chen, ChengBing Chu, YingMo Shen,
ZhenYu Zou and Xin Yuan

Abstract

The incidence of inguinal hernias in various age groups of children ranges from 0.8 to 4.4%. Pediatric indirect inguinal hernia is congenital, originating in the patent processus vaginalis. The inguinal hernia repair is one of the most common pediatric operations. The traditional high hernia sac ligation is the primary treatment for younger patients from 1 to 13 years of age and can correct the condition. The authors performed the high ligation of the hernia sac by the laparoscopic approach for the patients under 13 years old and achieved good therapeutic results in the last 10 years. However, through our clinical study, the authors found that the simple high ligation of hernia sac is inadequate for patients from 13 to 18 years of age, who had a longer medical history, larger diameter of the internal inguinal ring, and more serious defects of the transverse fascia. Pediatric inguinal hernias are prone to postoperative recurrence if the patients were only treated with the high ligation of hernia sac. To repair the transverse fascia and strengthen the posterior wall of the inguinal canal, Lichtenstein hernioplasty with a biological patch was performed for the patients from 13 to 18 years in the authors' department. The aims of this chapter are to narrate the individualized treatment of inguinal hernia in children and try to provide relatively reasonable operative methods.

Keywords: hernia, inguinal, children, herniorrhaphy, laparoscopic, biological patch, individualized

1. Introduction

The incidence varies from 0.8 to 4.4% for inguinal hernia in children less than 18 years [1]. A unilateral hernia is approximately 85% of children with an inguinal hernia. The incidence of incarceration ranges from 6 to 18% for the untreated hernias in infants and young children, but it is about 30% in infancy [2]. A surgical intervention for inguinal hernia is one of the most common operations performed in children [3]. The individualized treatment program was established for pediatric inguinal hernia in the authors' department and provided a relatively reasonable surgical treatment. This chapter was mainly to describe the individualized treatment program applied to pediatric inguinal hernia.

2. Etiology

Indirect inguinal hernias in children are basically caused by embryologic development, which is mainly composed of patency of processus vaginalis (**Figure 1**). At the early stage of gestation, the testes begin to descend from retroperitoneum and remain at the level of the internal inguinal rings as the kidney ascends into its usual position. The final descent of testes into the scrotum through canalis inguinalis occurs between gestation weeks 28 and 36 [4], combining peritoneum, transversalis fascia, and abdominal wall muscles. The testes descent is "guided" by the gubernaculums. Descending peritoneum ultimately forms the processes vaginalis, and the distal portion of the processus vaginalis wrapped around the testes becomes the tunica vaginalis. In the normal development, the processus vaginalis closes between 36 and 40 weeks of gestation or even shortly after birth [5]. The rate of patency is inversely proportional to the age of children, approximately 80% close to 2 years of age [4]. The left testis descends before the right one and the closure of the patent processus vaginalis on the left also precedes closure on the right, therefore, indirect inguinal hernia occurs more on the right side.

Though the embryology has been widely described, the cell-molecular mechanism is still unclear. Inguinal hernias most probably are inherited [6]. Zhang et al.'s [7] team have found that the functional sequence variants of some genes may be a risk factor for indirect inguinal hernia, such as gene TBX1, gene TBX3, gene SIRT1, and gene GATA6. These variants may affect the differentiation and proliferation of human skeletal muscles and fibroblasts [7–10].

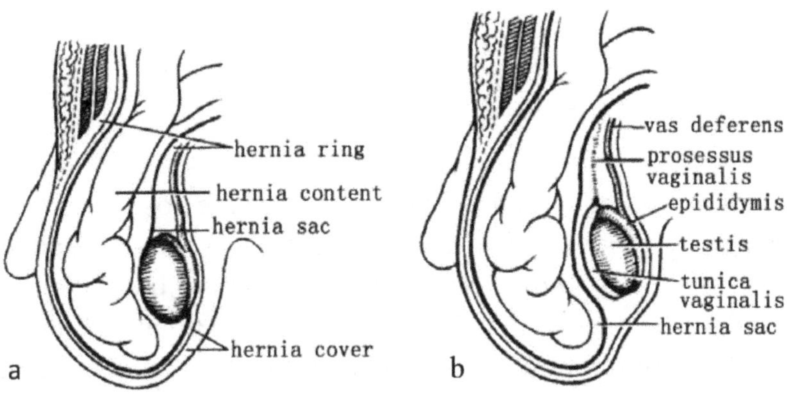

Figure 1. (a) Congenital indirect inguinal hernia and (b) acquired indirect inguinal hernia.

3. Clinical manifestation

A reducible bulge or mass in the inguinal region or unilateral or bilateral enlargement of the scrotum (**Figure 2a** and **b**) is the main diagnostic finding in most groin hernias. These symptoms can occur when abdominal pressure increases, such as while standing, coughing, crying, constipation, and playing, and disappears when patients lie down or fall asleep. Children less than two years of age will express themselves only by crying and screaming, so if children continue crying without obvious reasons, groin hernia should be considered.

There may be associated pain or vague discomfort in the region. Groin hernias are usually not extremely painful unless incarceration (**Figure 2c**) or strangulation has occurred [11]. The bowels inside the hernia sac being incarcerated or strangulated may cause intestinal obstruction, and the testis may turn red gradually. At this time, the spermatic cord is oppressed and the testicle may be diagnosed with ischemic necrosis. As the age increases, the size of hernia sac will gradually increase. The falling bowels pull down the mesentery and cause not only abdominal pain, nausea, and other gastrointestinal symptoms but also walking inconvenience. In addition, the spermatic cord being pressed continuously by the hernia sac will cause spermatic vessel reflux disorder and blood supply reduction as well as spermophlebectasia and testicular atrophy.

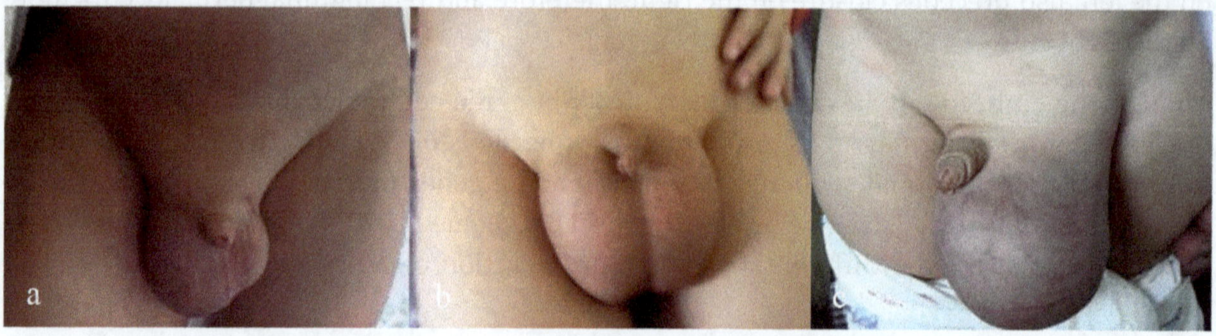

Figure 2. Pediatric hernias. (a) Right inguinal hernia, (b) bilateral inguinal hernia, (c) incarcerated left inguinal hernia.

4. Physical and accessory examination

The inguinal region is examined with the child in the standing position or with the infant held in the vertical position by parents. The examiner visually inspects and palpates the inguinal region, looking for asymmetry, bulge, or a mass [11]. Having the patient cough or cry can facilitate in the identification of a hernia. The examiner puts a fingertip into the external inguinal ring by invaginating the scrotum to detect a small inguinal hernia. If a bulge moves from lateral to medial in the inguinal canal, an indirect hernia is suspected. A bulge progressing from the deep to superficial through the inguinal floor suggests a direct hernia [11].

Ultrasound is very useful in the diagnosis, which can avoid the adverse effects of radiation in CT on children's development. There is a high degree of sensitivity and specificity for ultrasound in the detection of occult hernias [11]. An ultrasound can determine the hernia sac, the defect, the hernia contents (the bowel, the omentum, or the bladder), and complications such as hydrocele, guiding the surgical treatment.

5. Diagnosis and differential diagnosis

The diagnosis of inguinal hernia in children is mainly suggested by the history of the bulges or masses in groin area, usually found in children crying or regular physical examination. For slightly older children, blowing bubbles, tickling them to make them laugh, or having them blow up balloons (e.g., examination gloves) will increase intra-abdominal pressure and the hernias may appear. When they are in supine position, the bulges or mass may reduce by itself or by hands, which is called reduction.

For typical cases, it is generally not difficult to make the diagnosis, while for the unclear inguinal abnormalities, doctors can combine with the results of ultrasonic testing or further examination just like CT or MRI if it is necessary. Mainly depending on the different degree and level of processus vaginalis obliteration failure, these methods may help to find the abnormality of inguinal canal, including various types of hydrocele (communicating, non-communicating, funicular), spermatic cord cyst in males, hydrocele of the canal of Nuck in females, cyst of the round ligament of uterus, and indirect inguinal hernias [12]. Communicating hydrocele results from the patent processus vaginalis throughout its length. The fluid collection communicates with the peritoneal cavity and the scrotum. Non-communicating hydrocele happens at the time processus vaginalis obliterates and some fluid accumulates between the cavities of the tunica vaginalis enclosing the testis. Spermatic cord hydrocele results from an abnormal closure of the processus vaginalis, leading to fluid accumulation alongside the spermatic cord, which is separated from and located above the testis. A transillumination test, an ordinary means to distinguish the hydrocele and hernia, is widely used in clinical works. The scrotum is exposed in a dark room with a flashlight under it. If it contains fluid, light is allowed to go through. When it is opaque, a hernia will be detected. Hydrocele and cyst of the canal of Nuck are caused by the incomplete obliteration of the processus vaginalis in girls, which is unusual. The hernia of the canal of Nuck is also an uncommon condition in females, which is homogenous to the indirect inguinal hernia in males. The distinction of these abnormalities, facilitating diagnosis for early surgical intervention, needs to be paid much attention in specific conditions.

6. Treatment

6.1. Indications for surgery

The processus vaginalis is a finger-like projection of peritoneum that typically closes between the 36th and 40th week of gestation. It is thought that 40% closes in the first few months after birth and an additional 20% by the age of 2 [4]. Congenital inguinal hernia is a common malformation in children that requires operative treatment [13]. Surgery is indicated for all pediatric patients in whom the diagnosis of inguinal hernia has been made. The hernia in infants younger than 6 months should be operated as soon as possible due to high incidence of incarceration. Surgical treatment can be booked selectively for older children with few symptoms [14, 15]. Surgical procedure is provided for inguinal hernia to avoid the complications such as incarceration and obstruction, potentially resulting in ischemia/necrosis of the hernia contents and surrounding cord structures. In females, it is also possible that torsion/ischemia of the ovary can happen [16, 17].

Repair of inguinal hernias is one of the most common pediatric surgical procedures. Indirect inguinal hernias are congenital in origin due to a patent processus vaginalis. In recent years, with the development of materials technology and minimally invasive surgical techniques, surgical treatments of inguinal hernia in children were transitioned from the traditional open surgery to the laparoscopic high ligation of hernia sac and the use of biological patch in open surgery. The different techniques have their own indications and advantages. The authors carried out the individualized treatment of inguinal hernia in children, receiving significant clinical results.

The high hernia sac ligation is the primary treatment for younger patients from 1 to 13 years old. These patients had shorter medical history, smaller diameter of the hernia ring, and less serious defects of the transverse fascia or the inguinal canal posterior wall, therefore, the traditional high ligation of hernia sac can correct the condition. In the last 10 years, the authors have performed laparoscopic hernia sac ligation for the patients younger than 13 years old and have obtained satisfactory results.

According to the results of our clinical study [18], the authors found that the simple high hernia sac ligation is inadequate for adolescents (13 to 18 years old) with a longer medical history, larger diameter of internal inguinal ring, and more serious transverse fascia defects. The inguinal hernia treated with simple high hernia sac ligation in adolescents is prone to postoperative recurrence; therefore, the procedure, similar to the treatment of adult inguinal hernia, should be taken, for example, repairing the transverse fascia and strengthening of the posterior wall of the inguinal canal.

The therapy for pediatric inguinal hernia was carried out by the individualized treatment program in authors' department, which can provide a relatively reasonable surgical treatment. Individualized treatment programs consisted of three kinds of surgical procedures as described below.

6.2. Modified open pediatric inguinal hernia repair

The etiology of pediatric inguinal hernia is a patent processus vaginalis; therefore, inguinal hernias were generally repaired with open simple high ligation of the hernia sac for the patient younger than 13 years. The traditional open technique with high ligation of hernia is the classic surgical treatment method for pediatric inguinal hernia. An inguinal approach is taken for the traditional open technique of inguinal hernia repair. A 3–4-cm-long inguinal incision is made on the same side as the inguinal hernia that is to be corrected. The procedure includes the slit of external oblique aponeurosis, the isolation of the hernia sac from the surrounding cord structures which consist of the cremasteric muscle, vas deferens, and the testicular vessel surrounding the ligament. A high ligature is located on the proximal separated sac. The distal sac is divided and resected. The external inguinal ring is reconstructed. Although the traditional open inguinal approach is effective for hernia repair in the pediatric population [19–21], it carries numerous risks, including immediate and long-term postoperative complications [22–24]. Postoperative pain, surgical trauma, local swelling usually last 3–5 days for children. In addition, visualization of possible contralateral defects is limited and there remains a risk of hernia recurrence [25].

For the patients with a small hernia sac, the modified open operation of inguinal hernia repair with a small incision in the external inguinal ring could be performed to correct this pathological condition without slitting of the external oblique aponeurosis and ligating highly the hernia sac. This modified approach can maintain the normal anatomy of the inguinal canal to reduce complications. The modified open operation is widely used in Chinese primary hospitals at present, where it is relatively easy to do operations with low recurrence rate but has not been done for a long time in the authors' department.

6.2.1. Operative steps for the modified open pediatric inguinal hernia repair

A small skin incision of about 1–1.5 cm is made along the skin crease, which is located on the surface projection of external inguinal ring supra pubic tubercle. Incision is carried down through the dermis to expose the subcutaneous fat, Camper's fascia. Using sharp and blunt dissection, Scarpa's fascia is identified, grasped, and incised in the direction of the external inguinal ring. A gentle retraction is needed to maintain excellent exposure. Cremaster muscle is dissected to expose spermatic cord and the hernia sac within the external inguinal ring. The external inguinal ring is not opened. The hernia sac is elevated off the inguinal floor and isolated from the surrounding tissue with a blunt dissection in the internal inguinal ring. The hernia sac is opened (**Figure 3a**). If the hernia sac is small, it is directly ligated at its neck where extraperitoneal fat can be seen. If it is large, it is cut to about 2 cm, away from its neck, and then sutured and ligated at its neck (**Figure 3b**). The internal inguinal ring is sutured for 1–2 stitches for repair, if it is large. Subcutaneous tissue and skin are subsequently closed after hemostasis is done carefully.

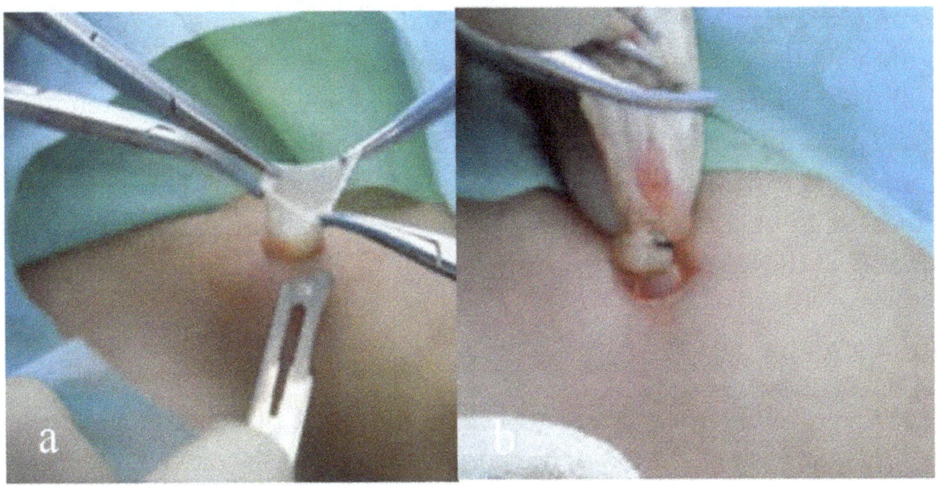

Figure 3. (a) The hernia sac was opened and (b) the hernia sac was sutured and ligated at its neck.

6.3. Laparoscopy high hernia sac ligation assisted with a needle-type grasper

In the last 2 decades, the advent of minimally invasive surgery has completely changed the management of pediatric inguinal hernias [26, 27]. Laparoscopic surgery, since its advent in the early 1990s, is increasingly being preferred by the surgeons and patients worldwide due to its overall benefits, evident by operative results and patient satisfaction [28]. Montupet is credited with performing the first intracorporeal laparoscopic pediatric hernia repair in 1993 [26]. The authors treated pediatric inguinal hernia with laparoscopy high ligation of the hernia sac with the aid of a needle-type grasper (**Figure 4**) [29]. With almost similar results to open mesh repair, laparoscopy provides an alternative to inguinal hernia repair especially in bilateral or recurrent cases [30].

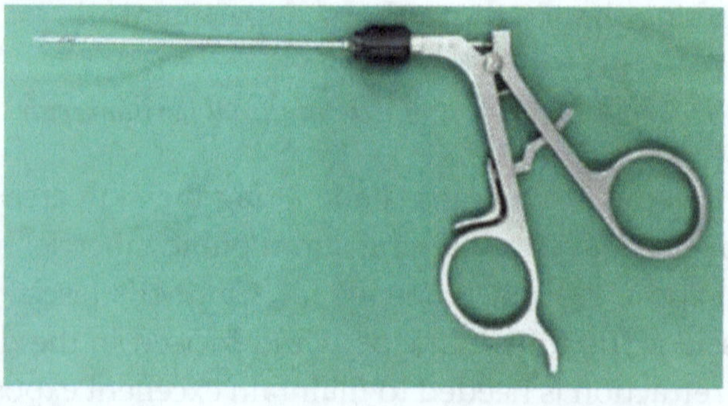

Figure 4. Needle-type grasper.

6.3.1. Preoperative preparation

Preoperative preparation includes fasting for 6 h. To be intraoperatively better exposed and minimize the risk of bladder injury, the bladder should be emptied before surgery.

6.3.2. Patient and team position

All patients underwent general anesthesia. The patient is positioned supine with both arms tucked (**Figure 6a**). To remove the intestine away from the operative area and to improve exposure of the working area, the patients are changed in 15–20° of the Trendelenburg position during the procedure (**Figure 6b**). The surgeon is on the opposite side of the defect to be repaired. The assistant with the camera is on the same side as the hernia to be treated, and surgical nurse should be located on the right side of the patient near the patient's knee. The monitor is placed at the foot of the operating bed.

6.3.3. Surgical procedures

An incision at the infra or supra umbilicus is then made for placement of a 5-mm trocar (we use a 5-mm 30° laparoscope). Access of the peritoneal cavity is achieved using standard techniques with a Veress needle to create the pneumoperitoneum. The pneumoperitoneal pressure was maintained at 8–10 mmHg. Once access to the peritoneal cavity has been established, an inspection of bilateral internal inguinal ring is made in search of hernia defects. A 1.5-mm incision at or above the linea alba midpoint between the umbilicus and pubic symphysis is made for entering the needle-type grasper. Another 1.5-mm small incision is made at the 12 o clock surface projection of internal inguinal ring. Through it, the endo-closure device (**Figure 5**) with No. 4 polyester thread was rotated back and forth and entered into the pre-peritoneal space at 11 (right side) or 1(left side) o clock of the internal inguinal ring under laparoscopic monitoring. The endo-closure device was then advanced along the lateral side of inferior epigastric vessels within the extraperitoneal space and around the internal inguinal ring and bypassed the vas deferens and spermatic vessels with the aid of needle-type grasper (**Figure 6d–f**). The tip of endo-closure device was pierced the peritoneum into the abdominal cavity at 6 o clock of internal inguinal ring. No. 4 polyester thread was pulled out from the endo-closure device with a needle-type grasper and cleaved into the abdominal cavity (**Figure 6g**), and the endo-closure device was pulled out of the body. The endo-closure device was inserted into the same skin incision again. From 12 o clock of internal inguinal ring to the beginning, the endo-closure device was rotated back and forth and advanced along the lateral side of internal inguinal ring beneath the peritoneum. The endo-closure device entered into the abdominal cavity at the same peritoneal hole as the No. 4 polyester thread had gone through (**Figure 6h**). The endo-closure device was then taken and the No. 4 polyester thread was taken out of the body. After squeezing the air out of the scrotal and groin area, No. 4 polyester thread was then tightened and tied, and the knot was subcutaneously buried. The high ligation of hernia sac was finished (**Figure 6i**). Bilateral indirect hernia was treated the same way. An inspection of the abdominal cavity is made before ending operation. The needle-type grasper is removed under laparoscopic monitoring. A 5-mm trocar was removed after the abdominal cavity air was emptied. Umbilical incision was sutured, and skin incision was intradermally sutured and stuck together with glue.

The manipulation of laparoscopy high hernia sac ligation with the aid of the needle-like grasper is easy to bypass the structure of the vas deferens and spermatic vessels under direct vision and does not injure it. Laparoscopic approaches offer the superior visualization to potentially avoid trauma to the vas deferens and spermatic vessels and the opportunity to accomplish a safe high ligation of the hernia sac at the internal ring [23, 31–33].

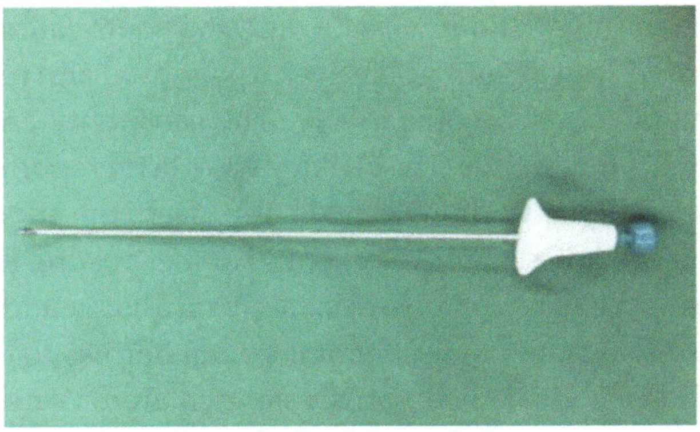

Figure 5. Endo-closure device (COVIDIEN).

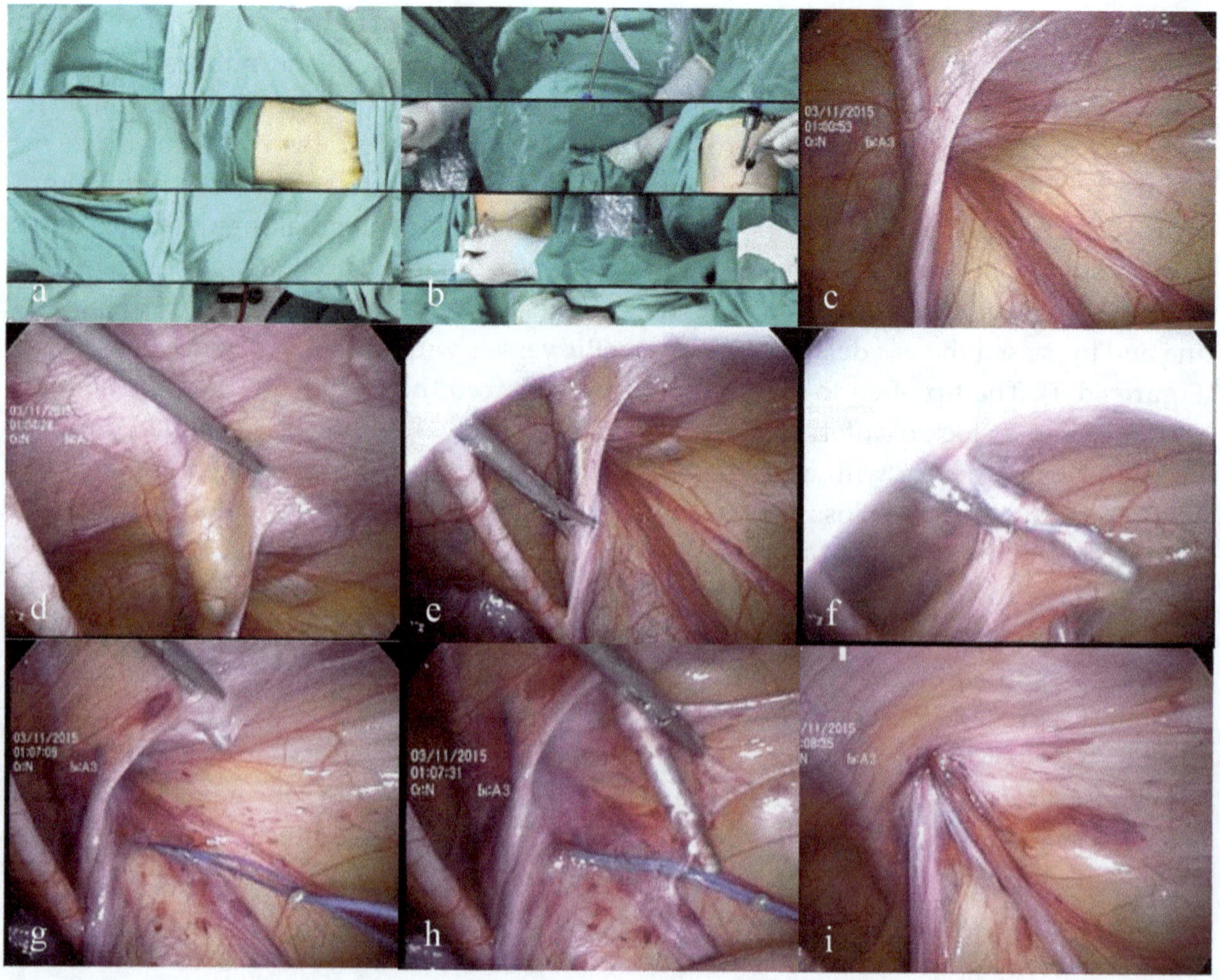

Figure 6. (a) The child with inguinal hernia has been disinfected and draped, (b) intraoperative location of the laparoscopic, needle-type grasper, and endo-closure device with the thread, (c) indirect inguinal hernia, (d) and (e) endo-closure device with No. 4 polyester thread entering into the pre-peritoneal space and then advanced along the lateral side of inferior epigastric vessels and around internal inguinal ring, (f) with the aid of needle-type grasper, the tip of endo-closure device bypassed the vas deferens which was under the tip of endo-closure device in this picture, (g) and (h) the endo-closure device advanced along the lateral side of internal inguinal ring beneath the peritoneum and entered into the abdominal cavity at the same peritoneal hole as the No. 4 polyester thread had gone through, and (i) high hernia sac ligation was finished.

Laparoscopic approaches offer the opportunity to visually inspect the contralateral canal for the presence of an occult hernia without incision, and the contralateral hernia, hiding hernia (**Figure 7**), or other affections can be intraoperatively diagnosed and repaired at the same time while diagnosing unilateral cases, preoperatively. The sensitivity and specificity of laparoscopic examination for detecting hidden PV patency have been reported to be 99.4 and 99.5%, respectively [1]. Compared to the traditional open approach, the advantages of laparoscopic hernia repair include minimal dissection, excellent visual exposure, less complications, comparable recurrence rates, as well as improved cosmetic results. In addition, laparoscopic hernia repair also makes it possible for contralateral inguinal hernias to be defined and repaired in the same operation [34–36]. Up to now, no scrotal hematoma or effusion has been found in the authors' department. At present, laparoscopy high hernia sac ligation assisted with the needle-type grasper is more favorable than open pediatric inguinal hernia repair, which is

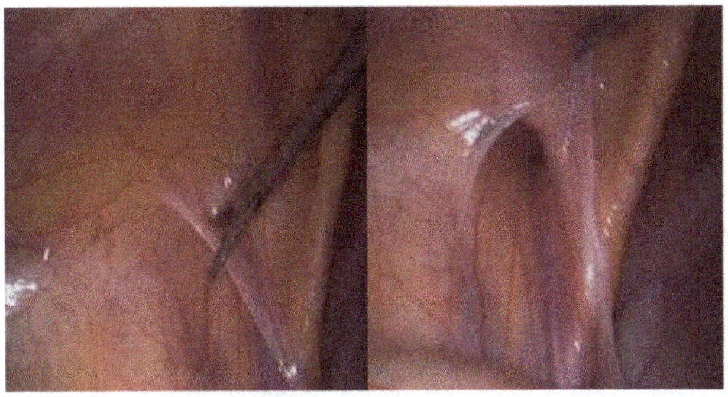

Figure 7. Hidden hernia was found with the aid of a needle-type clamp.

one of the most common surgical procedures in the authors' department. The operation could be implemented as long as there were no anesthetic or pneumoperitoneum contraindications.

The laparoscopic high inguinal hernia sac ligation must establish pneumoperitoneum, which can only be used in general anesthesia, which needs the endotracheal intubation and ventilator-assisted breathing and increases surgical costs and anesthesia-related problems. In addition, the families of children have some psychological concerns with the side effects of general anesthesia, which had a bad effect on surgical treatment.

6.4. Lichtenstein hernioplasty using a biological patch

As for the children from 13 to 18 years old, because simple hernia sac ligation surgery is not enough, the recurrence rate is high. The posterior wall of inguinal canal should also be repaired and strengthened in order to prevent recurrence. At present, it wasn't advocated for the children with hernia, from 13 to 18 years old, to be treated with non-biological synthetic patch (e.g., polypropylene) because they are still in the growth and development stage. Not stretching or contracting, the non-degradable patch can result in local postoperative obvious traction; local foreign body sensation and chronic pain may also cause spermatic cord adhesion and even affect fertility. For children and adolescents, their muscle and fascia tissue will gradually become strong in the growth and development stage. The absorbable biological materials can rely on their own characteristics to repair defects in the early stage and generate the new tissue plates through tissue replacement to prevent recurrence of hernia in the long term. After the biological materials are absorbed or degraded gradually, the biological patch will be replaced by autologous tissue without affecting the growth and development.

The authors found that the simple high hernia sac ligation is inadequate for adolescents who had a longer medical history, larger diameter of internal inguinal ring, and more serious transverse fascia defects and that the procedure similar to the treatment of adult inguinal hernias should be taken in order to repair the transverse fascia and strengthen of the posterior wall of the inguinal canal. The authors proposed the application of the biological patch to the treatment of the inguinal hernia of the patients who are 13–18 years old, and results show that compared with the traditional high ligation of hernia sac, the biological patch tension-free hernia repair surgery did not significantly increase the wound infection, male scrotal effusion, chronic pain or local foreign body sensation, and other complications.

Open "tension free" mesh repair technique, pioneered by Lichtenstein in 1984, is still considered the method of choice for primary inguinal hernia [37, 38]. For children from 13 to 18 years of age, inguinal hernia was treated with Lichtenstein hernioplasty with the biological patch, in which biological patch is placed in front of the transversalis fascia to reinforce the posterior wall of the inguinal canal.

6.4.1. Surgical procedures

The operative steps include dissection of the spermatic cord, dissection and resection of the hernia sac with high ligation (**Figure 8b–d**), and reconstruction of the floor of the inguinal canal. The inguinal canal is dissected to expose the shelving edge of the inguinal ligament, the pubic tubercle, and the sufficient area for biological patch. The biological patch must be large enough to overlap 1.5–2 cm medial to the pubic tubercle. The lateral portion of the patch is split into two tails such that the superior tail constitutes two-thirds of its width, and the inferior tail is the remaining one-third of its width (**Figure 8e**). The lateral tail of the biological patch passed through beneath the spermatic cord from medial to lateral and then sutured together with the medial tail using two vicryl 2/0 interrupted stitches, leaving a hole as large as the diameter of the spermatic cord, which was placed around the spermatic cord at the internal ring, but not too tight to strangulate it (**Figure 8f**). Two interrupted sutures with vicryl 2/0 thread were used to fix the inferior edge of the patch to the shelving edge of the inguinal ligament. The upper edge of the patch was then fixed to the inferior surface of external oblique aponeurosis with two vicryl 2/0 interrupted stitches. The tails were then placed on the surface of internal oblique muscle and fixed with glue. The medial edge of the patch was overlapped the pubic tubercle by 1.5–2 cm and fixed with medical glue in order to prevent medial recurrence. The reinforcement of the floor of the inguinal canal was finished

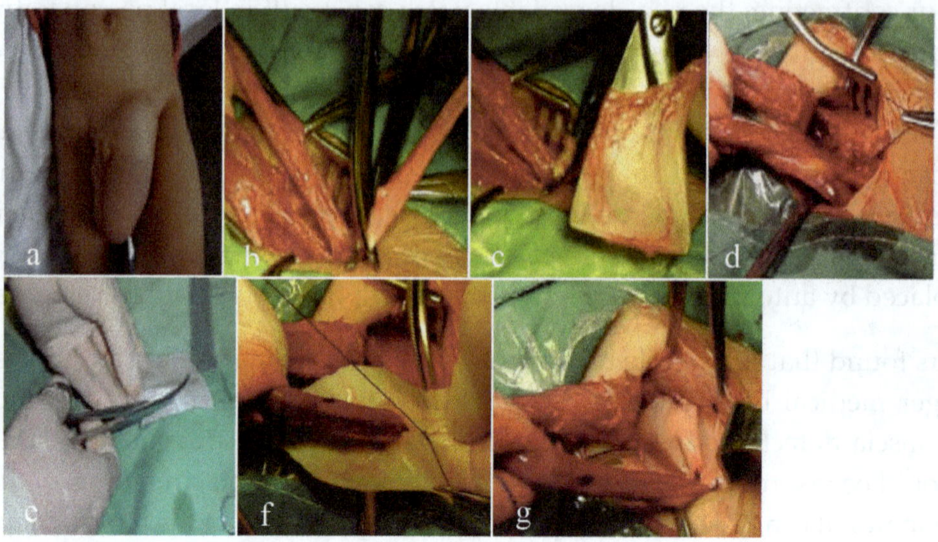

Figure 8. (a) The child with big indirect inguinal hernia, (b) and (c) the hernia sac was dissected and sheared, (d) the hernia sac was sutured and ligated at its neck, (e) a cellular tissue matrix patch (Grandhope Biotech Co., Ltd.) was prepared, (f) the two tails of the biologic patch were sutured together with 2/0 vicryl to surround the spermatic cord, (g) the fixation for the biological patch was finished.

(**Figure 8g**). External oblique aponeurosis was sutured with vicryl 2/0. Subcutaneous tissue is closed with vicryl 4/0. The skin incision was intradermally sutured with vicryl 4/0 and stuck together with medical glue.

Generally, it is not difficult to diagnose inguinal hernia in children; however, before surgery, there is no effective auxiliary examination to diagnose how much the hernia ring defect ranges, which is based on the options of individualized treatment of pediatric inguinal hernia. For some patients who are 13–18 years old, if the extent of hernia ring defect belonged to Gilbert type I or II, laparoscopic high hernia sac ligation could still be used. Preoperative non-invasive examinations, such as ultrasound, which can define the size of the hernia ring defect in most cases, are helpful to choose the surgery and carry out the individualized treatment program of inguinal hernia in children.

The individualized treatment of inguinal hernia in children is currently an effective and relatively reasonable treatment program to improve treatment of morbidity. However, it does not take a long time to use laparoscopic high hernia sac ligation and the biological patch repair. It must be further observed for the long-term effects and needs to be studied on the basis of the present in order to improve the clinical effects and reduce the postoperative complications.

Author details

Jie Chen*, ChengBing Chu, YingMo Shen, ZhenYu Zou and Xin Yuan

*Address all correspondence to: chenjiejoe@sina.com

Department of Hernia and Abdominal Wall Surgery, Beijing Chao-Yang Hospital, Capital Medical University, Beijing, China

References

[1] Miltenburg DM, Nuchtern JG, Jaksic T, et al. Laparoscopic evaluation of the pediatric inguinal hernia: A meta-analysis. Journal of Pediatric Surgery. 1998;**33**(6):874-879

[2] Parelkar SV, Oak S, Gupta R, et al. Laparoscopic inguinal hernia repair in the pediatric age group—experience with 437 children. Journal of Pediatric Surgery. 2010;**45**(4):789-792

[3] Lau S, Lee Y, Caty M. Current management of hernias and hydroceles. Seminars in Pediatric Surgery. 2007;**16**(1):50-57

[4] Brandt ML. Pediatric hernias. Surgical Clinics of North America. 2008;**88**:27-43

[5] Toki A, Watanabe Y, Sasaki K. Adopt a wait-and-see attitude for patent processus vaginalis in neonates. Journal of Pediatric Surgery. 2003;**38**(9):1371-1373

[6] Burcharth J, Pommergaard HC, Rosenberg J. The inheritance of groin hernia: A systematic review. Hernia. 2013;**17**:183-189

[7] Zhang Y, Han Q, Li C, et al. Genetic analysis of the TBX1 gene promoter in indirect inguinal hernia. Gene. 2014;**535**:290-293

[8] Han Q, Zhang Y, Li W, et al. Functional sequence variants within the SIRT1 gene promoter in indirect inguinal hernia. Gene. 2014;**546**:1-4

[9] Qiao Y, Zhang Z, Huang W, et al. Two functional sequence variants of the GATA6 gene promoter in patients with indirect inguinal hernia. Gene. 2014;**547**:86-90

[10] Zhao Z, Tian W, Wang L, et al. Genetic and functional analysis of the TBX3 gene promoter in indirect inguinal hernia. 2015;**554**:101-104

[11] Sabiston DC. Sabiston Textbook of Surgery: Hernias. 19th ed. Canada; Saunders' Elsevier Inc. 2012. pp. 1114-1119

[12] Sameshima YT, Yamanari MG, Silva MA, Neto MJ, Funari MB. The challenging sonographic inguinal canal evaluation in neonates and children: An update of differential diagnoses. Pediatric Radiology. 2017; **47**(4):461-472. [Epub ahead of print]

[13] Wiener ES, Touloukian RJ, Rodgers BM, et al. Hernia survey of the section on surgery of the American Academy of Pediatrics. Journal of Pediatric Surgery. 1996;**31**:1166-1169

[14] Gonzalez Santacruz M, Mira Navarro J, Encinas Goenechea A, et al. Low prevalence of complications of delayed herniotomy in the extremely premature infant. Acta Paediatrica. 2004;**93**(1):94-98

[15] Krieger NR, Shochat SJ, McGowan V, et al. Early hernia repair in the premature infant: Long-term follow-up. Journal of Pediatric Surgery. 1994;**29**(8):978-982

[16] Rajput A, Gauderer MW, Hack M. Inguinal hernias in very low birth weight infants: Incidence and timing of repair. Journal of Pediatric Surgery. 1992;**27**(10):1322-1324

[17] Uemura S, Woodward AA, Amerena R,et al. Early repair of inguinal hernia in premature babies. Pediatric Surgery International. 1999;**15**(1):36-39

[18] Shen YM, Chen J, Tian ML, et al. Lichtenstein repair of indirect inguinal hernias with acellular tissue matrix grafts in adolescent patients: A prospective, randomized, controlled trial. Surgery Today. 2014;**44**(3):429-435

[19] Nah SA, Giacomello L, Eaton S, et al. Surgical repair of incarcerated inguinal hernia in children: Laparoscopic or open? European Journal of Pediatric Surgery. 2011;**21**:8-11

[20] Boocock GR, Todd PJ. Inguinal hernias are common in preterm infants. Archives of Disease in Childhood. 1985;**60**:669-670

[21] Kozlov Y, Novozhilov V, Kovalev V, et al. Laparoscopic Inguinal Preperitoneal Injection (LIPI)—Novel Experimental Technique for Inguinal Hernia Repair in Children. Croatia: In Tech; 2014. pp. 71-84

[22] Esposito C, Montinaro L, Alicchio F, et al. Technical standardization of laparoscopic herniorraphy in pediatric patients. World Journal of Surgery. 2009;**33**:1846-1850

[23] Schier F. Laparoscopic inguinal hernia repair—A prospective personal series of 542 children. Journal of Pediatric Surgery. 2006;**41**:1081-1084

[24] Wilson JM, Aaronson DS, Schrader R, et al. Hydrocele in the pediatric patient: Inguinal or scrotal approach? Journal of Urology.2008;**180**(l4 Suppl):1724-1727

[25] Mollen KP, Kane TD. Inguinal hernia: What we have learned from laparoscopic evaluation of the contralateral side. Current Opinion in Pediatrics. 2007;**19**:344-348

[26] Esposito C, Escolino M, Farina A, Settimi A. Two decade of history of laparoscopic pediatric inguinal hernia repair. Journal of Laparoendoscopic & Advanced Surgical Techniques. Part A. 2014;**24**(9):669-670

[27] Ostlie DJ, Ponsky TA. Technical options of the laparoscopic pediatric inguinal hernia repair. Journal of Laparoendoscopic & Advanced Surgical Techniques. Part A. 2014;**24**(3):194-198

[28] Rao A, Kynaston J, MacDonald ER, et al. Patient preferences for surgical techniques: Should we invest in new approaches? Surgical Endoscopy. 2010;**24**:3016-3025

[29] Liu SJ, Wang F, Zhu YL, et al. Clamp type needle assisted single hole laparoscopic treatment in pediatric patients with inguinal hernia. Chinese Journal of Hernia and Abdominal Wall Surgery (Electronic Edition). 2014;**8**:16-17

[30] Feliu X, Clavería R, Besora P, et al. Bilateral inguinal hernia repair: Laparoscopic or open approach? Hernia. 2011;**15**:15-18

[31] Lukong CS. Surgical techniques of laparoscopic inguinal hernia repair in childhood: A critical appraisal. Journal of Surgical Technique and Case Report. 2012;**4**(1):1-5

[32] Chang YT. Technical refinements in single port laparoscopic surgery of inguinal hernia in infants and children. Diagnostic and Therapeutic Endoscopy. 2010;**2010**:392847

[33] Montupet P, Esposito C. Fifteen years experience in laparoscopic inguinal hernia repair in pediatric patients. Results and considerations on a debated procedure. Surgical Endoscopy. 2011;**25**(2):450-453

[34] Lee Y, Liang J. Experience with 450 cases of microlaparoscopic herniotomy in infants and children. Pediatric Endosurgery and Innovative Techniques. 2002;**6910**:25-28

[35] Schier F, Montupet P, Esposito C. Laparoscopic inguinal herniorrhaphy in children: A three-center experience with 933 repairs. Journal of Pediatric Surgery. 2002;**37**(3):395-397

[36] Schier F. Laparoscopic surgery of inguinal hernias in children; initial experience. Journal of Pediatric Surgery. 2000;**35**(9):1331-1335

[37] Lichtenstein IL, Shulman AG, Amid PK, Montllor MM. The tension-free hernioplasty. American Journal of Surgery. 1989;**157**:188-193

[38] Antoniou SA, Pointner R, Granderath FA. Current treatment concepts for groin hernia. Langenbeck's Archives of Surgery. 2014;**399**:553-558

11

Surgical Anatomy of the Groin

Kamer Tomaoglu

Abstract

Most surgeons are familiar with the inguinal anatomy from the anterior perspective. With the advent of laparoscopic techniques for inguinal hernia repair, it became important to understand the inguinal anatomy from the preperitoneal view for a posterior approach to the inguinal region. The purpose of this chapter is to describe the anatomic landmarks of the groin region.

Keywords: anatomy, groin, surgery

1. Introduction

The inguinofemoral region extends to above and under the line of Malgaigne. It composes the borderline region between anterolateral abdominal wall and upper portion of the triangle of Scarpa [1, 2]. It represents an important structure, which is a passage zone between the abdominal area, the external genital region, and the root of lower extremity. Two pedicles, the spermatic cord (or the round ligament of uterus) and the iliofemoral vascular pedicle cross the inguinofemoral region. It is equally a zone of embryologic importance, characterized by the evolution of peritoneo-vaginal channel, the testicular descent, and rarely an ectopic engagement of ovaries [2–4].

The groin is the region where most hernias of the abdominal wall occur. Inguinal hernia repair is the most commonly performed operation worldwide. Approximately 75% of abdominal wall hernias occur in the groin [5, 6]. Its surgical interest is evident which we understand easily by the consecutive diverse technical discussions after the apparition of the Shouldice Hospital technique, considered by many authors as a return to the "starting point" [7, 8].

2. History

In the sixteenthcentury, Fallope described the "inguinal ligament." Later on, Ambroise Paré tried to classify different hernias. In theeighteenthcentury, Poupart and Littre summarized the knowledge on hernia anatomy. Littre described the hernia of intestinal diverticulum (Meckel's diverticulum), which was called Littre's hernia later on. Scarpa, in 1812 published the famous "Traité des hernies" first in Italian language and later in French with illustrations of the inguinofemoral triangle. From surgical point of view, "Traité des hernies" was very rudimentary, only the hernias with failure of taxis were operated on. Intestinal interminable fistulas were frequently present in survived patients. The cauterization was sometimes used, without any considerable amelioration of the results [2, 3, 6].

Modern history of hernia cure begins with Bassini who described in 1886, the anatomic procedure of radical cure of inguinal hernia [9]. This was the first modern operation, based on a perfect anatomic analysis of the region. In the twentieth century, the modifications of Bassini's operation and McVay and Anson [16] revised the ideas of Lotheissen and insisted on the interest of low fixation, to the Cooper's ligament, underlying the importance of anatomic unity of the region while performing the surgical treatment of both inguinal and femoral hernias simultaneously [1–3].

Beginning from 1953, the Shouldice technique emerged in Toronto, which realized a retrofunicular suturing of the transversalis fascia, thus claiming to obtain maximum solidity [10].

Fruchaud, in 1956, published the classic "Anatomie des hernies de l'aine", which was based upon the structural unity of the inguinofemoral region which was centered on myopectineal orifice. Nyhus and Condon published the book "Hernia" in 1978.

In the early 1980s, Lichtenstein popularized the tension-free repair, supplanting the tissue-based repairs with prosthetic materials for inguinal floor reconstruction [11].

With the advent of minimally invasive surgery, since the initial description by Ger, inguinal hernia repair underwent its most recent transformation.

3. Embryology

Very early during the embryonic development, the peritoneal cavity presents two inferior diverticula, which protrude through the inguinal canal and become the processus vaginalis. They extend toward the scrotal draft or the major labium preceding the topographic gonadal evolution, which explains the possibility of congenital hernias associated to gonadal ectopies. During the normal course of development, the testes descend from the intra-abdominal space into the scrotum in the third trimester, a relative movement which is closely linked to the development of scrotal and lumbar ligaments. The gonads slide to the posterior of the peritoneo-vaginal canal to be placed under its inferior border, thus realizing the draft of the vaginal serosal layer.

As a rule, the peritoneo-vaginal canal closes before birth. The closure abnormalities of the peritoneo-vaginal canal or the equivalent Nuck's canal may explain the different modalities of intrafunicular indirect hernias predominant in young patients. The partial permeability of the proximal portion of the canal explains the congenital hernias found at birth or becomes evident during the first crisis. A total permeability results in a communicating hernia in which the visceral organs may be engaged descending to the testicular level, even contacting the testicle. Residual or "suspended" permeability explains the frequency of small hernia accompanying cordon cysts.

Indirect hernias frequently appear following an effort as a late manifestation of a congenital abnormality. In certain cases, the peritoneo-vaginal canal descends to the testicular level without communicating with the vaginalis.

The ductus deferens conserves its close relationship with the serous diverticulum, so it is mandatory to be vigorous during the resection of the indirect hernia sac, especially in infants. The ovaries exceptionally may be engaged into the inguinal trajectory, or even may be present in the major labium, giving rise to an intraparietal ectopy. So, one should be prudent not to blindly resect an inguinal mass in a female patient, misdiagnosing it as a simple lipoma.

According to Russel (1906), all indirect hernias are in fact congenital abnormalities. This opinion was controverted, many authors admitting that the simple fossa at the origin of the peritoneo-vaginal canal on the abdominal side, under the influence of parietal insufficiency may distend into the spermatic cord. On the other hand, in some male or female patients, the persistent permeability of peritoneo-vaginal canal may exist without any manifestation of hernia.

4. Architecture

The inguinofemoral region is constructed "around an orifice", which is named the Fruchaud's orifice. Fruchaudemphasized the fact that all hernias of the groin originate within a single weak area, the myopectineal orifice, which is subdivided as inguinal and femoral by the inguinal ligament representing the terminal part of the aponeurosis of the external oblique muscle. The muscles of the anterolateral abdominal wall are arranged in two layers, the aponeurosis of external oblique muscle anteriorly and the transversalis fascia and its reinforcements posteriorly [1, 2, 12].

Fascia transversalis is the principal structure of regional stability. The opening of the deep inguinal ring of the inguinal canal is at this level. The inguinal canal has three passages—the deep inguinal ring situated above and laterally, the myopectineal orifice in the middle, and the superficial inguinal ring (annulus superficialis) situated below and medially, thus forming a chicane first described by Ombredane. Each one of these three passages plays an important role in visceral contention. The importance of this chicane is even ameliorated by its transverse location in space, the ectomorph (longilineal), slender individuals being more prone to the development of inguinal hernias compared to the endomorph (brevilineal) ones, both in males and females [1, 3, 4].

5. The myopectineal orifice

The myopectineal orifice is bounded below by the anteroinferior part of the coccyx, the horizontal part of pubic bone, lined in its upper part by the ligament of Cooper; above by the conjoint tendon of internal oblique and transverse muscles; and medially by the lateral border of rectus abdominis and the overlying pyramidalis muscles (**Figure 1**). The myopectineal orifice is subdivided into two regions, femoral below and inguinal above by the inguinal ligament. So, there is a relationship between direct and femoral hernia, one pushing anteriorly and the second one inferiorly [13].

5.1. The bony construction

The inguinofemoral region is constructed at the anterior border of the iliac bone, which presents from above to downward the anterior superior iliac spine, an unnamed notch; the anterior inferior iliac spine, the iliopubic eminence, and the pectineal surface of the superior ramus of the pubic bone, bounded behind by the pecten of the pubis and medially by the pubic tubercle. The pubic bone is lined in its upper part by the pectineal ligament of Cooper [14].

The pelvic skeleton plays an important role in the occurrence of hernia by its general morphology, besides participating in the constitution of the myopectineal orifice. As already mentioned, ectomorph (longilineal) individuals are more predisposed to hernia

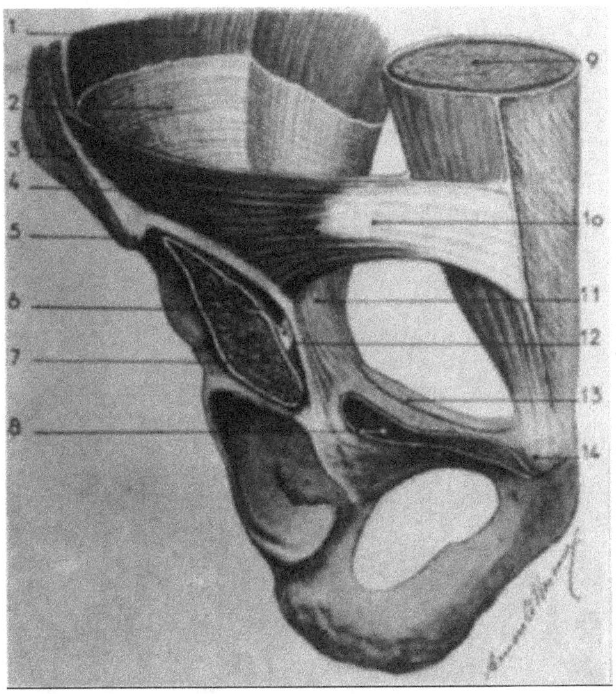

Figure 1. The myopectineal orifice: 1 = iliacus muscle; 2 = fascia iliaca; 3 = external oblique muscle; 4 = internal oblique muscle; 5 = superior iliac spine; 6 = femoral nerve; 7 = iliopsoas muscle; 8 = pectineus muscle; 9 = rectus muscle; 10 = internal oblique muscle; 11 = iliopectineal tract; 12 = fascia iliaca; 13 = Cooper's ligament; 14 = pubic tubercle.

formation. The angle of Radojevic is formed by the intersection of the line of Malgaigne and the horizontal line uniting both the anterior superior iliac spines (**Figure 2**). This angle differs between 25and 35°, the more the value of the angle, the more is the possibility of hernia formation. The distance between the superior border of pubic symphysis and the bi-spinal line may be substituted though, for example, 6 cm of distance giving approximately an angle of 30° [14].

5.2. Inferior attachments

These are in fact the anatomic structures on which we rely habitually for passing the sutures while performing hernia surgery.

5.2.1. Inguinal ligament

The inguinal ligament was initially described as an autonomous ligament uniting the anterior superior iliac spine to the pubic spine and winding around a center constructed by autonomous fibers of the lower part of the external oblique muscle aponeurosis. The question is that whether this is a true or discrete fibrous structure. The existence of the inguinal ligament was questioned by many authors, especially by Winckler, who demonstrated that the so-called inguinal ligament was only the inferior folded border of aponeurosis of the external oblique muscle. It may frequently be weakened, the direction of fibers constituting it are parallel to each other and may be frayed under the tension of sutures [15].

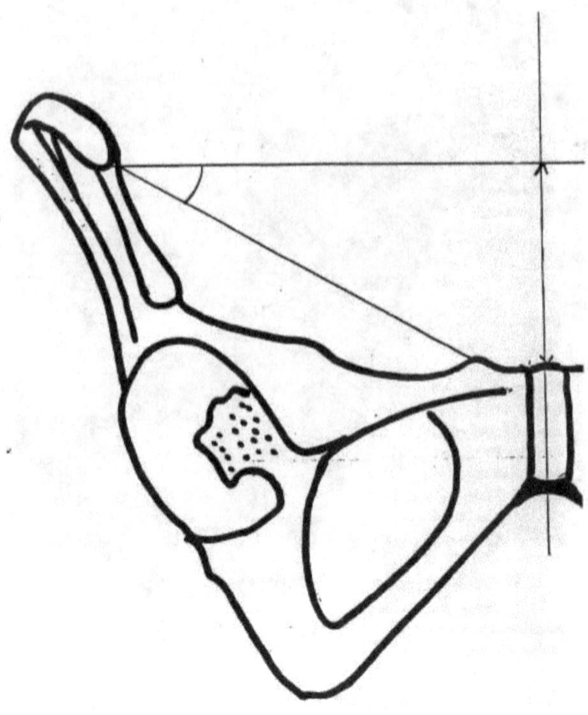

Figure 2. Radojevic angle.

5.2.2. The iliopubic tract (bandelette of Thomson)

Under the name "bandelette of Thomson" is described as the fibrous structures situated posterior to the lower free margin of the inguinal ligament, which are in fact the condensations of the transversalis fascia. It is to Alex Thomson that we owe the description of this fibrous structure. This tract is nearly parallel to the anterior aspect of the thigh. The fibers of the bandelette are parallel to the superior border of the anterior vascular sheath, enlarging considerably posteriorly and superiorly to attach between two bundles of the ligament of Cooper on the internal third of the crest of the pubic bone and on the lateral half of the anterior border of the superior aspect of the body of the pubis. This bandelette, with its own fibers of the lateral half of the iliofemoral-vascular fascia, is named the iliopubic tract (**Figure 3**).

For certain authors, these are the structures that we should rely on while passing the stitches more than the inguinal ligament, such as the conception of McVay and Anson [16].

5.2.3. The annexes of inguinal ligament: Iliopectineal bandelette, ligament of Gimbernat

The iliopectineal tract extends from one-third external part of the inguinal ligament to the iliopectineal (iliopubic) eminence of the pubic bone. This structure does not have any direct relationship with the inguinal ligament, it is a reinforcement of the internal border of iliac fascia, which slides under the inguinal ligament to which it closely adheres. The iliopectineal ligament separates the two passages situated under the inguinal ligament. The femoral nerve passes just lateral to it, whereas the femoral artery and the vein pass medially. Thus, the iliopectineal ligament separates the femoral nerve from the femoral artery.

The ligament of Gimbernat is placed medial to this vascular gap.

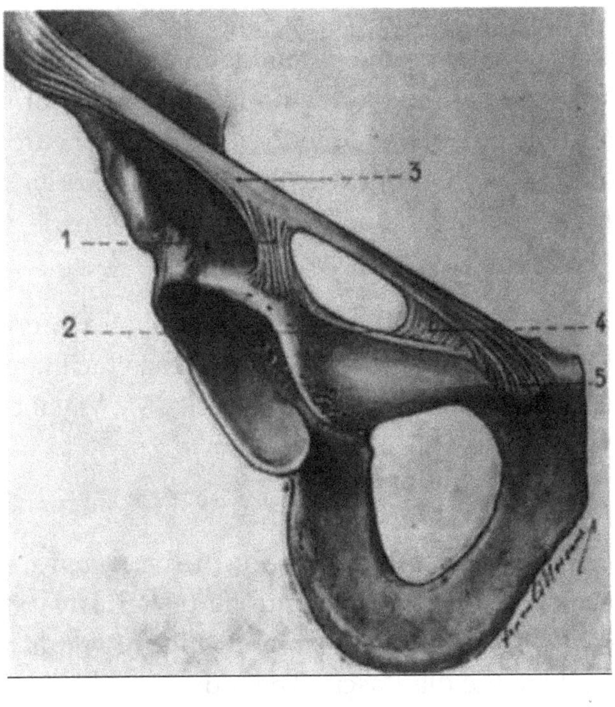

Figure 3. Anterior border of the iliac bone: 1 = iliopectineal tract; 2 = Cooper's ligament; 3 = iliopubic tract; 4 = Gimbernat's ligament; 5 = pubic tubercle.

This ligament presents a resistant external border, important in strangulation of femoral hernias. Between the femoral vein and the ligament of Gimbernat, extends a fibrous layer into which passes the lymphatics of the inferior extremities. This structure is called the femoral septum, which in fact is the inferior expansion of the transversalis fascia [15, 16].

5.2.4. *Cooper's ligament (pectineal ligament)*

The Cooper's ligament lines the superior border of the pubic bone between the pubic spine and the iliopectineal eminence. This ligament joins the inguinal ligament medially where it forms the lacunar ligament of Gimbernat but diverges laterally from it when runs in a much deeper position. The pectineal ligament is a heterogeneous structure comprising of three layers. It is formed by a superficial fibrous layer where the vertical fibers of the aponeurosis of the pectineal muscle and transverse fibers are running along the innominate line of the pelvis overlap. The middle, muscular layer is formed by the fibers of the pectineus muscle. The deep layer is in continuity with the periosteum of the superior pubic ramus.

Very thick and displaying an extreme degree of mechanical resistance medially, weakens while passing under the femoral vein. At this point, it becomes dangerous to pass stitches because of the close relationship with the femoral vein. The sutures that are sufficiently strong, passing from the Cooper's ligament, placed near the contact of pubic bone may virtually lift up the whole body. The Mc Vay procedure relies on this resistance, which automatically closes the inguinal and femoral passages when the sutures are in place [1, 16].

5.3. Internal border of the myopectineal orifice

The rectus abdominis muscle of the abdomen, very large, superiorly narrows until 4 cm at the inferior part just above the pubis terminating by a short tendon extending from the pubic symphysis to the pubic tubercle. At this level, the muscle does not contain any fibrous intersections. On its anterior face, habitually it is covered by the pyramidal muscle of the abdomen, which extends from the middle part of the median line to the horizontal branch of the pubis. The sheath of the rectus abdominis muscle is constituted anteriorly by the aponeurotic layers of the external oblique, internal oblique, and transverse muscles whereas posteriorly, below the level of the arc of Douglas, the posterior sheath consists of only the transversalis fascia, which is thickened at this level [17].

The rectus muscle may be mobilized and lowered laterally and inferiorly either to the inguinal ligament or to the Cooper's ligament. This maneuver is facilitated by incisions of relaxation on the anterior face of the rectus abdominis muscle (Mc Vay incision).

5.4. Superior border

The conjoint tendon (*tendo conjunctivus*) is made up of the transverse fibers of the internal oblique muscle anteriorly and the transverse muscle posteriorly extending from one-third external part of the inguinal ligament to the anterior face of rectus abdominis muscle. This muscle plan is fixed laterally to the iliac fascia. The muscular fibers, which are detached from the infero-external part wrap up the spermatic cord constituting the cremaster muscles, considerably thickening the origin of the spermatic cord [15].

5.5. Weak points of the myopectineal orifice

The myopectineal orifice is subdivided by some anatomic structures, such as the inguinal ligament, the inferior epigastric vessels, and the umbilical artery, into four regions, of which three of them are above and one is below the inguinal ligament.

Above the inguinal ligament, inside the umbilical artery, a hernia may be present between the posterior face of the rectus abdominis muscle and the umbilical artery. These are very rare hernias called the internal oblique hernias.

Between the umbilical artery and the epigastric vessels, the myopectineal orifice makes a gap. The only anatomic structure which may resist at this level is the transversalis fascia. This is the site of direct hernia frequently seen after 50 years of age.

Outside the epigastric vessels, passes the spermatic cord where a patent peritoneo-vaginal canal may exist, the site of development of external (indirect) hernias.

Below the inguinal ligament, between the vessels and the ligament of Gimbernat is located the femoral weak point, where femoral hernias are encountered [18].

6. The transversalis fascia

The transversalis fascia covers the totality of the myopectineal orifice, leaving just enough space for the passage of grand pedicles.

The transversalis fascia is not a true muscular aponeurosis, but in fact a fibrous layer situated between the deep face of the transverse muscle to which it adheres strongly and in front of the fatty tissue of fascia propria separating it from the peritoneal serosal layer.

The transversalis fascia is insignificant in the superior part of the abdomen, it becomes thicker below the layer of the arc of Douglas, where it gets the qualities of a true aponeurosis. Below the conjoint tendon level, the transversalis fascia continues to be frequently reinforced by the arciform fibrous bands, which are parallel to the transverse muscle fibers. It occupies the inguinal triangle of the myopectineal orifice and continues toward the posterior face of the rectus abdominis muscle. Outside and upward it forms a fibrous layer on which the cremaster muscles are attached. Likewise the deep inguinal ring is formed under which the inferior epigastric vessels pass. The fascia transversalis attaches to the posterior border of the inguinal ligament laterally and continues downward to form the femoral septum, and finally attaches strongly to the deep layer of the Cooper's ligament [16].

6.1. The reinforcements of the transversalis fascia

6.1.1. The ligament of Hesselbach

The ligament of Hesselbach or the interfoveolar ligament is a reinforcement of the transversalis fascia, which makes an upward-looking curve at the inferior border of the deep inguinal ring. Medially, it begins from the arc of Douglas, passes under the deep inguinal ring and ascends laterally to be vanished in the deep face of the transverse muscle toward the anterosuperior iliac spine. The internal part of the ligament interferes with the fibrous sheet of the epigastric vessels. The ligament stretches by the contraction of the transverse muscle thus narrowing the deep ring of the inguinal canal opposing to the protrusion of visceral organs. It is probably a residual muscle because it is accompanied by some muscle fibers.

6.1.2. The ligament of Henle

The ligament of Henle is composed of fibers, which leave the external border of the rectus abdominis muscle and cover the internal part of the inguinal ligament. It continues below by the ligament of Gimbernat. Frequently, the ligament of Henle is not well identified. It is probably a residual muscle, like the ligament of Hesselbach [2, 15–18].

6.2. Aponeurotic layer of the external oblique muscle

The external oblique muscle extends from the posteroinferior costal intersections to the anterosuperior iliac spine. At the inguinal level, the muscle is represented only by an aponeurotic layer, which by its inferior border constructs the inguinal ligament extending from the anterosuperior iliac spine to the pubic spine. The fibers which are attached to the pubic spine are thicker and they form the lateral edge of the superficial ring of the inguinal canal (lateral crus). Other fibers, separated from the lateral edge of the superficial ring attach to the pubic symphysis and even transverse the midline. This is the internal edge or the medial crus. Between these two pillars opens the superficial orifice (superficial annulus) into which passes the spermatic cord.

Incisions performed in the direction of fibers of this aponeurosis of external oblique a little above the level of inguinal ligament and opening the superficial inguinal ring is indispensable for anterior approach of myopectineal orifice and the spermatic cord. The during hernia cure, the closure of the external oblique aponeurosis in front of the spermatic cord reestablishes the inguinal chicane. Certain authors (Jaboulay) place the sutures of external oblique aponeurosis in retrofunicular position, leaving likewise the spermatic cord under the skin [3, 16].

6.3. The skin and the subcutaneous tissue

The subcutaneous fascia of Camper lies in front of the external oblique aponeurosis, which is a lamellar organization of adipose tissue forming the suspensor ligament of penis in the midline.

In the same adipose tissue is found the superficialis fascia, which sometimes may be well organized to be mistaken as external oblique aponeurosis. Between the subcutaneous fascia and the superficialis fascia, an arterial network made up of small branches of arteries and specially, a venous network which converges toward the saphenous vein are present.

6.4. Posterior structures: Fascia propria, prevesical umbilical aponeurosis, peritoneum

The transversalis fascia layer is separated from the peritoneum by an adipose space, more or less thicker depending on the individual. This layer extends laterally to the Retzius space.

This space which is opened during the incision of the transversalis fascia above the Cooper's ligament is called the Bogros's space (**Figures 4, 5**). This space contains bulky anastomotic veins between the external iliac vein and the inferior epigastric vein. Hemorrhages during the dissection of this area may be quite difficult to control. The arteries named "corona mortis" may follow the ligament of Cooper posteriorly, which may be a cause of hemorrhages [3, 13, 19].

On the midline, the adipose tissue may hide the superolateral part of the urinary bladder, which may be engaged in a direct hernia or a femoral hernia.

Posterior to the fatty layer on the midline suspends the residual cords of ourach, in general well identified on the one-third inferior part, but tapering toward the umbilicus and the umbilical artery (corda arteria umbilicalis), which is located just lateral to it. These structures converge toward the umbilicus and unite by an aponeurosis called the umbilico-prevesical aponeurosis.

The parietal peritoneum covers these structures to form three fossae, which are important in the laparoscopic or the posterior approach of the groin region.

Between the ourach and the umbilical artery, the "internal inguinal fossa" where very rare internal inguinal hernias may occur; between the umbilical artery and the epigastric vessels or the "middle inguinal fossa" (fovea inguinalis medialis) where direct inguinal hernias may occur; and finally lateral to the epigastric vessels the "external inguinal fossa" (fovea inguinalis lateralis) where indirect inguinal hernias may occur.

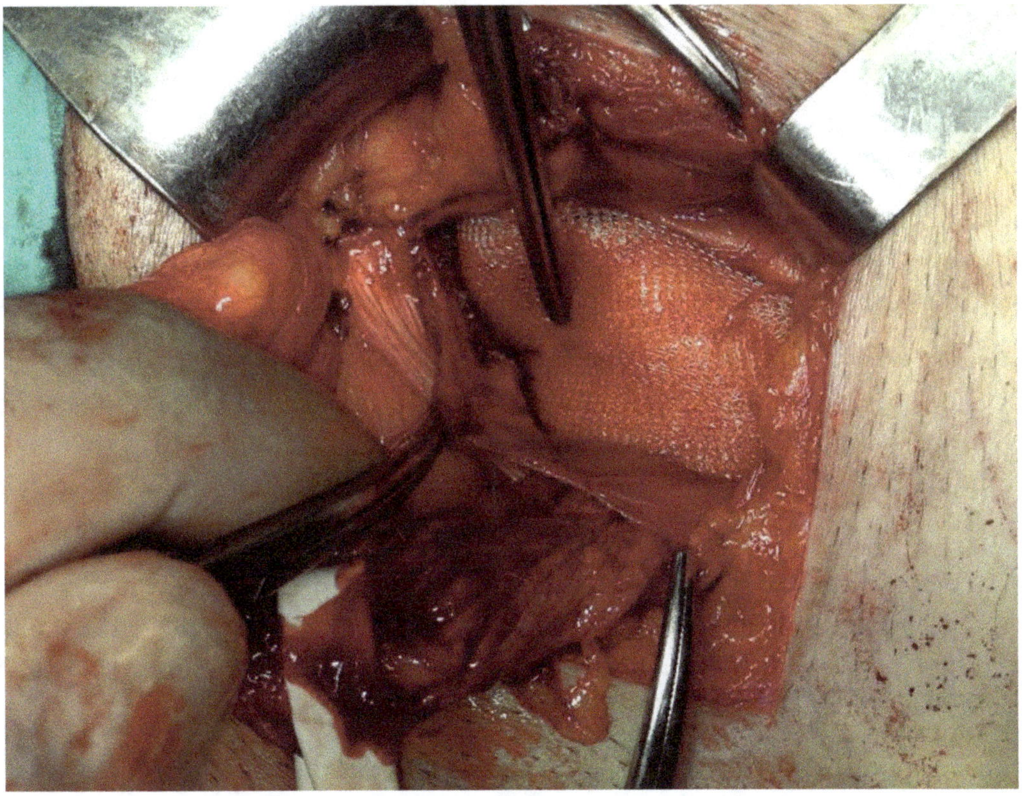

Figure 4. Mesh placement in preperitoneal space by anterior approach.

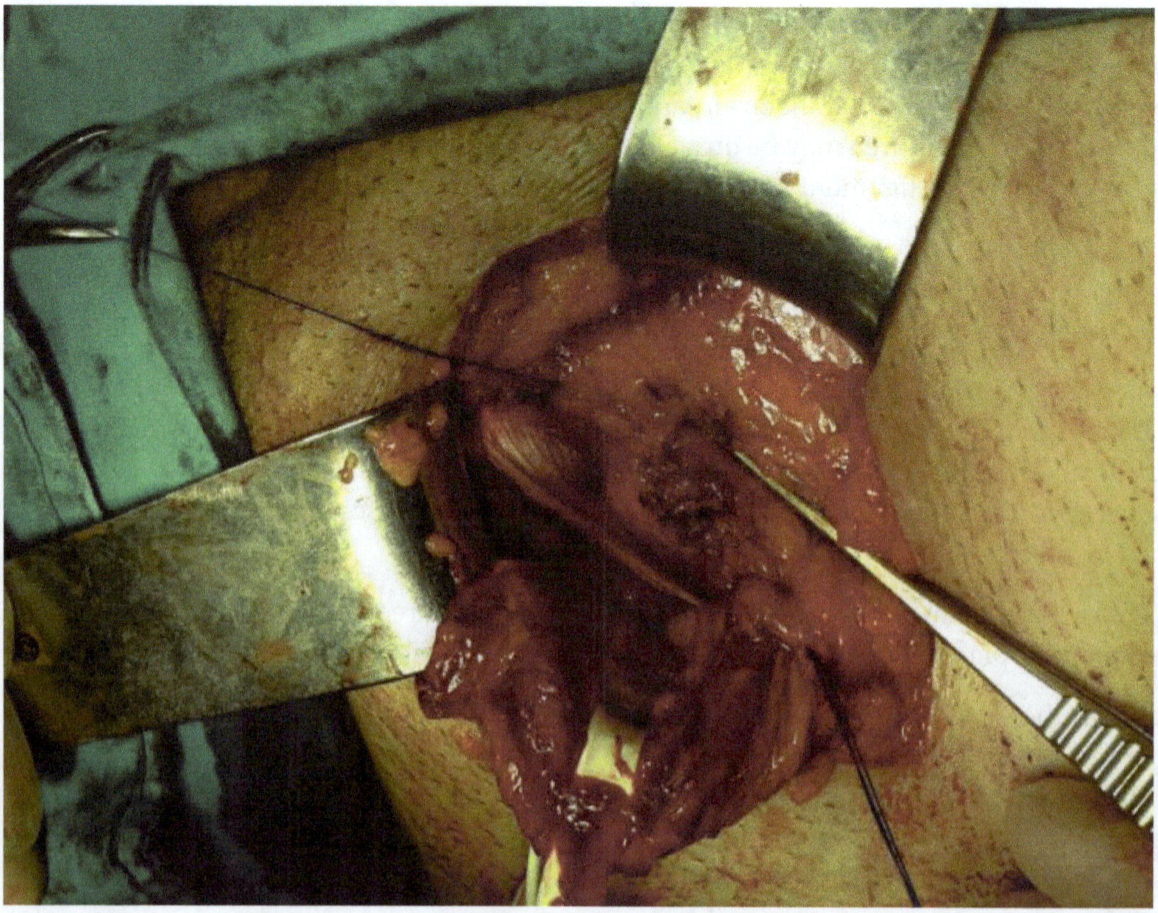

Figure 5. Closure of transversalis fascia after mesh placement in the preperitoneal space.

7. Vascularization

The vascularization of the superficial layers is abundant, which is supplied by the ramification of the superficial iliac circumflex vessels and the superficial epigastric vessels. The veins in the subcutaneous adipose tissue are particularly abundant. They join the saphenous vein inferiorly.

The lymphatic drainage of the anterolateral abdominal wall, the umbilical region, and sometimes even the mammary glands is toward the inguinal ganglions. This fact may explain some minimal lymphatic infections, which may be encountered after surgical cure of inguinal hernia.

The arterial blood supply of deep layers emerges from the deep circumflex iliac artery, the epigastric artery, and its branches, obturatrice-epigastric anastomoses connected to the descending branch of the epigastric artery, which follows the posterior face of the rectus abdominis muscle below the arc of Douglas.

The vascularization at the femoral level is reassured by the external pudendal arteries emerging from the femoral artery which are directed toward the internal and superior thigh, scrotum, or the labium majus.

The inferior epigastric vein, which is separated internally from the inferior epigastric artery before joining the femoral vein forms a unique trunk of about 3 cm. The femoral vein constitutes the principle surgical danger in this region [4, 12, 15].

8. Innervation

Numerous nerves exist in the inguinofemoral region. Their injury or capture between the sutures explains the relative frequency of the extremely invalidating postoperative pain. The reoperations or the attempt of neurolysis do not always ameliorate the situation. The two principle nerves of the region are the abdominogenital and the genitofemoral nerves.

8.1. Abdominogenital nerves

Iliohypogastric and ilioinguinal nerves arise from the lumbar plexus (level L1), follow a path between the external oblique and transverse muscles. Both nerves arrive the inguinal region just inside the anterosuperior iliac spine, they pierce the internal oblique muscle and follow a course parallel to the superficial fibers of the conjoint tendon. The anastomotic branches may exist between the two nerves. The ilioinguinal nerve, following the anterosuperior part of the spermatic cord, exits through the superficial inguinal ring and descends to the testicles. It supplies somatic sensation to the skin of the upper and medial thigh and innervates the base of the penis and labium majus in females. The nerve or one of its branches may be injured or entrapped between the sutures during hernia surgery [2, 4, 13].

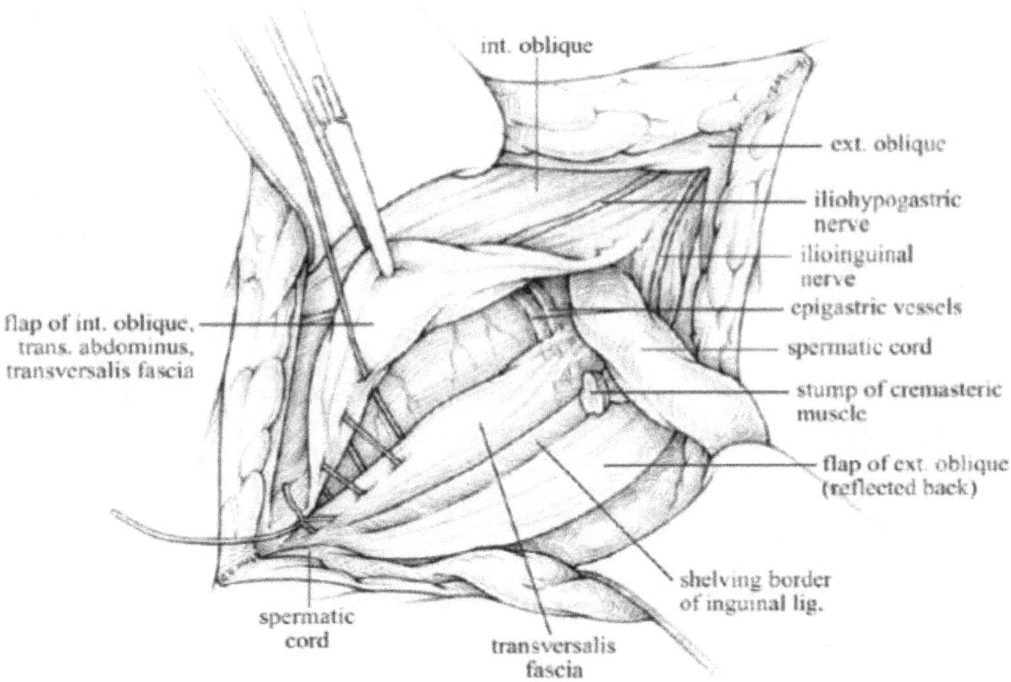

Figure 6. Inguinal anatomy anterior view.

8.2. Genitofemoral nerve

The genitofemoral nerve arises from L1-L2, follows the sheath of the psoas muscle, and divides into two branches. The femoral branch courses along the femoral sheath, descends to the thigh, supplying the skin of the upper anterior thigh. The genital branch reaches the spermatic cord at the level of the deep inguinal ring, lateral to the inferior epigastric vessels. During the dissection of the upper part of the spermatic cord, this nerve may be injured. Below, the nerve follows the inferior and deep part of the spermatic cord and finally gives branches to genital teguments. It may be injured during the dissection of the hernia sac or the cremaster muscle, which itself is innervated by the nerve [2, 4, 13].

8.3. Other nerves of the region

The lateral femoral cutaneous nerve, the femoral nerve, and the obturator nerve are exceptionally injured during hemostatic maneuvers in the adipose tissue of the space of Bogros. The lateral femoral cutaneous nerve arises from L2-L3, emerges lateral to the psoas muscle toward the anterior superior iliac spine. It then passes inferior to the inguinal ligament (**Figure 6**) [2, 4, 13].

9. The Nyhus classification system

The Nyhus classification categorizes hernia defects by location, size, and type [1].

Type I is an indirect hernia, the internal abdominal ring is normal, seen typically in infants, children, and young adults.

Type II is an indirect hernia, the internal ring is enlarged without impingement on the floor of the inguinal canal, which does not extend to the scrotum.

Type IIIA is a direct hernia, of which the size is not taken into account.

Type IIIB is an indirect hernia that has enlarged enough to encroach upon the posterior inguinal wall. The indirect sliding, pantaloon, or scrotal hernias are usually placed in this category because they are commonly associated with the extension to the direct space.

Type IIIC is a femoral hernia.

Type IV corresponds to recurrent hernia, modifiers A–D are sometimes added, which correspond to indirect, direct, femoral, and mixed, respectively.

10. Surgical approaches

10.1. Inguinal incision

Inguinal incision is placed on the half-distance between the external border of the rectus abdominis muscle and the inguinal ligament. This incision may equally be made 2 cm above the line of Malgaigne. The inguinal incision permits the surgical treatment of all the varieties of inguinal or femoral nonstrangulated hernias. Likewise, the hernia sac is approached on the level above its collar. This approach is used in several operations, such as Mc Vay, Bassini, Shouldice, Lichtenstein, and so on (**Figures 6** and 7).

10.2. Vertical approach

Vertical approach is frequently used for femoral hernias. The incision is traced internal to the femoral vessels, which ascend a couple of centimeters above the inguinal ligament. The approach to the inguinal ligament, which may eventually be sectioned, or the Cooper's ligament is possible with this incision, which is the incision of choice for strangulated femoral

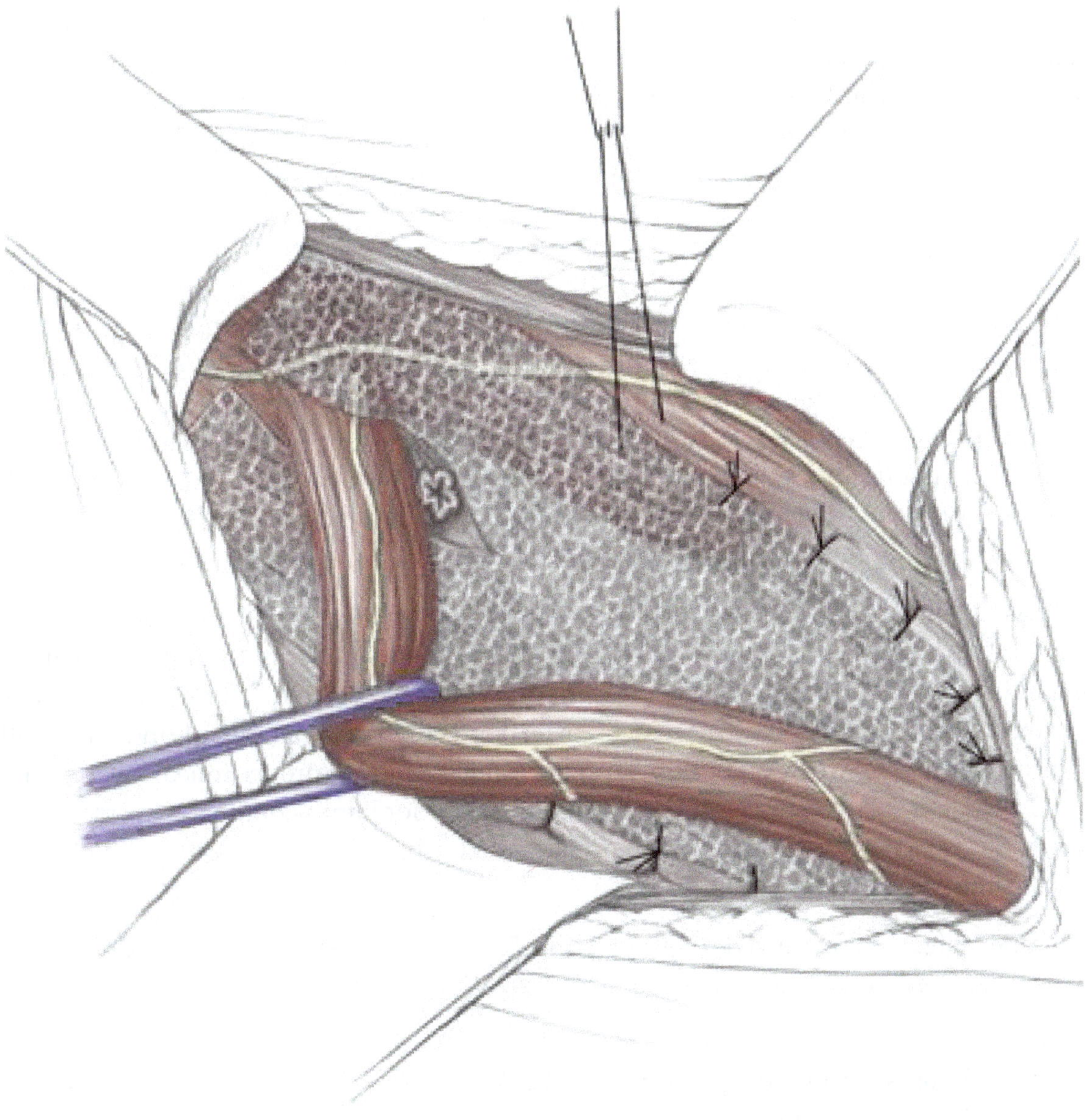

Figure 7. Lichtenstein's operation.

hernias. Direct approach of the hernia sac and verification of its contents and their reintegration in the abdominal cavity are possible.

10.3. Inguinal horizontal approach

The inguinal horizontal approach is comparable to the horizontalized Mc Burney incision, which gives rise to the direct approach of the peritoneum and dissecting the peritoneum inferiorly, the origin of the hernia sac may be identified facilitating its simple ligation without dissecting the spermatic cord. This approach is recommended in infants where the testicular pedicle is particularly fragile.

10.4. Infraumbilical extraperitoneal median incision

This longitudinal incision, after a blunt lateral dissection of preperitoneal space, makes it possible to see till the iliac vasculature. Likewise, the treatment of bilateral inguinal hernias is possible by ligation and section, to mobilize and dissect the spermatic cord and to place a synthetic mesh between the posterior face of the muscles and the peritoneum. This incision was introduced by Stoppafor the treatment of bilateral recurrences of inguinal hernias [20, 21].

10.5. Laparoscopic approach

The laparoscopic approach to hernia repair provides a posterior perspective to the peritoneal and preperitoneal spaces. The parietal peritoneum covers the deep layer of the abdominal wall above the inguinal ligament. On the midline suspends the residual cords of ourach or the *median umbilical ligament* which extends from the fundus of the bladder to the umbilicus. Corda arteria umbilicalis or the *medial umbilical ligament*, which covers the distal portion of the umbilical artery, is located just lateral to the precedent. The *lateral umbilical ligament* is the fold of peritoneum around the epigastric vessels.

These folds delineate three shallow fossae on either side of the midline: Supravesical, medial, and lateral fossae. Very rarely, internal inguinal hernias may occur in the supravesical fossa. The medial fossa is the region where direct hernias are encountered. The lateral fossa which lies lateral to the inferior epigastric vessels corresponds to the deep inguinal ring, the location of indirect hernias. Bogros's preperitoneal space, which contains preperitoneal fat and areolar tissue, is situated between the peritoneum and the posterior lamina of the transversalis fascia. The medial aspect of this space which corresponds to the superior region of the bladder is known as the space of Retzius.

The Cooper's ligament is viewed roughly in a horizontal direction. The bandelette of Thomson may be visualized in thin individuals after mobilization of the peritoneum.

The vascular space is situated between the posterior and anterior laminae of the transversalis fascia, and it houses the inferior epigastric vessels. The inferior epigastric artery supplies the rectus abdominis. It is derived from the external iliac artery, and it anastomoses with the superior epigastric, a continuation of the internal thoracic artery. The epigastric veins course parallel to the arteries within the rectus sheath, posterior to the rectus muscles. Inspection of the internal inguinal ring will reveal the deep location of the inferior epigastric vessels.

The nerves pass from under or through the bandelette of the Thomson lateral to the external inguinal fossa and the spermatic vessels. The nerves of interest in the inguinal region are the ilioinguinal, iliohypogastric, genitofemoral, and lateral femoral cutaneous nerves.

The preperitoneal anatomy seen in laparoscopic hernia repair led to the characterization of important anatomic areas of interest, known as the "triangle of doom," the "triangle of pain," and the "circle of death."

The triangle of doom is bordered medially by the vas deferens and laterally by the vessels of the spermatic cord, the summit of the triangle corresponding to the deep inguinal ring. The contents of the space include the external iliac vessels, the deep circumflex iliac vein, the femoral nerve, and the genital branch of the genitofemoral nerve.

The triangle of pain is a region bordered by the iliopubic tract above and the gonadal vessels below. The lateral femoral cutaneous, femoral branch of the genitofemoral, and femoral nerves may be injured in this region.

The circle of death (corona mortis) refers to the anastomotic branches of vasculature in this region formed by the common iliac, internal iliac, obturator, inferior epigastric, and external iliac vessels.

Author details

Kamer Tomaoglu

Address all correspondence to: kamertom@hotmail.com

Department of General Surgery, S.P. Hospital, Istanbul, Turkey

References

[1] Nyhus LM, Condon RE, editors. Hernia. Philadelphia: JB Lippincott Company; 1995

[2] Skandalakis LJ, Colborn GL. Surgical anatomy of the abdominal wall. 14. ed Vol 1, Bölüm 9, PMP Co, Athens: 2004, s. 395-491

[3] Skandalakis LJ. Abdominal wall and hernias. In: Skandalakis JE, editor. Surgical Anatomy. 14th ed., Vol. 1, Bölüm 9. Athens: PMP Co; 2004. pp. 395-491

[4] Wantz GE. Atlas of Hernia Surgery. New York: Raven Press; 1991

[5] Skandalakis LJ. Modern Hernia Repair. Vol. 1. London: Catagologing Publishing; 1992

[6] Wantz GE. Abdominal wall hernias. In: Schwartz SI, editor. Principles of Surgery. 7th ed., Vol. 2, Bölüm 34. Singapore: McGraw Hill Co; 1999. pp. 1585-1611

[7] Glassow WF. A comparison of the Shouldice and Cooper ligament repair for adult inguinal hernias. The American Journal of Surgery. 1976;**131**:306-311

[8] Nordin P, Bartelmess P, Jansson C, Svensson C, Edlund G. Randomized trial of Lichtenstein versus Shouldice hernia repair in general surgical practice. British Journal of Surgery. 2002;**89**:45-49

[9] Bassini E. Nuovo metodo sulla cura radicale dell' ernia inguinale. Archives of Italian surgical society 1887;**4**:80

[10] Shouldice EE. The treatment of hernia. Ontario Medical Review. 1953;**96**:1-14

[11] Lichtenstein IL, Shulman AG, Amid PK, et al. The tension free hernioplasty. American Journal of Surgery. 1989;**157**:188-192

[12] Cooper A. The Anatomy and Surgical Treatment of Abdominal Hernia. London: Longman and Co.; 1804

[13] Fruchaud H. Anatomie chirurgicale des hernies de l'aine. Paris: G. Doin; 1956

[14] Radojevic S. Anatomie chirurgicale de la region inguinale. Acta Anatomica. 1962;**50**: 208-263

[15] Gray FJ. The applied anatomy of the inguinal region. Australian and New Zealand Journal of Surgery. 1961;**30**:183-190

[16] Mcvay CB, Anson BJ. Aponeurotic and fascial continuities in the abdomen, pelvis and thigh. Anatomical Record. 1940;**76**:213-231

[17] Romanes GJ, editor. Cunningham's Textbook of Anatomy. 10th ed. London: Oxford University Press; 1964. p. 302

[18] Chandler SB, Schadewald M. Studies on the inguinal region. I. The conjoined aponeurosis versus the conjoined tendon. Anatomical Record. 1944;**89**:339-343

[19] Masereeuw J. Contributions to the structural anatomy of the inguinal region. Acta Anatomica. 1966;**64**:179-197

[20] Stoppa R. Traitement par voie prépéritonéale des hernies de l'aine de l'adulte. Encycl Medico Chir Tech Chir. 2000;**1**:40-115

[21] Wantz GE. Une technique de hernioplastie propéritonéale. Le renforcement unilatéral du sac viscéral par grande prothése de Mersiléne. Chirurgie. 1993-1994;**119**:321-326

12

Significance of Autologous Tissues in the Treatment of Complicated, Large, and Eventrated Abdominal Wall Hernias

Gábor Martis and László Damjanovich

Abstract

Repair of complicated, large, or eventrated abdominal wall hernias poses a considerable challenge. Not infrequently, synthetic grafts implanted earlier become infected, entero- or subcutaneous fistulas appear, or emergency conditions like mechanical ileus or peritonitis develop. In such cases, direct closure of the abdominal wall with sutures or reinforcement with synthetic grafts is not recommended. Not many surgical techniques are capable of creating a low tension state. One is bridging of the abdominal wall defects; another is mobilization of the musculo-aponeurotic elements of the abdominal wall (components separation). In this chapter, the use of autologous double-layer dermal grafts and the technique of bilateral rectus muscle turnover allowing reconstruction of eventrated hernias in a tension-free way are discussed. In both procedures, only autologous tissues are used for reconstruction. With autologous dermal grafts, the rate of surgical complications is 4%, recurrence in the first 24 months is 11%, and the quality of life is significantly improved. With bilateral rectus muscle turnover, surgical complications occur at a rate of less than 2%, 24-month recurrence is 0%, and the quality of life is significantly improved. The technique of the interventions, their indications and contraindications, as well as their feasibility, advantages and disadvantages are described.

Keywords: infected and complicated abdominal wall hernia, eventrated hernia, autologous reconstruction, double layer dermal grafts, rectus turning over, recurrence, quality of life

1. Introduction

Repair of complicated, large, or eventrated abdominal wall hernias poses a considerable challenge for surgeons. Conditions characterized by the presence of an eventrated scar hernia and an extensive abdominal wall defect developed from an initially small ventral abdominal wall hernia are not infrequent in the surgical practice. Progression of incisional hernias in laparotomy scars may lead to a similar condition. Reconstruction of abdominal wall hernias accounts for 3–11% of all surgeries performed in general surgical wards, depending on the type and profile of the institute. Incisional hernias have a special significance in the surgical practice for two reasons: first, they develop as a consequence of an earlier intervention and have to be corrected, preferably in a definitive way, also satisfactory to the patient; second, abdominal wall hernias cannot always be resolved definitively despite all efforts. Scar hernias may recur for various reasons. They may be the consequence of inadequate surgical technique; in many cases, however, they are due to lack of compliance and discipline (strain exerted too early and not in a gradual fashion) on the patient's part. The question whether scar hernias are complications or natural corollaries of surgical interventions has been asked by several authors [1]. Whatever the reason, flat abdominal muscles lose their adherence partly or completely along the linea alba in the midline of the abdominal wall, and a progressive, well-defined, and well-known vicious circle is started. Since the reconstructed abdominal wall must resist, as much as possible, the intra-abdominal pressure—which often rises abruptly—as well as tension due to physical strain, reinforcement of the abdominal wall is a key factor in the surgery of abdominal wall hernias. Four kinds of techniques, each fundamentally different from the other, have evolved for the repair of abdominal wall hernias. The *first* is direct abdominal wall suture, with a synthetic mesh implanted in one of the following positions: epifascial (onlay), interfascial (inlay), or subfascial (sublay) [2, 3]. The *second* is the so-called components separation technique, in which closure of the defect is achieved by specific release of individual muscular components in the abdominal wall [4]. The *third* is laparoscopic abdominal wall reconstruction, in which a synthetic mesh is used to reinforce the abdominal wall [5]. The *fourth* technique involves bridging or replacement of the abdominal wall defect using synthetic or biological substances [6–8]. The common objectives of all these techniques are reducing the incidence of surgical complications, lowering recurrence rate, and improving the patients' quality of life.

Infected/compromised and eventrated abdominal wall hernias account for 1–8% of all (ventral and incisional) abdominal wall hernias in various institutes [9–10].

Treatment of complicated, large, or infected incisional hernias places a considerable burden on the patient, the hospital staff, the GP, as well as the social insurance [11–15].

The common objectives of all procedures performed in such cases are: (1) *elimination of contamination* in the abdominal wall environment; (2) *closure* of the abdominal wall *defect* with as little tension as possible; (3) maintenance of near-*normal intraabdominal pressure*; (4) *reduction* of postoperative surgical *complications*; (5) *reduction* of hernia *recurrence*; and last but not the least (6) *improvement of the quality of life*.

1.1. Definition, terminology

The use of a unified and unequivocal terminology is essential in the surgery of abdominal wall hernias. The nomenclature follows the recommendations of the European Hernia Society (EHS) [16]. *Ventral abdominal wall hernias* are defined as abdominal wall defects of nonsurgical origin, through which intraabdominal tissues and organs leave the abdominal cavity and enter among subcutaneous tissues. Ventral hernias are located in an area bordered by the bilateral anterior axillary line, the costal arches, and the pubic bone. *Incisional abdominal wall hernias* are defined as abdominal wall defects developing in the scars of an earlier surgical intervention allowing tissues and organs to leave the abdominal cavity and enter among subcutaneous tissues. *Medial abdominal wall hernias* are defined as hernias between the medial margins of the bilateral rectus abdominis sheaths; they can be M1: xyphoidal, M2: epigastric, M3: umbilical, M4: infraumbilical, and M5: suprapubic hernias. *Lateral abdominal wall hernias* are defined as abdominal wall defects located lateral of the outer margin of the rectus abdominis sheath, with L1 being subcostal, L2: iliac, L3: lumbar, and L4: inguinal. In small abdominal wall hernia, the longest diameter of the abdominal wall defect is less than 2 cm. In medium-sized abdominal wall hernia, the longest diameter of the abdominal wall defect is between 4 and 10 cm. In large abdominal wall hernia, the shortest diameter of the abdominal wall defect is at least 10 cm. *Midline scar hernias* are defined as incisional hernias developed in the scars of median laparotomies. *Lateral scar hernias* are defined as incisional abdominal wall hernias located lateral of the rectus abdominis sheath. *Recurrent abdominal wall hernias* are defined as scar hernias that have been repaired at least once in an earlier surgery. They consist of two basic components: the abdominal wall defect and the hernia sac with the hernia contents. It should be borne in mind that an abdominal wall protuberance is not an abdominal wall hernia by definition. A *seroma* is a circumscribed, encapsulated pocket of interstitial noninfected fluid developing between the abdominal wall fascia and the subcutis in the operative area. A diffuse, unencapsulated collection of fluid is not to be interpreted as a seroma. An *enterocutaneous fistula* is an abnormal passage allowing chronic communication between two epithelial surfaces (e.g., the small or large intestine and the skin). A *subcutaneous fistula* is a chronic abnormal communication system connecting the abdominal wall superficial fascia and the implanted synthetic/biological material. *Graft* is a fixed synthetic or biological material without blood supply of its own implanted over, under, or among the abdominal wall fascia. *Flap* is a tissue with its own blood supply transferred from another area of the body to cover or replace the abdominal wall defect. *Synthetic grafts* are man-made substances (polyethylene, polypropylene, and teflon) used to reinforce the abdominal wall. *Xeno- and allografts* are specially prepared biological substances of animal (porcine, bovine) or human origin used for reinforcement and/or replacement of the abdominal wall in special cases. *Autografts* are tissues collected from the patient's own body, suitable for replacement and/or reinforcement of abdominal wall defects. A *superficial wound infection* is an inflammatory process at the site of the operation affecting exclusively the skin and the subcutaneous fatty tissue. A *deep wound infection* is an inflammatory process at the site of the operation affecting the skin, the subcutaneous fatty tissue, the abdominal wall fascia, the muscles, as well as the implanted mesh. The abdominal cavity is not affected by this process. *Wound dehiscence* is partial, clean, or clean-contaminated rupture of continuity affecting the skin and the subcutaneous tissue. *Centers for Disease Control and Prevention (CDCP) wound environment*: classification of wounds by cleanliness into four categories. CDCP 1: clean, sterile; CDCP 2: clean but contaminated; CDCP 3: infected; CDCP 4: severely contaminated, necrotic. An *infected abdominal wall hernia* is defined as confirmed bacterial infection of the implanted synthetic graft or biological substance with simultaneous recurrence of the hernia. Earlier reconstructive surgery and recurring hernia are both assumed. *Compromised graft*: current or earlier bacterial infection of a synthetic graft. At best, it means a potentially contaminated environment (CDCP 2). The term *complicated* is used for incisional abdominal wall hernias which have recurred once or several times, featuring a compromised, or infected, synthetic graft and/or enterocutaneous fistula, with its hernia gate at least 10 cm in diameter. Abdominal wall incisional hernias with hernia sacs corresponding to at least 50% of the volume of the abdominal cavity, or chronically containing more than 50% of intraabdominal organs as defined by some authors [17], are called *eventrated*. The terms "loss of domain" and "loss of abdominal wall domain" are commonly used in the literature.

1.2. Aim of the chapter

1. Presentation of the technical details of reconstructive surgery using autologous double-layer dermal grafts in large recurrent infected abdominal wall hernias.
2. Discussion of short- and long-term outcomes and the results of quality of life studies following surgery with dermal grafts.
3. Computed tomographic (CT) examination of the musculoaponeurotic elements of the abdominal wall and discussion of its importance in the design of full midline giant abdominal wall hernia operations.
4. Presentation of the technical details of bilateral release and turnover of the rectus abdominis muscle and subsequent midline recreation, a surgical technique developed for the resolution of eventrated midline abdominal wall hernias.
5. Discussion of the short- and long-term outcomes of rectus turnover and changes in the quality of life following surgery.

2. Use of autologous double-layer dermal grafts in infected/recurrent large abdominal wall incisional hernias

2.1. Surgical technique

The intervention is performed under general intratracheal anesthesia in a state of complete muscle relaxation. A wide laurel-leave-shaped skin incision is made crosswise (never median!) between both spina iliaca anterior superior. The cutaneous-subcutaneous panniculus is removed (dermolipectomy), with the greater omentum carefully spared. The synthetic mesh implanted earlier is completely removed. The abdominal wall edges left behind should be strictly intact. The hernia sac should be spared if possible. In the case of multiple hernia gates, individual intact abdominal wall bridges are not opened into each other.

2.1.1. Preparation of the dermal grafts

The retained panniculus is stretched in all directions, and the epidermis is completely removed (**Figures 1** and **2**). The next step is removal of the subcutaneous adipose tissue (**Figure 3**). The prepared dermal graft is stored in a 2:1 solution of H_2O_2-povidone iodine until being used. An adequately prepared dermal graft contains the reticular and vascular layers, as well as a small amount of adipose tissue, without epidermal elements, hair follicles, sebaceous, or sweat glands on its surface (**Figure 4**). The dermal graft is then cut to size in a way that its margins extend beyond the margins of the abdominal wall defect by at least 5 cm. On the basis of our own measurements, a dermal graft can be expanded to 130–135% of its original size when stretched.

2.1.2. Crucial steps of the procedure

The graft is placed in the abdominal cavity with its original surface facing outward. Two procedures may be used here, depending on the status of the greater omentum (intact or not). In case there is no greater omentum, the spared hernia sac and the peritoneum are circularly separated from the inner surface of the abdominal wall, corresponding to the size of the implanted graft. The hernia sac and the peritoneum are closed with 3/0 absorbable thread, and then the graft is placed over the closed peritoneum. The first graft complements the abdominal wall defect. The edges of the abdominal wall are fixed to the graft circularly using 3/0 nonpenetrating, knotty, nonabsorbable stitches (**Figure 5**).

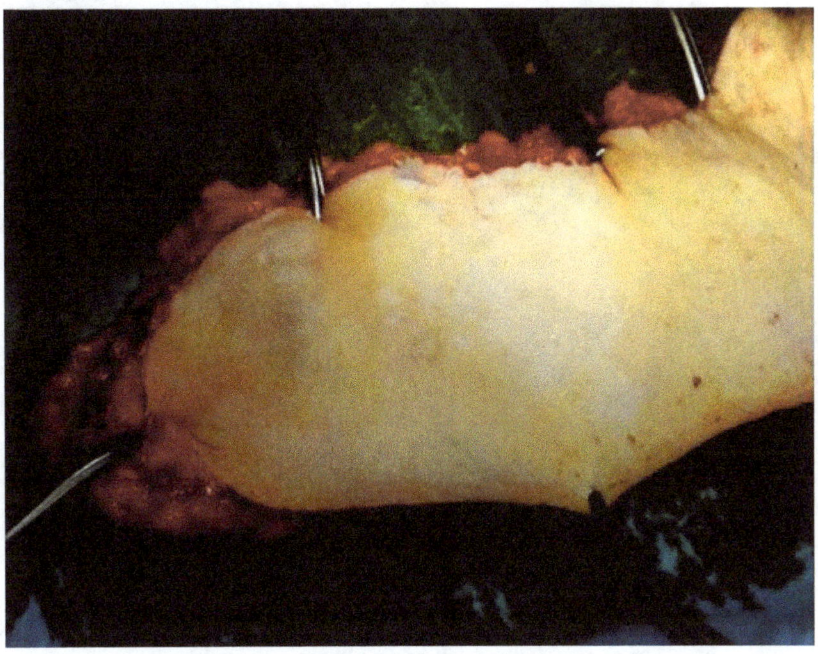

Figure 1. An appropriately stretched panniculus. The subcutis is not yet removed. The dermis is homogeneous without visible scars.

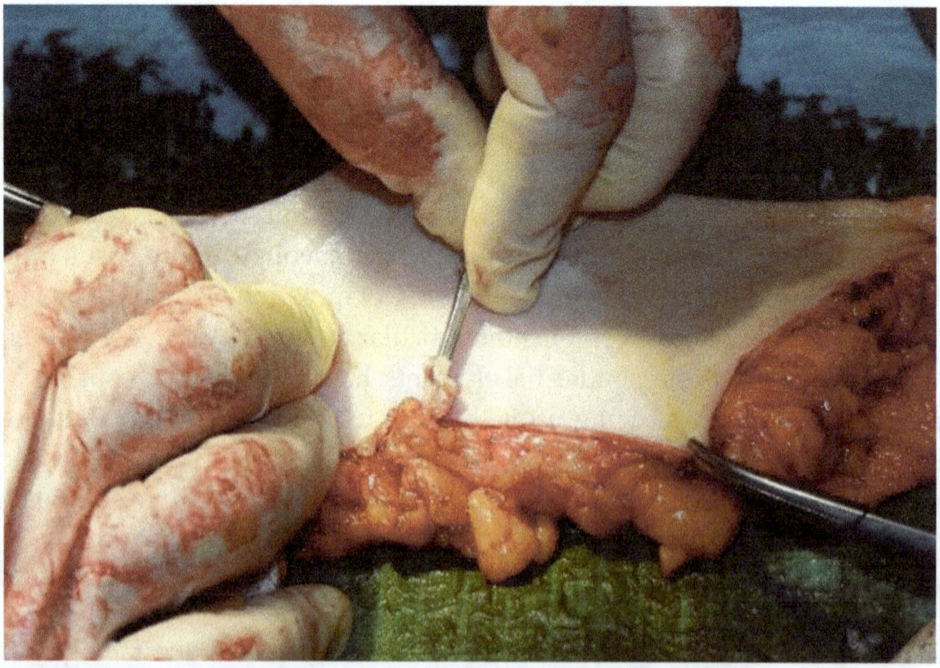

Figure 2. Removal of the epidermis. You can see removed epidermal elements on the blade. The blade is held tilted at approximately 30°. The lighter and darker sections of the dermis are clearly visible. The lighter section corresponds to the graft without the epidermis, while the darker section still contains the epidermis. The dermis must not be damaged during removal. Make sure that all epidermal elements are removed.

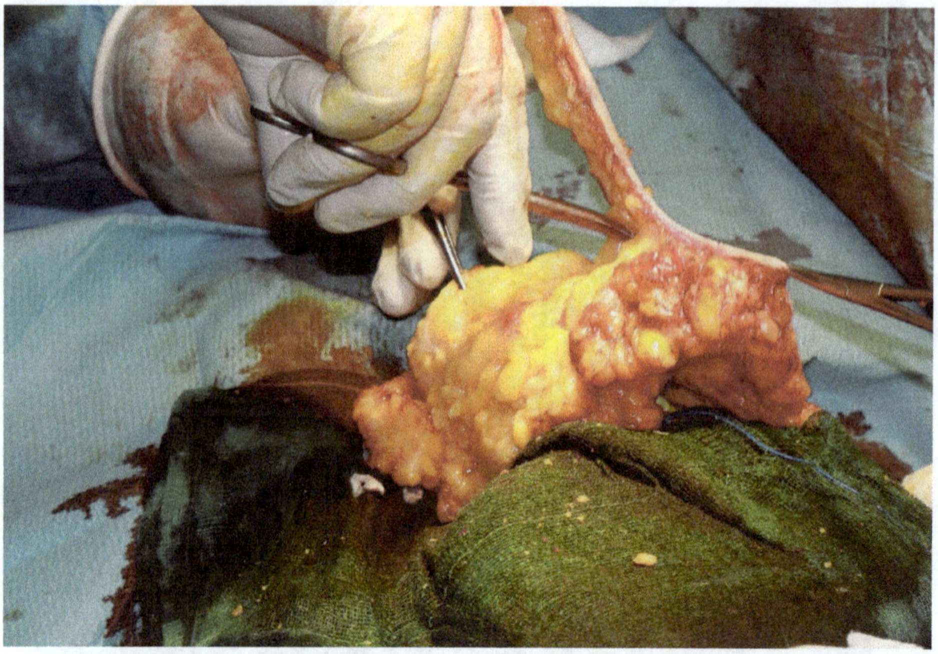

Figure 3. Removal of the adipose tissue. It is not necessary to remove the whole adipose tissue element. The numerous viable ADSCs in the adipose tissue (≈250,000–400,000 cells/5 ml homogenized adipose tissue) play an important role in the integration of the dermal graft.

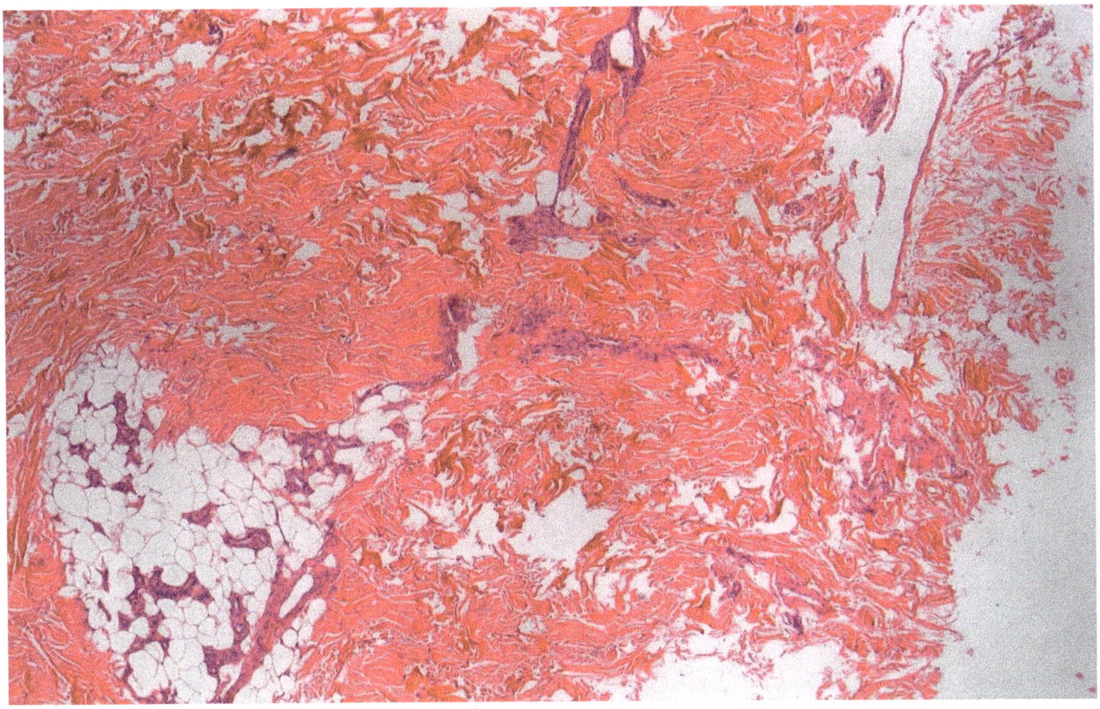

Figure 4. Histological picture of an adequately prepared dermal graft. There are no epidermal elements or signs of penetrating or partial dermal lesions. HE stain 100×.

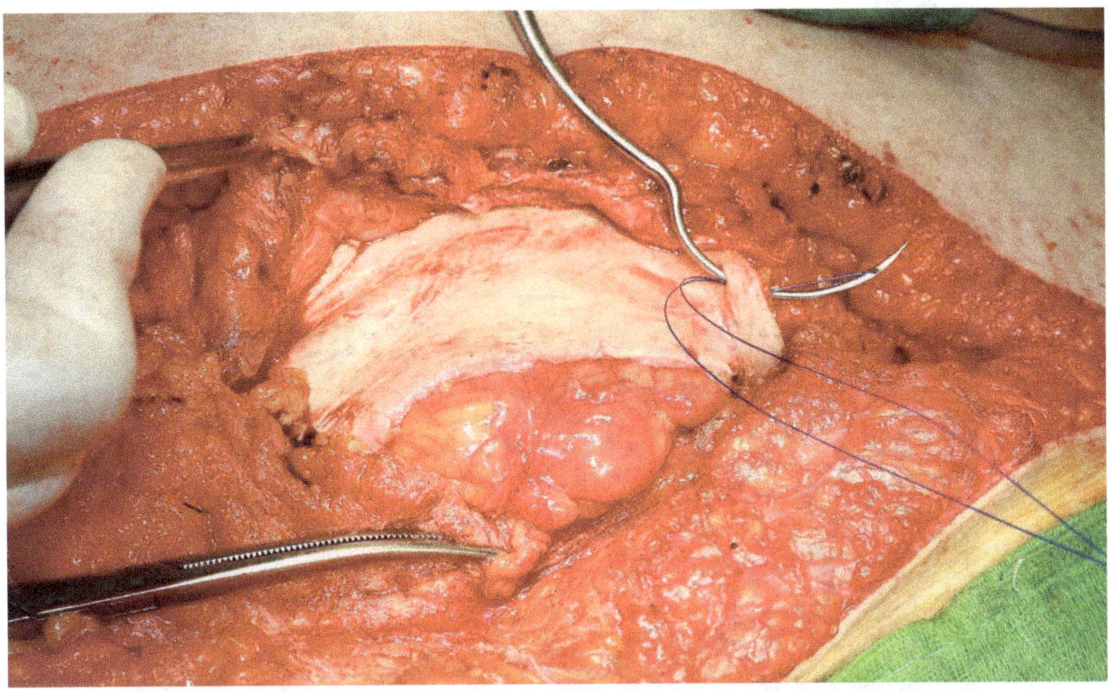

Figure 5. Placement of the first dermal graft. The inner graft is fixed with knotty, nonabsorbable 2/0 stitches with an overlapping margin of at least 5 cm. Intact abdominal wall edges must be constructed. These edges should then be fixed to the dermal graft with knotty, nonpenetrating stitches. There is no direct abdominal wall suture. The area of the abdominal wall defect is 168 cm^2. The placement of remote stitches is considerably easier when an instrument specifically designed for the purpose is used.

In the next step, the second graft is cut to size with its margins extending beyond the margins of the abdominal wall by approximately 2 cm. The graft is placed with its original surface facing inward. This way, the original epidermal surfaces face each other. Like the first one, the second graft is fixed to the abdominal wall fascia with nonabsorbable knotty stitches, in a nonfully stretched state (**Figure 6**). The outer dermal graft can also be applied perforated (**Figure 7**). The surgical area is rinsed with a 2:1 solution of H_2O_2-povidone iodine, with two or three suction drains left behind. The subcutis is "anchored" to the abdominal wall fascia with 8–10 absorbable stitches. The wound must be closed tension-free, using double-layer nonabsorbable subcutaneous and knotty or intracutaneous skin sutures (**Figure 8**).

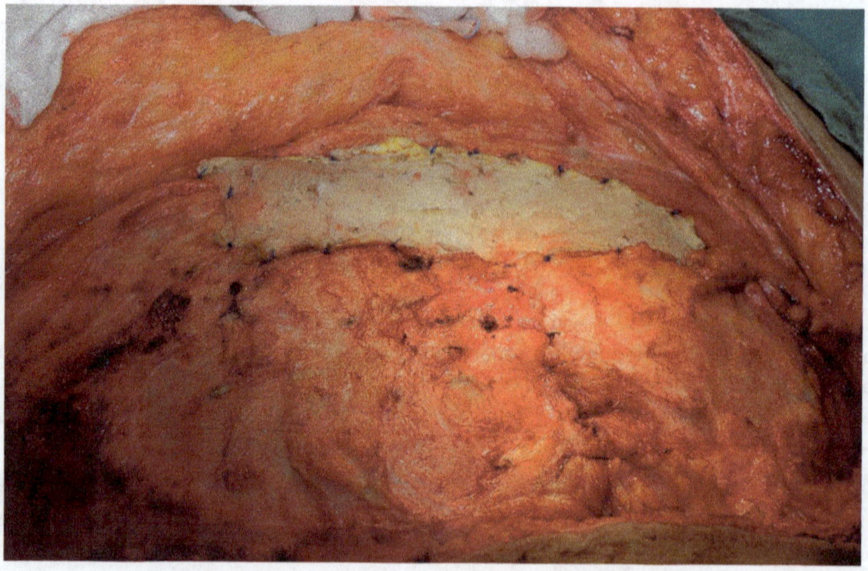

Figure 6. The second dermal graft (two pieces) in a fixed state. The hernia had an extension of 178 cm². The knotty stitches used for fixing are clearly visible. The original dermal surface looks inward.

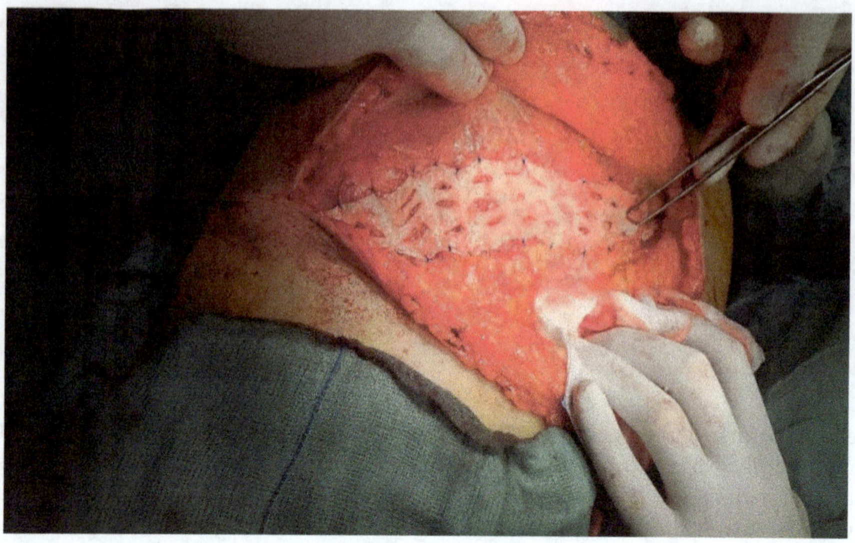

Figure 7. Reconstruction of L_1 recurrent infected abdominal wall hernia using a double-layer dermal graft. The outer graft is perforated as seen. Integration is probably faster with perforated grafts.

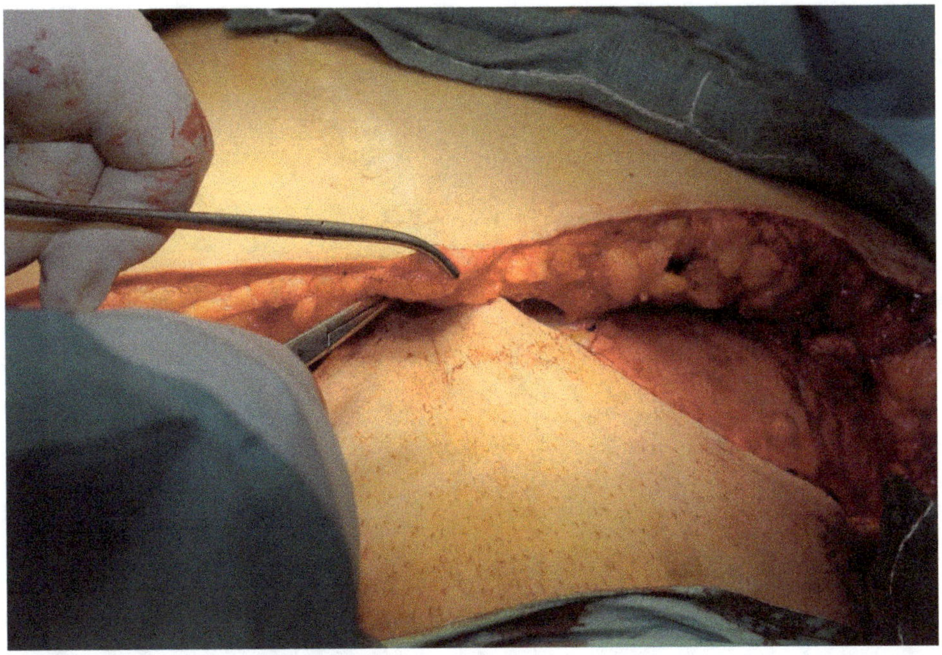

Figure 8. The wound must be closed tension-free. To achieve this, the skin-subcutis must be mobilized to the required extent. The sufficiently thick adipose tissue layer, a key factor in the integration of the second graft, is clearly visible. The adipose tissue should be protected as much as possible during surgery. It should be raised with a wet wipe, without using sharp, traumatizing hooks. Any worn-out adipose tissue particles are removed at closure.

2.1.3. Complications, recurrence and quality of life following abdominal wall reconstructions with autologous double-layer dermal grafts

Reconstructions with autologous double-layer dermal grafts are not free from complications. Hematomas (2.5%), superficial wound infections (3%), and deep wound infections (2.5%) are the most frequent complications in the early postoperative stage. In the late postoperative period, diffuse fluid build-up is the most common complication (17%). These fluid collections, however, are not circumscribed real seromas and can be successfully treated by percutaneous or ultrasound-guided puncture. Genuine subcutaneous seromas are very rare and require surgical exploration. Deep infection in the surgical area may lead to the formation of subcutaneous fistulas (2.5%), which must be removed surgically as they are not likely to resolve spontaneously. Inadequate preparation of the dermal grafts (epidermal elements, such as sebaceous glands or hair follicles, left on the surface) may also lead to complications. An adequately prepared dermal graft should contain nothing but the stratum reticularis and the stratum vascularis of the dermis, with a minimum amount of subcutaneous fatty tissue islands, but without *any* epidermal structures. Dermal grafts have no blood supply of their own. The grafts serve as a kind of connective tissue "scaffolding" for integration and remodeling. Neovascularization starts partly from the subcutaneous adipose tissue and partly from the greater omentum. The process takes 4–5 weeks. Adipose-derived stem cells (ADSCs), present in large quantities in the fatty tissue, play an important role in angiogenesis and connective tissue remodeling (**Figure 9**). Without remodeling and integration, the hernia will recur. Recurrence is invariably preceded by the dermal graft becoming lax, followed by recurrence of the hernia. Abdominal wall laxity occurs in 10–15% of the cases after such operations. Laxity develops in the first 12 months, and recurrences occur in the first 2 years.

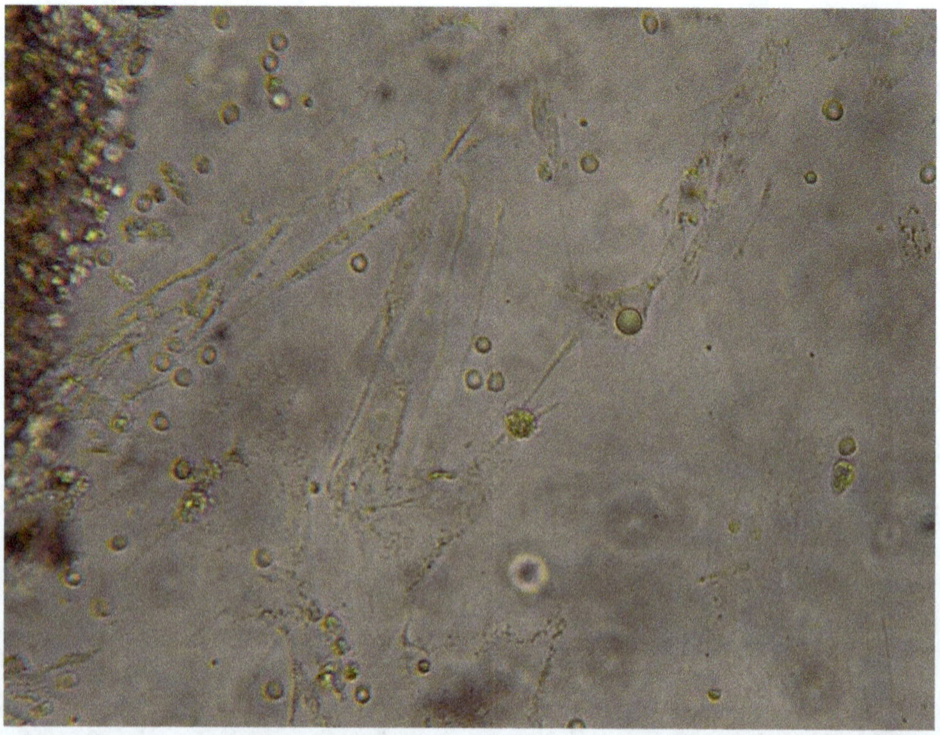

Figure 9. ADSC *in vitro* culture can be seen in the picture. The cells are derived from the abdominal subcutaneous adipose tissue harvested during dermal graft reconstructive surgery. The cells have vital role in the integration and restructuring of autologous dermal grafts. ADSC cells are the elongated rice-grain forms in the picture. (No stain, native photograph of the cell culture, 300×, the author's own research, photogpaphed by Máté Rózsahegyi).

Predisposing factors include smoking, diabetes mellitus (DM), chronic obstructive pulmonary disease (COPD), negligence of the use of elastic trusses, and physical activity too intensive or started too early following surgery (**Table 1**). The rate of recurrence can be reduced provided the patients wear the hook-and-loop elastic truss for long enough and in the right way, properly fitted. Medium or heavy physical load should be avoided during this period. Patients are recommended to follow a regimen of light meals several times a day, avoid foods that cause bloating, and lose weight. If the hernia recurs, further dermal graft reconstruction is usually no longer feasible, as grafts of the required quality and quantity are no longer available after the previous operation. In such cases, components separation, rectus muscle turnover, reinforcement with a synthetic or biological graft, or reconstruction using pedicled or free musculoaponeurotic flaps may be considered.

In case the surgical intervention is performed in a complicated CDCP 2–3 (infected synthetic mesh, enterocutaneous, or subcutaneous fistulas) or CDCP 4 (peritonitis, necrotic abdominal wall) environment, the patient should receive antibiotics. The recommended regimen is i.v. amoxicillin-clavulanic acid 1.2 g three times a day for 5 days (or i.v. cephalosporin 2 g once a day or i.v. clindamycin 600 mg three times a day in case of hypersensitivity to penicillin) and i.v. metronidazole 15 mg/kg/day. No antibiotic is required for surgeries in CDCP 1 environment, unless the operation lasts longer than 180 minutes [18, 19]. To prevent deep venous thrombosis and pulmonary embolism, subcutaneous enoxaparin 0.6–0.8 ml once a day should be administered prophylactically for 3 weeks from the second postoperative day. Mobilization should

Recurrence after double-layer dermal graft reconstructions														
	Gender	Age	BMI (kg/m²)	DM	COPD	Smoking	Omentum	Peritoneum closure	Fluid accumulation	Time to laxity (month)	Time to recurrence (month)	Previous reconstructions (n)	Previous fitula formation	Physical activity	Elastic bandage with Velcro*
1	Female	54	36.9	+	+	+	–	–	+	3	13	3	+	+	2
2	Female	47	37.5	–	+	+	–	–	+	5	17	2	+	+	2
3	Female	63	41.9	+	+	+	–	–	+	6	19	2	+	+	3
4	Male	57	27.5	–	+	+		–	+	–	21	3	+	+	Continuous

Notes: One patient had M_1, two patients had M_3, and one patient had M_4 hernia. The size of the abdominal wall defects was 275, 103, 78, and 153 cm^2 (mean: 152.3 cm^2), in order of magnitude. There is no significant difference between the mean size of the abdominal wall defects of all patients (145.9 cm^2) and the mean size of recurrent hernias (0.657, ns, Student's t-test). Recurrence was more frequent in women, all the patients were severely overweight, and all of them were active smokers. In none of the cases could the hernia sac be spared and a peritoneal layer created. None of the patients had the greater omentum. Abdominal wall reconstructions at the same site have been performed twice or three times earlier. Surgery was performed in a CDCP 3 environment in all patients. At the time of recurrence (12–24 months after surgery) all patients were physically active and only one of them wore an elastic truss

Abbr: DM: diabetes mellitus, BMI: body mass index, COPD: chronic pulmonary obstructive disease. *: how long he/she wore the elastic bandage?

Table 1. Data of recurrent abdominal wall hernias following reconstructive surgery with double-layer dermal grafts.

start on day 2 following the operation, assisted by a physiotherapist, with loading applied in a stepwise fashion. First, the patient is allowed to sit up from a supine position, and then stand up with help in the beginning. Gradual mobilization without the risk of overexertion is one of the most important postoperative rules to be observed in these cases. Postoperative pain gradually subsides (measured on a 10-point numerical rating scale, RNS). On day 1 following surgery, the mean score of pain intensity was 5.9 ± 1.7, which decreased to 3.4 ± 0.76 by day 5. Ninety percent of the patients reported that the intensity of pain was significantly lower following surgery with dermal grafts compared to earlier abdominal wall reconstruction(s), and 100% would prefer reconstruction with dermal grafts if allowed to choose.

With regard to the quality of life, 30 months after the operation, 84% of the patients are satisfied with the result of the intervention and their load capacity. They have had no significant difficulty sitting or standing up from a supine position since the third postoperative month and more than 82% of the patients would opt for dermal graft surgery as opposed to earlier interventions. Recurrences generally occur at months 12–24. Return to presurgery activities should be gradual. In the first 4 weeks, the patients are allowed nothing but light strolls while wearing their elastic trusses; they must avoid carrying any load. In the second 4-week period, light physical load is permitted: the patients may lift loads of 2–7 kg, walk or stroll, or go for a light swim. At weeks 9–12, they may return to their earlier activities but should wear the elastic truss during the day. Cycling is allowed. To protect the reconstructed abdominal wall and prevent it from becoming lax again, the patients should continue wearing the truss in case of major physical strain (**Table 2**). Subcutaneous or enterocutaneous fistulas are

Quality of life statistical data

Month	**1**	**3**	**6**	**9**	**12**	**18**	**24**	**30**
Avg. satisfactory score (1–3)	2.2 ± 0.31	2.3 ± 0.38	2.6 ± 0.13	2.7 ± 0.31	2.4 ± 0.52	2.4 ± 0.1	2.1 ± 0.23	2.3 ± 0.42
Avg. pain score (1–10)	5.3 ± 0.51	4.2 ± 0.30	3.9 ± 0.44	4.1 ± 0.10	3.0 ± 0.19	2.3 ± 0.28	3.2 ± 0.2	2.8 ± 0.46
Which procedure would you choose if you decided now? (1–2)	1.0 ± 0.0	1.0 ± 0.0	1.2 ± 0.2	1.4 ± 0.21	1.35 ± 0.43	1.45 ± 0.23	1.37 ± 0.21	1.47 ± 0.54
Do you wear the elastic bandage regularly? (1–2)	1.0 ± 0.0	1.0 ± 0.0	1.2 ± 0.11	1.25 ± 0.36	1.19 ± 0.45	1.67 ± 0.67	2.0 ± 0.0	2.0 ± 0.0
How difficult to sit up? (1–3)	1.78	1.9	2.36	2.53	2.73	2.83	2.73	2.76
How difficult to stand up? (1–3)	1.59	1.77	2.36	2.5	2.62	2.58	2.56	2.65
Have the daily routine been affected by the procedure? (1–2)	1.8	1.9	1.9	1.9	1.8	1.6	1.7	1.7

Abbr: Avg: average.

Table 2. Changes in quality of life between months 1 and 30 following surgery.

invariably eliminated by adequately performed surgery, a fact appreciated by patients much more than the repair of the recurrent hernia itself. The use of double-layer dermal grafts improves the quality of life in both the early and the late postoperative periods. Since the intraabdominal pressure is low following the interventions (12.1 ± 2.3, 11.3 ± 3.1, 9.5 ± 1.3 8.7 ± 2.2, and 7.2 ± 1.9 mmHg on days 1–5 after surgery), pain is less intense, making mobilization significantly easier and more successful. Patients should be checked every 6, then every 12 months in the first 2 years; follow-up visits should include physical examination in supine and standing position, as well as abdominal ultrasonography.

3. Bilateral rectus abdominis muscle release, turning-over and recreation of the midline gap in the cases of eventrated loss of abdominal wall domain hernias

Complete lack of the midline, with the bilateral rectus abdominis muscles moved further away from each other, leading to medial abdominal wall hernia and eventration, is a well-known phenomenon following serial intraabdominal surgeries (**Figures 10** and **11**).

Following open abdomen treatment or intraabdominal serial surgeries, the medial section of the abdominal wall usually heals *per secundam intentionem* between the medial margins of the dynamically lateralizing rectus abdominis muscles [20, 21]. This state makes the patients disabled not only in an aesthetic sense but also functionally. The procedure consists in a tension-free

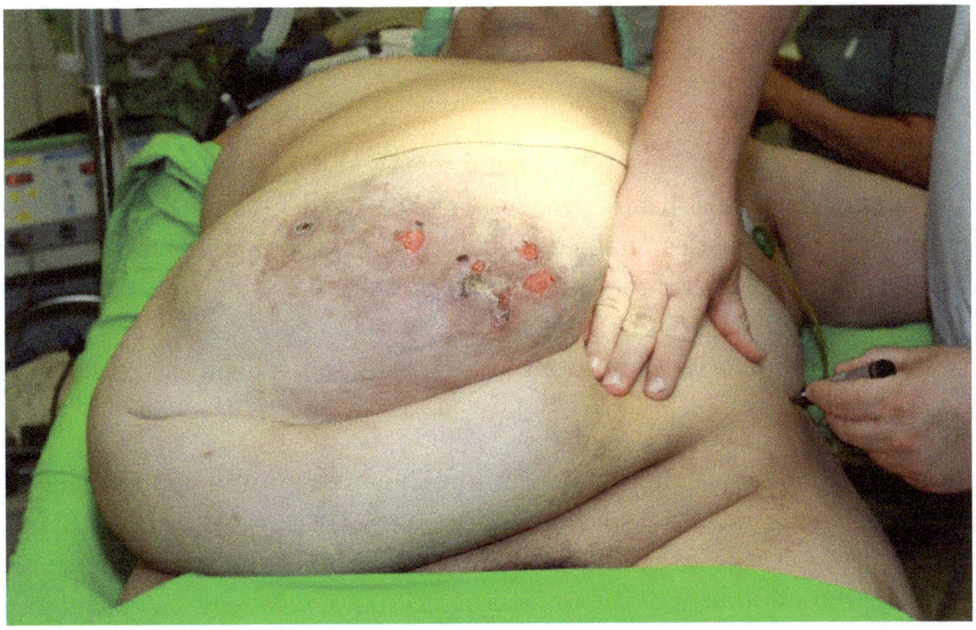

Figure 10. Eventrated, loss of abdominal wall domain, complicated hernia having recurred four times. The skin shows signs of contact dermatitis and fistula ducts. The fistulas started from the level of the infected synthetic mesh. The BMI is 57.1 kg/m^2. Primarily, the 62-year-old male patient underwent surgery for necrotizing pancreatitis and extensive retroperitoneal necrosis. The area of the abdominal defect, 19 cm wide at its largest extension, was 676 cm^2. The medial margin of the rectus abdominis muscle was located at the medioclavicular line. The main complaint in such cases, apart from the aesthetic aspect, is the abdominal wall's lack of loading capacity. The incision line is precisely marked out on the operating table, right before the operation.

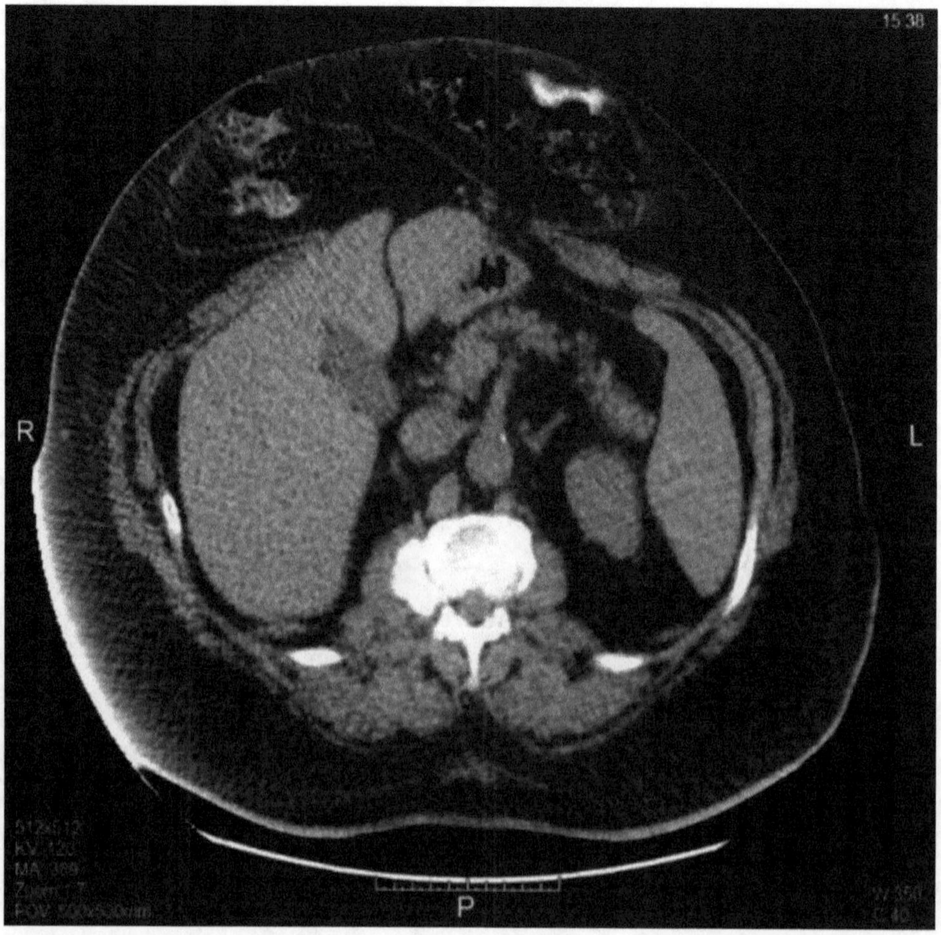

Figure 11. Changes in the size of the midline gap and the combined width of the bilateral rectus muscles in cm. As can be seen clearly, the two lines intersect at month 12 and the combined width of the turned-over bilateral rectus muscles can cover the gap until about month 18.

recreation of the *midline* and the linea alba, lateral release of both *rectus abdominis muscles* from the posterior fascia of the rectus sheath, their *turning-over* at a degree of 180° toward the midline, with blood supply to the muscles retained. Only the spared hernia sac and the intact bilateral rectus abdominis muscles are used for the reconstruction.

3.1. Significance of preoperative computed tomography to perform the rectus muscle turning-over procedure

The evolution of abdominal wall hernias (including dynamics, time course, and changes in the size of the bilateral rectus muscle) after intraabdominal serial surgeries and/or open abdomen treatment follows a typical course [22]. The combined width of the bilateral rectus muscles is sufficient to cover the midline abdominal wall defect in a tension-free way, but performance of the intervention has an "optimal" time interval (**Table 3** and **Figure 12**). Detailed and precise evaluation of the musculoaponeurotic elements of the abdominal wall is essential before reconstructive surgery with the rectus muscles. Feasibility of the intervention must be assessed by CT/MR imaging prior to surgery. The bilateral rectus muscles will be able to cover the complete midline abdominal wall defect free of tension if their *combined* width is nearly the same.

	T_0	T_3	T_6	T_{12}	T_{18}	T_{24}
Avg. midline gap (cm)	3.94	5.57	9.2	14.1	16.3	19.7
Avg. rectus sheath thickness (cm)	1.38	1.28	1.24	1.2	1.09	0.98
Righ rectus sheath width Th-XI, (cm)	7.36	7.27	7.08	6.89	6.7	6.49
Left rectus sheath width Th-XI (cm)	7.46	7.34	7.25	6.99	6.55	6.23
Righ rectus sheath width L-II (cm)	7.72	7.7	7.36	7.12	7.01	6.93
Left rectus sheath width L-II (cm)	7.8	7.85	7.43	7.2	7	6.85
Righ rectus sheath width L-IV (cm)	5.16	5.02	4.89	4.83	4.69	4.57
Left rectus sheath width L-IV (cm)	5.27	5.13	4.87	4.83	4.68	4.63

Abbr: Avg: average, $T_{(0-24)}$: $Time_{(month)}$, Th: Thoracal, L: Lumbar.

Table 3. Mean sizes of the rectus muscle and of the abdominal wall defect at various time points. Width of the rectus sheath was measured at three altitudes, as the rectus muscle width is not the same at various altitudes, featuring characteristic anatomical morphologies.

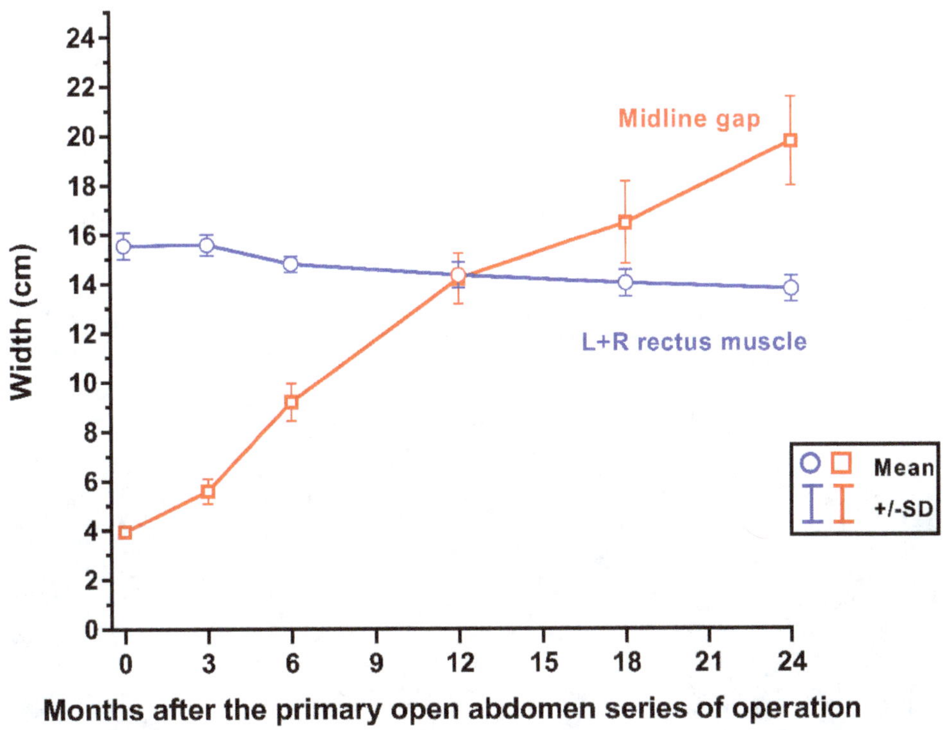

Figure 12. Characteristic CT image of an eventrated, loss of abdominal wall domain. The edge of the liver also reaches into the hernia sac. The bilateral intact rectus muscles (combined width 17.3 cm) and the midline abdominal wall defect (16.15 cm wide) are clearly visible. The size of the abdominal wall defect was 529 cm^2.

3.2. Surgical technique

The operation is performed under general anesthesia in a state of complete muscular relaxation. Preoperative antibiotic prophylaxis is not necessary [18, 19]. Following a full median or transverse skin incision, the intact hernia sac is not removed, only in case it is severely damaged. The choice of a median or transverse incision depends on the quality of the midline skin. In the case of relatively intact skin in the midline, the transverse "bay-leaf" form excision between the two iliac crest is superior to median incision. The aim is to spare as much as possible of the hernia sac, which will be the inner layer of the recreated abdominal wall. The next step is identification of the lateral margin of the bilateral rectus abdominis muscle. After this, the anterior rectus muscle fascia is incised from the origin to the adhesion of the muscle, to reveal the rectus abdominis muscle (**Figure 13**).

Starting from its lateral margin, the full length of the muscle, except its 2-cm medial margin, is prepared off the posterior wall fascia. During mobilization, at least three minor perforant segmental arteries and veins are revealed; each of them is dissected and tied up. The origin of the muscle is separated from the seventh and eighth rib cartilages. The medial half of the muscular origin (processus xiphoideus, fifth and sixth rib cartilages) is left intact. The arteria epigastrica superior and inferior vessels are carefully spared. Release of the lateral half of the muscular adhesion from the symphysis is also performed. The arteria and vena epigastrica inferior vessels are spared. The released muscle is turned over in the direction of the midline at a degree of 180° (**Figure 14**).

The abdominal wall defect is reconstructed in the following way: the spared hernia sac is precisely cut to size and closed in the midline with 3/0 absorbable monofilament running stitches (**Figure 15**). The released rectus muscle is turned over medially at a degree of 180°. The fascia (originally anterior, becoming posterior when the muscle is turned over) is closed with 3/0 absorbable, monofilament running stitches at a distance of 1 cm from each other (**Figure 16**). The rectus muscles laid next to each other are closed in the midline with 3/0 absorbable,

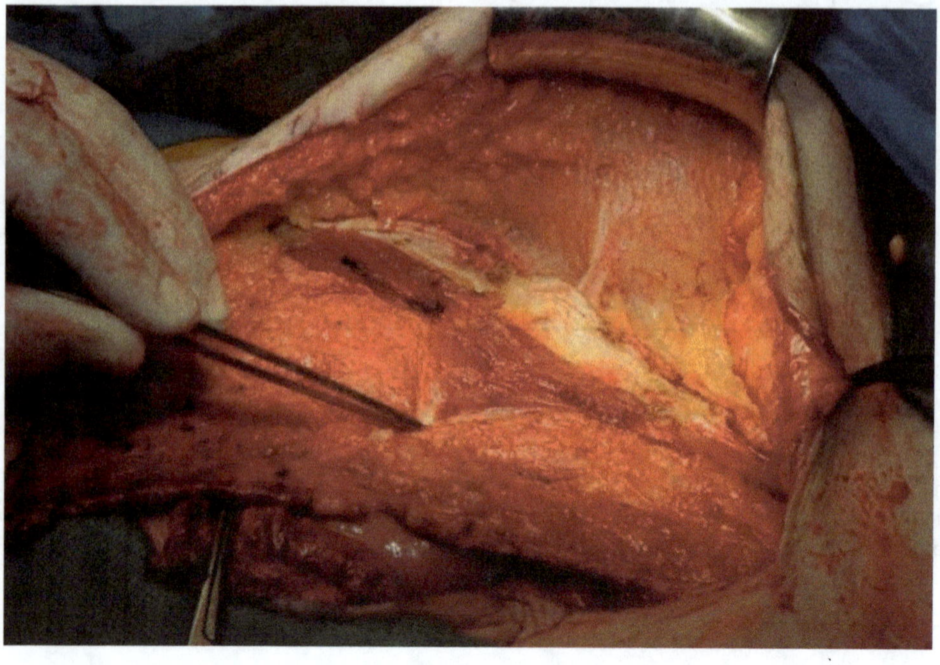

Figure 13. First step of rectus muscle release. The rectus fascia is incised full length 1 cm of the lateral margin of the muscle in a medial direction and the rectus abdominis muscle is revealed.

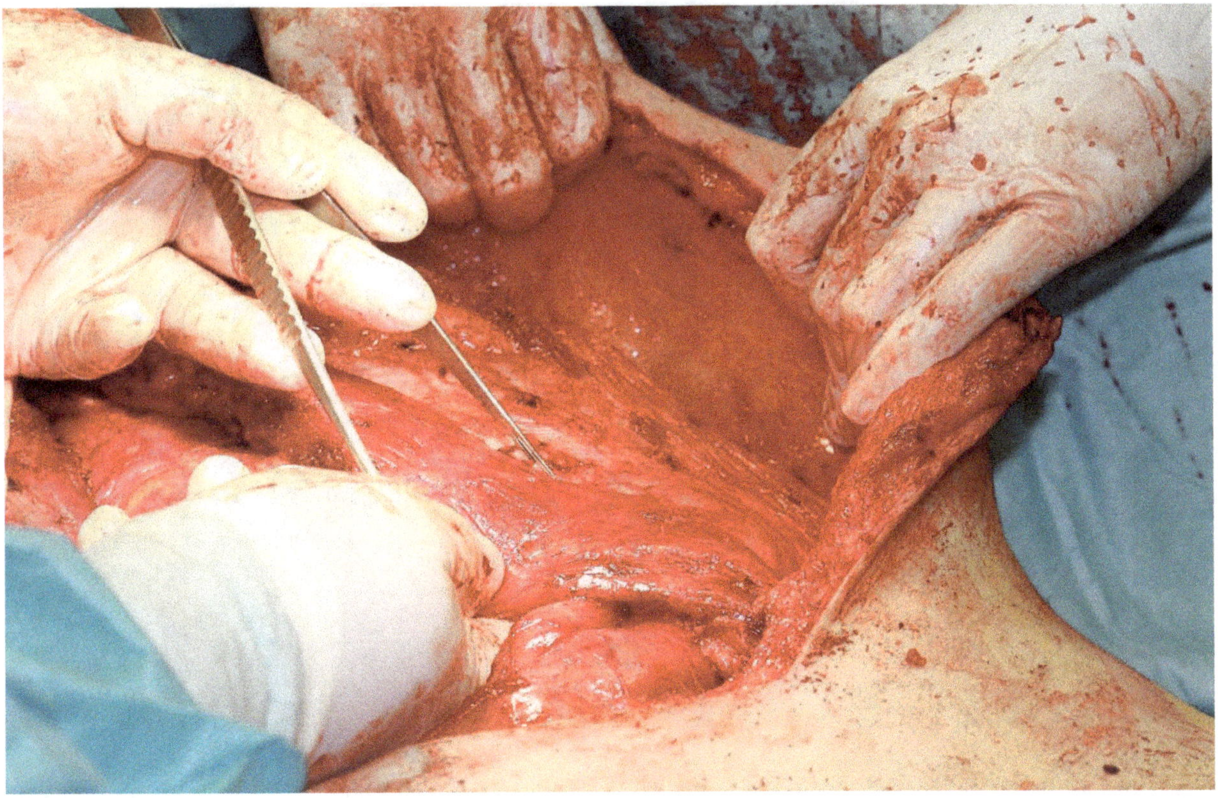

Figure 14. The left-side rectus muscle can be seen properly released and turned over medially. The right hand holds the turned-over, good-quality muscle, which has good blood supply. The forceps indicate the width of the rectus muscle, 1.32 cm thick and 7.24 cm wide.

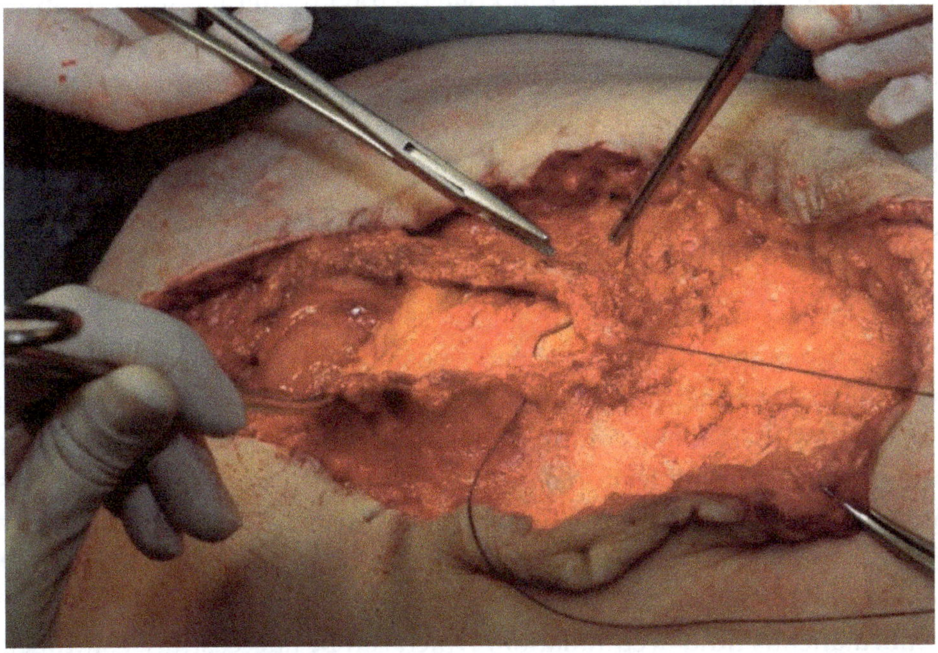

Figure 15. First step of midline recreation, closure of the peritoneum. After closing the peritoneum, the posterior (anterior before the turnover) fascia of the rectus sheath is closed.

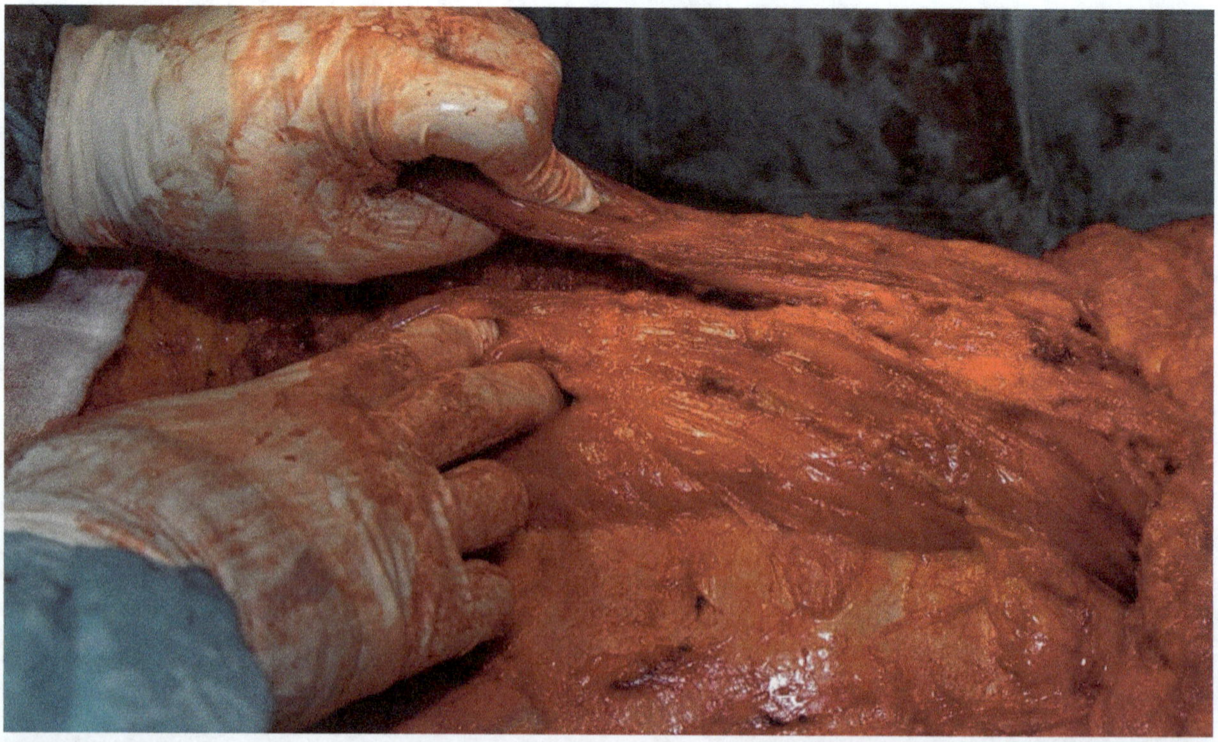

Figure 16. Last step of midline recreation. The two rectus muscles of good quality and blood supply are turned facing each other and are tension-free. The closure is performed using knotty stitches along the full length of the muscle.

monofilament knotty stitches placed at a distance of 2 cm from each other. Laterally, the fascia of the obliquus externus and internus muscles is sewn to the posterior wall fascia with running 3/0 absorbable monofilament stitches (**Figure 17**). Three suction drains are left behind in the operative area, one in the midline and one each with lateral outlets (**Figure 18**). Before skin closure, the subcutis is fixed to the fascia with 8–10 absorbable, knotty 3/0 subcutaneous anchor stitches. The midline is closed with 3/0 interrupted subcutaneous stitches and 2/0 interrupted nonabsorbable monofilament skin stitches. After the operation, *before extubation*, an adjustable elastic abdominal wall bandage must be placed on the abdominal wall.

3.3. Complications, recurrence, and quality of life following rectus muscle turning-over procedure

The rate of surgical complications in the early postoperative stage following rectus muscle turnover is less than 2%. Superficial wound infections and wound dehiscence requiring local treatment are the most frequent complications. Normally, there is no need for antibiotic administration. Deep wound infection occurs in less than 1% of the patients. In such cases, empiric antibiotic therapy (i.v. amoxicillin-clavulanic acid 1.2 g three times daily or, in the case of hypersensitivity to penicillin, i.v. clindamycin 300 mg three times daily for 5 days) or antibiogram-based targeted antibiotic administration is required, in addition to open wound treatment. Subcutaneous fluid accumulation, which can be successfully controlled by percutaneous tapping, develops in less than 10% of the cases. Genuine seromas are very rare. In the early postoperative stage, necrosis of the turned-over rectus muscle may theoretically occur.

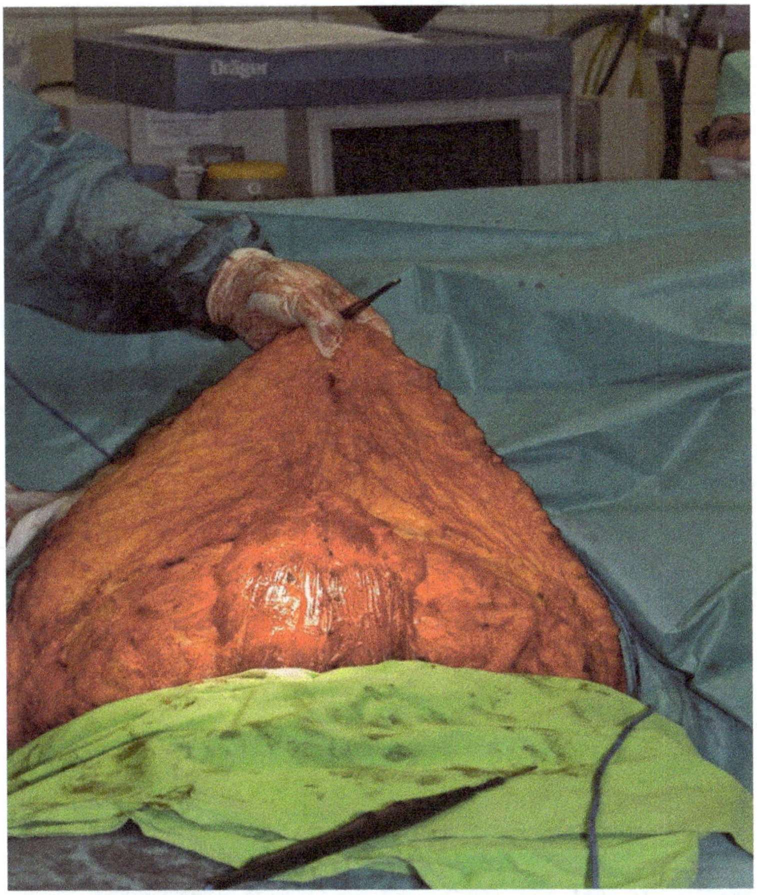

Figure 17. The intervention is complete. The muscle covers the midline and is in a fully closed, turned-over position. Blood supply to the muscle is maintained, it has the proper colour, nonlivid. The bilateral lateral segments, original sites of the rectus muscles, can be seen clearly. The posterior wall of the rectus sheath and the medial margin of the externus abdominis muscle are also clearly visible.

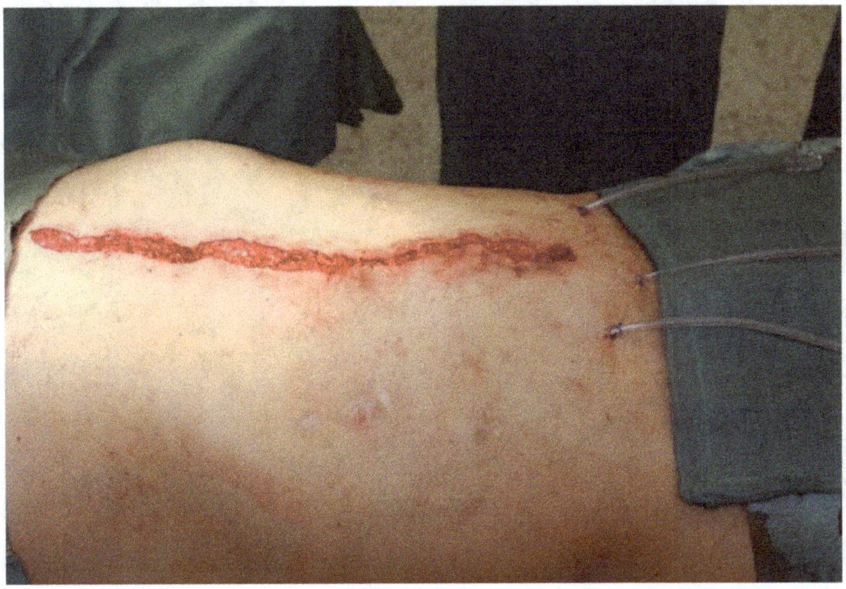

Figure 18. The reconstructed abdominal wall. Three drains are left behind, draining the medial and lateral areas.

It happens when blood supply to the muscle stops during turning-over. Prevention is paramount: the arteria epigastrica superior and inferior vessels must be spared applying extreme caution. Should the vessels be damaged, reconstruction should preferably be performed by a vascular surgeon. A circumscribed dark purple discoloration may develop on the surface of the turned-over muscle during surgery; it does not require any intervention and causes no complications.

The operation does not require antibiotic administration, except when reconstruction of the eventrated abdominal wall hernia is performed as an emergency for mechanical ileus or peritonitis. To prevent deep venous thrombosis or pulmonary embolism, the patients are given s.c. enoxaparin prophylactically in a dose of 0.4–0.8 ml once daily, depending on body weight, for 3 weeks. On the first 5 days following the operation, the mean scores of pain intensity on the NRS scale were 6.9 ± 2.4, 6.1 ± 1.64, 6.2 ± 0.99, 5.5 ± 1.1, and 4.7 ± 0.67. Intraabdominal pressure gradually falls during the first 5 postoperative days (13.5 ± 2.5, 12.9 ± 1.7, 10,.2 ± 2.6, 10.1 ± 0.3, and 8.2 ± 2.4 mmHg). Abdominal wall laxity following reconstructions with the rectus muscle develops in 2% of the cases; recurrence of the abdominal wall hernia, however, was not observed during a mean follow-up of 24 months (**Figure 19**). Elimination of eventrated hernias leads to a marked improvement in the quality of life. There is a significant difference in the quality of life when the periods before and after the surgery are compared. By the evidence of a quality of life test performed after the first 30 days, the

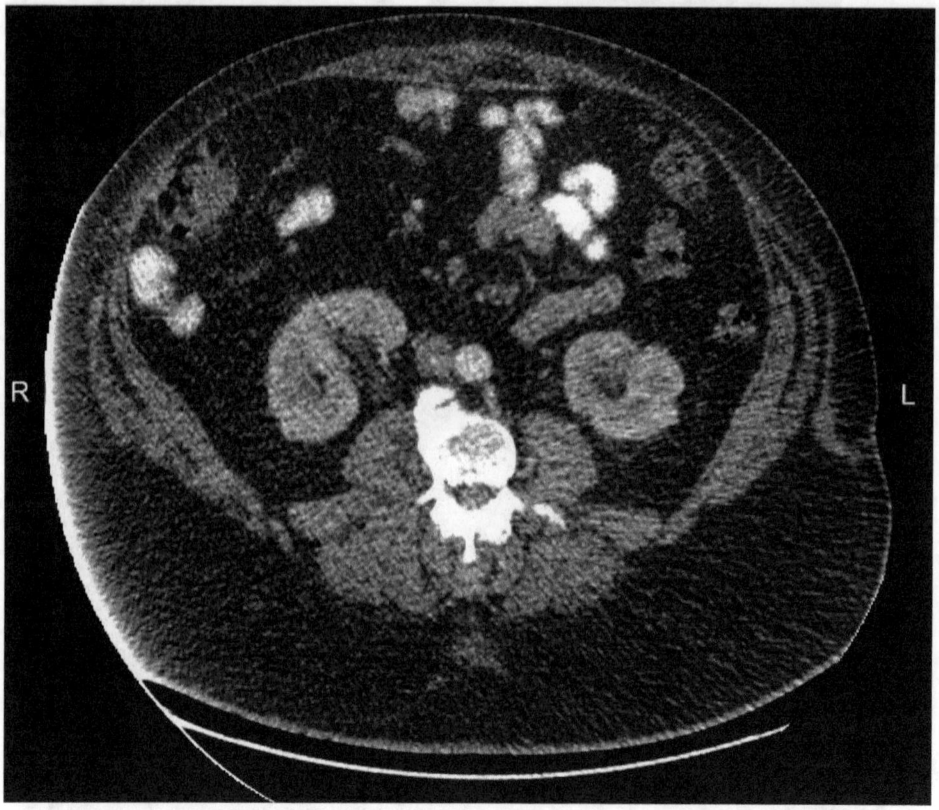

Figure 19. CT image taken one year after the intervention. There is no recurrence. The rectus muscle is hypertrophic, a phenomenon typically occurring in all patients. Its cause is unknown.

patients were completely satisfied with the outcome of the surgery (satisfactory score: 6.0 ± 0.0) (**Figure 20**). In our study, the mean QoL score (measured by the Ferrans-Power quality of life test adapted to the study) [23] was 23.3 ± 13.59 before the reconstructive surgery, which increased to 46.7 ± 6.38 by day 30 following the intervention. The difference was statistically significant, $P = 0.0013$, Student's unpaired t-test. The mean QoL scores at months 6, 12, 18, 24, and 30 were 47.1 ± 4.2, 45.2 ± 5.3, 48.0 ± 2.9, 47.4 ± 4.5, and 46.4 ± 4.8; the differences were not significant (p: ns, Student's unpaired t-test).

3.4. How and when to apply the rectus muscle release and turning-over procedure? Terms of application

CT morphometric analyses suggest that availability and intact state of the bilateral rectus muscle confirmed by CT is a fundamental criterion of applicability. Indication or contraindication of the procedure must be based on the assessment of the size of the abdominal wall defect and the condition of the bilateral rectus muscle at its full length. Patients with COPD or having a high body mass index (BMI) will particularly benefit from the procedure, as there is no risk of significant increase in intraabdominal pressure following surgery. Due to the complex nature of the procedure and the fact that applicability must be determined (on the basis of physical examination and evaluation of the CT images) preoperatively, the intervention should be indicated and performed by an experienced surgeon. Maintaining blood supply to the rectus muscle is the most critical element of the procedure. Release of the muscle from the lateral direction leads

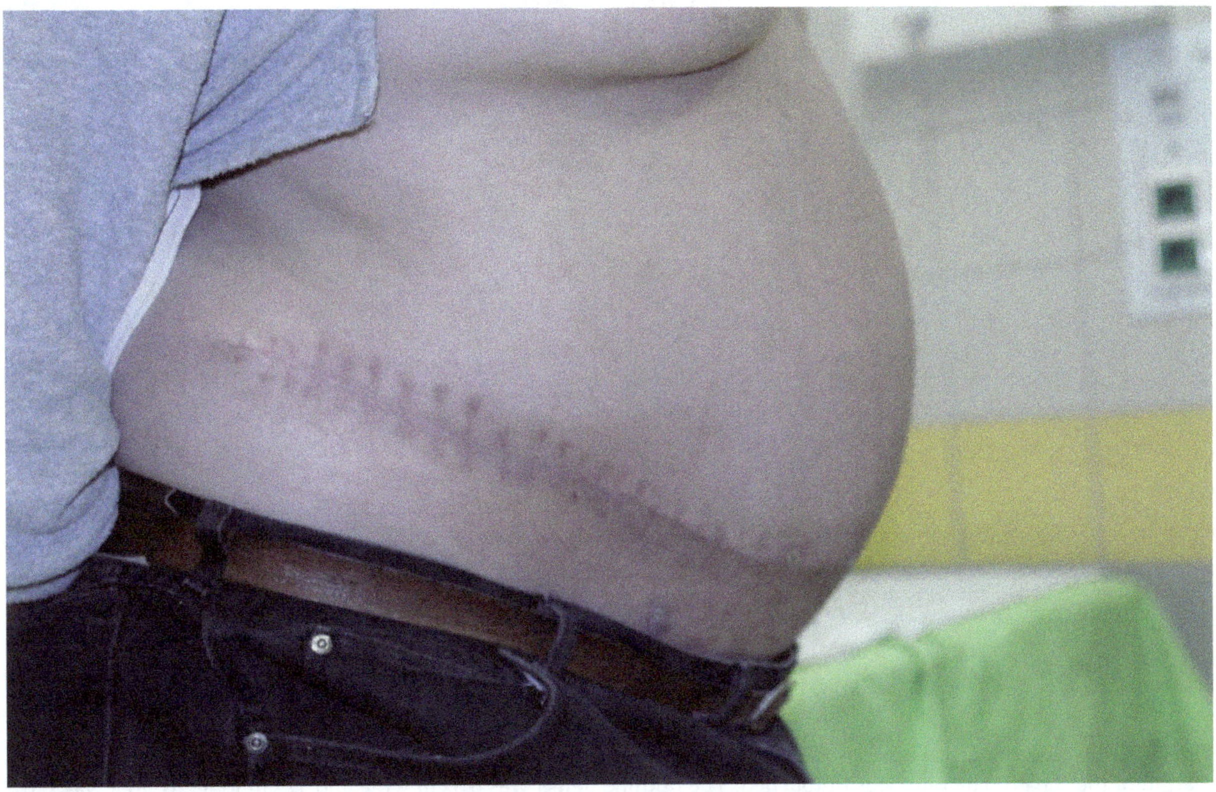

Figure 20. Three months after the rectus muscle turning-over surgery. The BMI is 56.3 kg/m^2. The patient had an eventrated, giant hernia with four earlier recurrences and an abdominal wall defect of 621 cm^2.

to denervation of its lateral (becoming medial after the turnover) parts [24]. Although the outcome of abdominal wall reconstruction is not affected by denervation, patients should wear an adjustable elastic truss for at least 3 months following surgery to prevent midline laxity. After this period, they are still advised to wear their elastic abdominal wall bandage with Velcro™ when doing activities involving medium or more intensive physical strain. The function of the turned-over rectus muscle is retained. From month 3, sitting up and standing up no longer cause difficulty for the patient.

4. Rectus sheath anterior fascia release for large (not eventrated) midline incisional hernias

Autologous tissues can also be used for the reconstruction of large midline (noneventrated) hernias. If the width of the midline defect is not larger than 6–8 cm in a relaxed, supine position (which corresponds to the width of a unilateral rectus muscle, see **Table 3**), the midline can be reconstructed free of tension by release of the anterior fascia of the bilateral rectus muscle. In such cases, release and turnover of the muscle are not necessary (**Figure 21**).

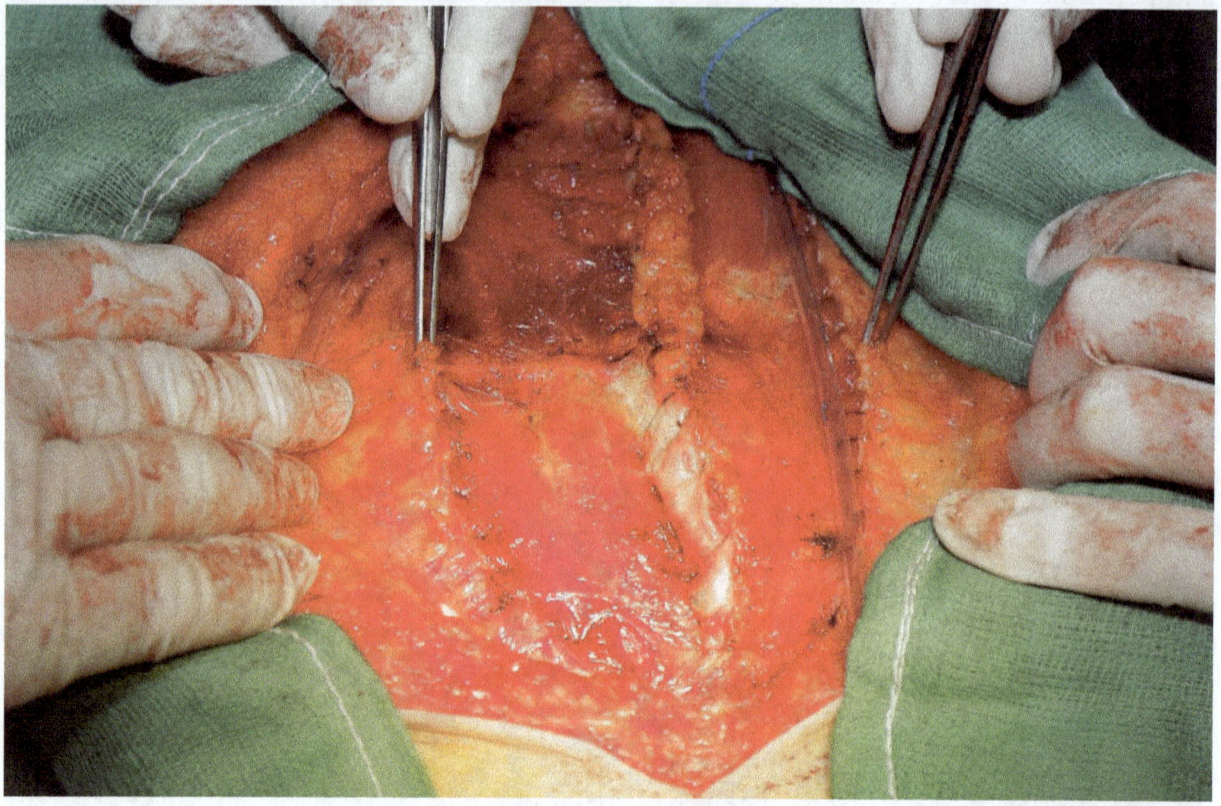

Figure 21. The anterior fascia is released from the anterior surface of both rectus sheaths. The forceps indicate the lateral margin of the sheath. The muscle is untouched. The midline defect was 6.5 cm wide and 17 cm long, its area was 110.5 cm^2. The midline could be closed free of tension. There was no need for synthetic mesh implantation. The fascia plates turned over the midline and closed in the middle are clearly visible.

4.1. Surgical technique

Following a full median incision, the midline is carefully prepared. The hernia sac is spared and used for reconstruction of the peritoneal surface of the midline. The anterior fascia of the rectus sheath is incised full length along the lateral margin of the rectus sheath and prepared off the rectus muscle. The fascia plate is turned over toward the midline and fixed to the edge of the abdominal wall on the other side using 3/0 nonabsorbable running monofilament stitches. The same is repeated with the fascia plate of the other side so as to close the midline defect in two layers. Two drains are inserted. The adjustable elastic bandage is already applied on the operating table, before extubation.

4.2. How and when to use the rectus anterior sheath fascia turnover?

Rectus anterior sheath turnover was described by da Silva as early as 1979 [25–28]. Several modifications of the procedure are known. The procedure presented here is a tension-free modification of the original technique. The important difference is that it is used only when the midline abdominal wall defect is not wider than the width of a unilateral rectus muscle (about 6–8 cm), confirmed by abdominal CT prior to the intervention. If the defect is wider than the width of a unilateral rectus muscle, the rectus fascia turnover (the so-called "open-book" technique) is not recommended. Similarly, it is not recommended for repair of smaller abdominal wall incisional hernias, as these types of hernia can be successfully treated by less complicated procedures.

One of the advantages of the technique is tension-free reconstruction. Furthermore, less than 2% of the patients develop midline protuberance, provided the precise indication is observed. The recurrence rate is less than 3%. Subcutaneous fluid build-up (4–8%) and superficial wound infection (5%) are the most common complications. As with the other procedures, patients should wear an elastic truss for at least 3 months after surgery. Although minor or medium physical load is permitted, patients are advised to avoid heavy physical exertion even after this period. Should they perform any hard physical activity, patients must always wear an elastic truss.

5. Discussion

The presence of large, infected, or eventrated abdominal wall hernias is an intolerable condition for patients. Complicated, recurrent, and/or infected incisional hernias and eventrated giant abdominal wall hernias are considered to be the consequence of earlier surgical interventions [29]. We fully agree with Kohler et al. [2], who claim (when discussing the question whether complicated incisional hernias are a natural corollary or a surgical complication) that surgical technique and accuracy of abdominal wall closure are key factors in the development of these conditions. There are two other factors playing a role: these are the presence of *predisposing* factors, a phenomenon extensively researched, and the patients themselves, to the extent they comply with the instructions they are given following surgery [30]. The reason why ventral and incisional hernias are increasingly researched is their increasing incidence and the growing costs involved. In the USA, approximately 3.5 billion dollars are spent on the treatment of abdominal wall hernias each year [31]. Although prevention of recurrences and complications should be a major consideration at the very first intervention when doing reconstructive surgery in patients with abdominal wall hernia, the fact is that 20–37% of ventral hernias and 40–64% of incisional hernias recur and the number of complications increases with each intervention [32]. Infection of the synthetic material implanted during an earlier surgery (or surgeries) is the most significant complication [33]. The cost of hospitalization is doubled and, furthermore, there is a 6-time increase in the cost of dressing changes when the operative area and/or the mesh become infected [34]. We can agree with Sanchez, who claims that the treatment of infected/compromised grafts varies from case to case, with the mesh either spared or not in the end. Predisposing factors for mesh infection include a high BMI (≥25 kg/m^2), DM, COPD, infection of the site of an earlier operation, prolonged duration of surgery, opening of an intestine, and presence of enterocutaneous fistulas. The implanted mesh is removed in ≈5% of the cases, infection being the most common reason (69%) [35]. When repairing a recurrent and/or compromised incisional hernia, the surgeon usually faces two major problems: (1) the surgical environment is infected (CDCP 3–4) or contaminated (CDCP 2); (2) the abdominal wall defect is too extensive and cannot be closed free of tension. In such cases, most surgeons are understandably reluctant to implant another synthetic graft [36]. In cases requiring extensive abdominal wall replacement, the use of biological allo- and xenografts and various autologous tissues is the preferred choice in reconstructive surgeries. Of biological grafts, human, porcine, and bovine ADMs have been used [37–41]. In the vast majority of the cases, there is no question about the resolution of small or medium-size abdominal wall hernias. However, when faced with a *large, eventrated, complicated,* or *incarcerated* hernia and an *infected* (CDCP 3–4) *environment,* the surgeon must adopt a fundamentally different strategy. To choose the most appropriate surgical technique, the surgeon must have precise information on the condition of the musculoaponeurotic elements in the abdominal wall. The best way to obtain such information is abdominal CT/MR imaging [22], allowing assessment of the position of individual abdominal wall components, size of the hernia gate(s), and the volume of the hernia contents. In the case of eventrated hernias, determination of the size of the hernia sac is essential. Another important factor is knowledge of the various surgical techniques, necessary for the selection of the procedure that imposes the least possible stress in a *specific case.* Evaluation of literary data shows that the use of autologous tissues is indispensable in the repair of complicated, eventrated, or giant abdominal wall hernias [42]. There are procedures, which can be applied in certain cases only, and their use would be a mistake in any other case.

Direct abdominal wall sutures should never be used in *elective* or *acute* surgery of large, eventrated, or complicated hernias. Implantation of synthetic materials for abdominal wall reinforcement (but not replacement) is an option for elective surgeries in a CDCP 1–2 environment. Implantation of a synthetic substance in a CDCP 3–4 environment is associated with a high incidence of surgical complications in the operative area (25–65%), as well as a high recurrence rate (30–70%); for this reason, use of synthetic materials is not recommended in such cases. The use of ADMs may be an alternative; however, the high cost of the procedure, coupled with a high recurrence rate, is a limitation to its use. Generally, there are several options in each case; it is important, however, that the one involving the least possible stress should be selected and applied. Of autologous tissues, the use of dermal grafts is associated with the least strain during and after surgery; this is followed by rectus muscle turnover and the various component separation techniques, and finally by reconstructions with free or pedicled flaps.

The most important consideration when using autologous dermal grafts is the availability of tissues of adequate size and quality for reconstruction. To cover a defect of 10 cm in diameter (an area of 78.5 cm^2), the area of the dermal graft should be at least 220 cm^2. The 30–35% expansion capacity of a properly prepared graft should also be taken into account. All this means that grafts of adequate size and quality can only be obtained from obese patients. Prepared dermal grafts should not contain any epidermal elements or scar tissue.

Double-layer dermal grafts are preferred in cases of large medial or lateral incisional hernias having recurred at least once, in which a synthetic mesh was implanted during an earlier reconstructive surgery and CDCP 2–3 environment, compromised graft, deep wound infection, or subcutaneous and/or enterocutaneous fistulas developed in the postoperative period. In a CDCP 1 environment, this is the preferred choice if the hernia is large and a direct abdominal wall suture would lead to a significant increase in intraabdominal pressure. The procedure has obvious advantages in obese patients, where grafts are usually available in sufficient quantities, making synthetic grafts unnecessary. In patients with BMIs higher than 25 kg/m^2, the quantity and quality of dermal grafts are sufficient for the reconstruction of large hernias [43]. In patients with DM or COPD, conditions associated with a higher risk for recurrence and infection of the operative area, the use of autologous grafts is preferred to direct sutures or synthetic grafts. Perforated double-layer dermal grafts can successfully be used in CDCP 4 environments. Their advantages include faster integration and a significantly lower risk of infection at the site of operation. However, this procedure cannot be used in patients in whom dermal grafts of appropriate quantity and quality are not available. There are data, although limited, on the use of double-layer dermal grafts in CDCP 4 environments and in the case of extensive abdominal wall necrosis. Large abdominal wall defects can be repaired relatively quickly and cost-effectively without implanting synthetic or allo- or xenografts and without significant early postoperative tension even in CDCP 4 environments [44].

A precondition of bilateral rectus muscle turnover is the intact state of the bilateral rectus muscle confirmed by CT. A CT examination prior to surgery allows assessment of the size of the abdominal wall defect and the state of the bilateral rectus muscle, and serves as basis for the indication or contraindication of the intervention. In patients with COPD or having a high BMI, the procedure is clearly preferred, as there is no risk of increased intraabdominal pressure following surgery. Maintaining blood supply to the rectus muscle from the epigastric vessels is essential. In case of injury, the artery must be reconstructed. Maintaining blood supply to the rectus muscle is the most critical element of the intervention. Although release of the muscle from the medial direction leads to partial muscle denervation, the outcome of abdominal wall reconstruction is not affected and the turned-over muscle retains its function. To prevent the development of abdominal wall bulking, patients should wear an adjustable elastic abdominal wall binding with Velcro for at least 3 months following surgery and also later when exposed to physical load.

The procedure of bilateral rectus muscle release and turnover is used to reconstruct eventrations and midline abdominal wall defects developed after open abdomen treatments, retroperitoneal, and/or intraabdominal serial operations. The technique is also suitable for resolution of midline, recurrent, or neglected, primary medial giant abdominal wall hernias. The intervention can successfully be performed in patients with incarcerated eventrated hernias or in CDCP 3–4 environments. It is crucial that in case the rectus muscle was damaged or intersected during an earlier surgery, or the patient underwent transverse laparotomy (involving transverse intersection of the rectus muscle) earlier, the intervention cannot be performed. The width of the midline abdominal wall defect and the combined width of the bilateral rectus muscles along their full length must be carefully assessed. If the values "correspond" to each other, the intervention can be indicated from a morphological-anatomical point of view.

6. Conclusion

The statements related to the surgical procedures discussed in this chapter are summarized as follows:

1. Double-layer homogeneous dermal grafts can successfully be used in *large hernias* in *CDCP* 2–3 surgical environments. Quality of life significantly improves following surgery. If used accurately, the technique is capable of eliminating abdominal wall fistulas. The incidence of early and late complications is low. The recurrence rate is approximately 11%. The fact that grafts of sufficient quantity and quality can only be collected from overweight (BMI $\geq$ 25 kg/m^2) patients is a drawback of the procedure.
2. *In recurrent infected abdominal* wall hernias, *the infected synthetic mesh* should be *removed* completely. Partial removal fails to provide a permanent solution in most cases. In case the hernia has not recurred but the graft is infected, vacuum assisted closure (VAC) may be attempted. VAC is not recommended when recurrence and mesh infection occur simultaneously.
3. Double-layer dermal grafts can also be used in *CDCP* 4 surgical environments, provided that the outer graft is implanted perforated. *Perforated outer* grafts contribute to faster integration and remodeling.
4. The *greater omentum* and the *subcutaneous* adipose tissue are important factors in the integration of grafts. *Maximum caution* should be applied to *spare* them during surgery.
5. Patients should wear an adjustable *elastic truss* for 3 months following the intervention, even at night in the first month. Noncompliance increases the risk of recurrence.
6. The intervention is not recommended in patients with *eventrated* hernia or *extensive abdominal wall defect.*
7. Rectus muscle turnover is a method suitable for closure of wide midline abdominal wall defects and eventrated midline hernias. Lateral eventrated and large hernias can be repaired by unilateral rectus muscle release and turnover in the *lateral* direction.

8. Patients should wear an *elastic truss* for 3 (or 4, depending on the degree of physical activity) months following surgery. When doing activities involving medium or heavy physical load, patients are advised to continue wearing the truss to protect the abdominal wall.

9. The intervention is followed by a significant improvement in the quality of life.

10. The hernia recurrence rate is low. So far, no recurrence has occurred.

11. The procedure is recommended for reconstruction of repeatedly recurring midline (M_1–M_5) giant eventrated abdominal wall hernias developing after *open abdomen treatments* or retroperitoneal *serial surgeries*.

12. The procedure is also suitable for *emergency* operations (incarcerated hernia or CDCP 3–4). Before using the technique in emergency cases, however, surgeons should gain experience in elective interventions.

13. Abdominal CT allowing assessment of the volume of the hernia, the size of the midline abdominal wall defect and morphometry of the bilateral rectus *muscle* should be performed prior to the operation. An intact bilateral rectus muscle is a precondition of the procedure.

14. *Only* autologous tissues are used for abdominal wall reconstruction in the procedures discussed in this chapter. The procedures are cost-effective.

15. *Primary prevention* (increasing the proportion of minimally invasive intraabdominal penetrations) and *secondary prevention* (*lege artis* closure of laparotomies, use of a truss, and avoidance of overexertion following surgery) of abdominal wall incisional hernias may significantly reduce the incidence of large and complicated hernias.

16. The use of autologous tissues is *unavoidable* in the reconstruction of large, eventrated, or complicated abdominal wall incisional hernias in elective as well as acute interventions. Their application must be carefully weighed in these cases. Reconstruction of complicated abdominal wall hernias must be preceded by careful evaluation of the available techniques and selection of the one which is the most effective and the least stressful for the patient.

17. The use of autologous tissues requires further research to improve existing techniques and outcomes.

Author details

Gábor Martis* and László Damjanovich

*Address all correspondence to: gabor6911@gmail.com

Department of General Surgery, Institute of Surgery, Clinical and Health Science Center, University of Debrecen, Debrecen, Hungary

References

[1] Kohler A, Baldi G. Recurrence after hernia surgery: Complication or natural course? Chirurg. 2014;**85**(2):112-116

[2] Montgomery A. The battle between biological and synthetic meshes in ventral hernia repair. Hernia. 2013;**17**(1):3-11

[3] Rickert A, Kienle P, Kuthe A, Baumann P, et al. A randomized, multi-centre prospective, observer and patient blind study to evaluate a non-absorbable polypropylene mesh vs. a partly absorbable mesh in incisional hernia repair. Langenbeck's Archives of Surgery. 2012;**397**(8):1225-1234

[4] Ramirez OM, Ruas E, Dellon AL. "Component separation" method for closure of abdominal-wall defects: An anatomic and clinical sudy. Plastic and Reconstructive Surgery. 1990;**86**(3):519-526

[5] Suwa K, Okamoto T, Yanaga K. Closure versus non-closure of fascial defects in laparoscopic ventral and incisional hernia repairs: A review of the literature. Surgery Today. 2016;**46**(7):764-773

[6] Lu Y, Cao D, Guo F, et al. Abdominal wall reconstruction using a combination of free tensor fasciae latae and anterolateral thigh myocutaneous flap: A prospective study in 16 patients. The American Journal of Surgery. 2015;**201**(2):365-373

[7] Hill HL, Naha F, Vasconez LO. The tensor fascia lata myocutaneus free flap. Plastic and Reconstructive Surgery. 1978;**61**:517-522

[8] Blatnik J, Jin J, Rosen MJ, et al. Abdominal wall hernia repair with bridging acellular dermal matrix – an expensive hernia sac. The American Journal of Surgery. 2008;**196**:47-50

[9] Falagas ME, Kasiakou SK. Mesh related infections after hernia repair surgery. Clinical Microbiology and Infection. 2005;**11**(1):3-8

[10] Chung L, Tse GH, O'Dwyer PJ. Outcome of patients with chronic mesh infection following abdominal wall hernia repair. Hernia. 2014;**18**(5):701-704

[11] Bower C, Roth JS. Economics of abdominal wall reconstruction. Surgical Clinics of North America. 2013;**93**(5):1241-1253

[12] Funk LM, Perry KA, Narula VK, Mikami DJ, Melvin WS. Current national practice patterns for inpatients management of ventral abdominal wall hernia in the United States. Surgical Endoscopy. 2013;**27**(11):4104-4112

[13] Reynolds D, Davenport DL, Korosec RL, Roth JS. Financial implication of ventral hernia repair: A hospital cost analysis. Journal of Gastrointestinal Surgery. 2013;**17**(1):159-166

[14] Fischer JP, Nelson JA, Wes AM, Win KJD, et al. Complex ventral hernia repair using components separation with or without synthetic mesh: A cost-utility analysis. Plastic and Reconstructive Surgery. 2014;**133**(3):687-699

[15] Fernandez Lobato R, Ruiz de Adana Belbel JC, Angulo Morales F, et al. Cost-benefit analysis comparing laparoscopic and open ventral hernia repair. Cirugía Española. 2014;**92**(8): 553-560

[16] Muysoms FE, Miserez M, Berrevoet F, et al. Classification of primary and incisional abdominal wall hernias. Hernia. 2009;**13**(4):407-414

[17] Mancini GJ, Le HN. Loss of abdominal domain: Definition and treatment strategies 2016 (34) 358-369. in Hernia Surgery. Current principles. Editor: YW Novitsky ISBN 978-3-319-27468-3 DOI: 10.1007/978-3-319-27470-6.

[18] Bratzler DW, Dellinger EP, Olsen KM, Perl TM, Auwaerter PG, Bolon MK, Fish DN, Napolitano LM, Sawyer RG. Clinical practice guidelines for antimicrobial prophylaxis in surgery. American Journal of Health-System Pharmacy. 2013;**70**(3):195-283

[19] Bratzler DW, Dellinger EP. Antimicrobial prophylaxis for surgery: An advisory statement from the national surgical infection prevention project. The American Journal of Surgery. 2005;**189**:395-404

[20] Ross SW, Oommen B, Heniford BT, Augenstein VA. Component separation in complex ventral hernia repair: Surgical technique and postoperative outcomes. Surgical Technology International. 2014;**24**:167-177

[21] Winder JS, Behar, BJ, Juza RM, Potochny J, Pauli EM. Transversus abdominis release for abdominal wall reconstruction: Early experience with a novel technique. Journal of the American College of Surgeons. 2016;**223**(2):271-278

[22] Martis G, Laczik R, Damjanovich L. Significance of the computed tomography assisted morphometry in the surgical planning of eventrated abdominal wall hernias. Orvosi Hetilap 2017;**158**(7):266-272

[23] Ferrans CE, Powers MJ. Psychosomatic assessment of the quality of life index. Research in Nursing & Health. 1992;**15**:29-38

[24] Tessone A, Nava M, Blondeel P, Spano A. Avoiding complication in abdominal wall surgery: A mathematical model to predict the course of the motor innervation of the rectus abdominis. Annals of Plastic Surgery. 2016;**76**(2):227-230

[25] da Silva AL. Surgical correction of longitudinal median or paramedian incisional hernia. Surgery, Gynecology & Obstetrics. 1979;**148**:579-583

[26] Hope PG, Carter SS, Kilby JD. The da silva method of incisional hernia repair. British Journal of Surgery. 1985;**72**:569-570

[27] De Franco AJ, Kingman GJ, Sterchi JM, Marks MW, Throrne M. Rectus turnover flaps for the reconstruction of large midline abdominal wall defects. Annals of Plastic Surgery. 1996;**37**(1):18-23

[28] Kushimoto S, Yokota H, Kawai M, Yamamoto Y. Management of the open abdomen – usefulness of bilateral anterior rectus abdominis sheath turnover flap method for early fascial closure. Japan Medical Association Journal. 2008;**51**(4):272-277

[29] Hesselink VJ, Luijendijk RW, de Wilt JH, Heide R, Jeekel J. An evaluation of risk factors in incisional hernia recurrencies. Surgery, Gynecology & Obstetrics. 1993;**176**(3):228-34

[30] Schumpelick V. Incisional hernia: An unpleasant complication in surgery. Chirurg. 2010;**81** (3):185

[31] Poulose BK, Shelton J, Philips S. Epidemiology and cost of ventral hernia repair: Making the case for hernia research. Hernia. 2012;**16**(2):179-183

[32] Holihan JL, Alawadi Z, Martindale RG. Adverse events after ventral hernia repair: The vicious cycle of complications. The American Journal of Surgery. 2015;**221**(2):478-485

[33] Sanchez VM, Abi-Haidar YE, Itani KM. Mesh infection in ventral incisional hernia repair incidence, contributing factors, and treatment. Surgical Infections (Larchmt). 2011;**12**(3):205-210

[34] Weber G, Baracs J, Horvath OP. "Onlay" mesh provides significantly better results than "sublay" reconstruction. Prospective randomized multicenter study of abdominal wall reconstruction with sutures only, or with surgical mesh – results of a five-years follow-up. Magyar Sebészet. 2010;**63**(5):302-311

[35] Hawn MT, Gray SH, Snyder LW. Predictors of mesh explantation after incisional hernia repair. The American Journal of Surgery. 2011;**202**(1):28-33

[36] Nicholas J, Slater B, van der Kolk M. Biologic grafts for ventral hernia repair: A systematic review. The American Journal of Surgery. 2013;**205**:220-230

[37] Beale EW, Hoxworth RE, Livingstone EH. The role of biologic mesh in abdominal wall reconstruction: A systematic review of the current literature. The American Journal of Surgery. 2012;**204**:510-517

[38] Butler CE, Burns NK, Campbell KT. Comparison of cross-linked and non-cross-linked porcine acellular dermal matrices for ventral hernia repair. Journal of The American College of Surgeons. 2010;**211**:368-376

[39] Primus FE, Harris HW. A critical review of biological mesh in ventral hernia repairs under contaminated conditions. Hernia. 2013;**17**(1):21-30

[40] Kissane NA, Itani KM. A decade of ventral incisional hernia repairs with biologic acellular dermal matrix: What have we learned? Plastic and Reconstructive Surgery. 2012;**130** (5 Suppl. 2):194S–202S

[41] Lee L, Mata J, Landry T. A systematic review of synthetic and biological materials for abdominal wall reinforcement in contaminated fields. Surgical Endoscopy. 2014;**28**(9): 2531-2546

[42] de Vries Reilingh TS, Bodegom ME, van Goor H, et al. Autologous tissue repair of large abdominal wall defects. British Journal of Surgery. 2007;**94**(7):791-803

[43] Martis G, Damjanovich L. Use of double-layer autologous dermal flap in the treatment of recurrent and/or infected incisional hernias. Presentation of the surgical technique and the results of one-year follow-up. A prospective, consecutive cohort study. Hernia. 2016;**20**(3):261-270

[44] Martis G, Rózsahegyi M, Deák J, Damjanovich L. Incarcerated an eventrated abdominal wall hernia reconstruction with autologous double-layer dermal graft in the field of purulent peritonitis—A case report. International Journal of Surgery Case Reports. 2017;**30**:126-129

Permissions

All chapters in this book were first published in HERNIA, by InTech Open; hereby published with permission under the Creative Commons Attribution License or equivalent. Every chapter published in this book has been scrutinized by our experts. Their significance has been extensively debated. The topics covered herein carry significant findings which will fuel the growth of the discipline. They may even be implemented as practical applications or may be referred to as a beginning point for another development.

The contributors of this book come from diverse backgrounds, making this book a truly international effort. This book will bring forth new frontiers with its revolutionizing research information and detailed analysis of the nascent developments around the world.

We would like to thank all the contributing authors for lending their expertise to make the book truly unique. They have played a crucial role in the development of this book. Without their invaluable contributions this book wouldn't have been possible. They have made vital efforts to compile up to date information on the varied aspects of this subject to make this book a valuable addition to the collection of many professionals and students.

This book was conceptualized with the vision of imparting up-to-date information and advanced data in this field. To ensure the same, a matchless editorial board was set up. Every individual on the board went through rigorous rounds of assessment to prove their worth. After which they invested a large part of their time researching and compiling the most relevant data for our readers.

The editorial board has been involved in producing this book since its inception. They have spent rigorous hours researching and exploring the diverse topics which have resulted in the successful publishing of this book. They have passed on their knowledge of decades through this book. To expedite this challenging task, the publisher supported the team at every step. A small team of assistant editors was also appointed to further simplify the editing procedure and attain best results for the readers.

Apart from the editorial board, the designing team has also invested a significant amount of their time in understanding the subject and creating the most relevant covers. They scrutinized every image to scout for the most suitable representation of the subject and create an appropriate cover for the book.

The publishing team has been an ardent support to the editorial, designing and production team. Their endless efforts to recruit the best for this project, has resulted in the accomplishment of this book. They are a veteran in the field of academics and their pool of knowledge is as vast as their experience in printing. Their expertise and guidance has proved useful at every step. Their uncompromising quality standards have made this book an exceptional effort. Their encouragement from time to time has been an inspiration for everyone.

The publisher and the editorial board hope that this book will prove to be a valuable piece of knowledge for researchers, students, practitioners and scholars across the globe.

List of Contributors

Adrian Claudiu Ratiu
University of Medicine and Pharmacy "Victor Babes", Timisoara, Romania

Joanne Baerg, Arul Thirumoorthi and Rajaie Hazboun
Loma Linda University Children's Hospital, Loma Linda, CA, USA

Fatih Altintoprak and Enis Dikicier
Istinye University Faculty of Medicine, Department of General Surgery, Istanbul, Turkey

Emrah Akin and Kemal Gundogdu
Sakarya University Research and Educational Hospital, Department of General Surgery, Sakarya, Turkey

Ahmed Abdelghaffar Helal
Department of Pediatric Surgery, Faculty of Medicine, Al-Azhar University, Cairo, Egypt

Mohamed Abdelmohsen Bedewi
College of Medicine, Prince Sattam Bin Abdulaziz University, Alkharj, Kingdom of Saudi Arabia

Mohamed El-sharkawy
King Khalid University Hospital, King Saud University, Riyadh, Kingdom of Saudi Arabia

Kaylene Barrera, Paul Chung, Sarrina Shraga and Gainosuke Sugiyama
Downstate Medical Center, State University of New York, Brooklyn, New York, United States of America

Suleyman Utku Celik, Akin Firat Kocaay and Cihangir Akyol
Department of General Surgery, Ankara University School of Medicine, Ankara, Turkey

Ivan Šeparović
University Hospital Centre Zagreb, Zagreb, Croatia

Goran Augustin
University Hospital Centre Zagreb and School of Medicine, University of Zagreb, Zagreb, Croatia

Angelo Guttadauro, Matteo Maternini, Nicoletta Pecora and Francesco Gabrielli
Department of Medicine and Surgery, General Surgery Unit, Istituti Clinici Zucchi, University of Milano-Bicocca, Monza, Italy

Marco Chiarelli
General Surgery Unit, Ospedale di Lecco, Italy

Valentina Riggio
Department of Medicine and Surgery, University of Milano-Bicocca, Italy

Jie Chen, ChengBing Chu, YingMo Shen, ZhenYu Zou and Xin Yuan
Department of Hernia and Abdominal Wall Surgery, Beijing Chao-Yang Hospital, Capital Medical University, Beijing, China

Kamer Tomaoglu
Department of General Surgery, S.P. Hospital, Istanbul, Turkey

Gábor Martis and László Damjanovich
Department of General Surgery, Institute of Surgery, Clinical and Health Science Center, University of Debrecen, Debrecen, Hungary

Index

www.ingramcontent.com/pod-product-compliance
Lightning Source LLC
LaVergne TN
LVHW060548210926
848485LV00005B/1277